Healthcare Information Systems and Informatics:

Research and Practices

Joseph Tan
Wayne State University, USA

T0325047

Medical Information Science
REFERENCE

MEDICAL INFORMATION SCIENCE REFERENCE

Hershey · New York

Acquisition Editor: Kristin Klinger
Senior Managing Editor: Jennifer Neidig
Managing Editor: Jamie Snavely
Assistant Managing Editor: Carole Coulson
Development Editor: Kristin Roth
Copy Editor: Ashley Fails
Typesetter: Carole Coulson
Cover Design: Lisa Tosheff
Printed at: Yurchak Printing Inc.

Published in the United States of America by
        Information Science Publishing (an imprint of IGI Global)
        701 E. Chocolate Avenue
        Hershey PA 17033
        Tel: 717-533-8845
        Fax: 717-533-8661
        E-mail: cust@igi-global.com
        Web site: http://www.igi-global.com

and in the United Kingdom by
        Information Science Publishing (an imprint of IGI Global)
        3 Henrietta Street
        Covent Garden
        London WC2E 8LU
        Tel: 44 20 7240 0856
        Fax: 44 20 7379 3313
        Web site: http://www.eurospanbookstore.com

Library of Congress Cataloging-in-Publication Data

Healthcare information systems & informatics : research and practices / Joseph Tan, editor.
      p. ; cm.
   Includes bibliographical references and index.
   Summary: "This book addresses issues involving health information systems and informatics as innovative forms of investment in healthcare"--Provided by publisher.
   ISBN 978-1-59904-690-7 (hardcover) -- ISBN 978-1-59904-692-1 (ebook)
   1. Medical informatics. 2. Information storage and retrieval systems--Medical care. 3. Health services admin-istration--Data processing. I. Tan, Joseph K. H.
   [DNLM: 1. Medical Informatics. 2. Health Services Administration. W 26.5 H43454 2008]
   R858.H3843 2008
   651.5'04261--dc22
                          2008007906

British Cataloguing in Publication Data
A Cataloguing in Publication record for this book is available from the British Library.

Healthcare Information Systems and Informatics:

Research and Practices

Table of Contents

Preface

Over the past decade, the proliferation of e-technology, Internet-based data exchanges, and improved computing security has allowed the field of Health Information Systems & Informatics (HISI) to flourish and germinate an emergent body of theoretical frameworks, empirical research, and practitioner-based literature—all with the ultimate goal of improving HISI implementation, evaluation, and best practices while simultaneously enriching HISI policy formulation and the knowledge transfer processes. The active cross-pollination of ideas and fresh knowledge from various disciplines has gone beyond just healthcare computing, or even mobile and wireless networks, in bringing together various HISI sub-areas, from traditional hospital information systems to emerging patient-centered e-health and m-health. These efforts are already impacting the rapid growth and further development of a rich, expanding field.

Despite recent and continuing efforts among well-meaning researchers and practitioners to establishing HISI as a discipline, I still must repeat what I have noted in the inaugural issue of the International Journal of Healthcare Information Systems & Informatics, that is, the HISI field is still in its infancy, and much of the published work has previously been scattered in a myriad of disciplined-based outlets. Indeed, the evolving HISI discipline still lacks directing frameworks, reliable and well-tested measurement tools, and formalized research methodologies to guide future medical and health informatics researchers and practitioners. Accordingly, this series of compiled works serve to provide a focal point for key contributions in emerging HISI conceptualization, methodologies and applications that would further evolve the field, whether it is from the perspective of building relevant theories or applying and adapting rigorous and established methodologies to the field. Some of the works even suggest innovative strategies and models for improving HISI implementation and best practices, while others attempt to concentrate on HISI evaluation, or policy formulation and knowledge transfer processes.

As a timely testament to the sheer diversity of conceptual, methodological, evaluative, and practical breakthroughs that eager researchers and practitioners are trying to cross-fertilize in HISI, the contributions within this volume may be sequenced into four interconnected sections. Section I, comprising Chapters I through III, provides a sampling of newer HISI theoretical development by identifying some of the knowledge gaps requiring further attention from current and future HISI researchers and practitioners. These chapters focus selectively on concepts and constructs awaiting theoretical development and policy formulation—concepts and constructs that will eventually define the different sub-areas of the emerging HISI discipline, including mobile health (M-Health), the acceptance and diffusion of clinical-based information and communications technology (ICT), and a HIPAA-compliant framework for detailing health web privacy and security policy. These chapters also illustrate how new questions specific to key HISI research areas may be conjured by highlighting some of the challenges faced when working in a rapidly emerging field. Section II, encompassing Chapters IV through XII, concentrates on various methodological approaches to, and applications of, extracting data empirically so that specific HISI research questions can be answered. The highlighted methodologies range from quantitative approaches, including rigorous statistical modeling, secondary data analysis, and survey-based instrumentation to more qualitative techniques, such as interviews and the use of cases to triangulation, which combines both qualitative and quantitative approaches. Section III, covering Chapters XIII through XVI, emphasizes the practicality of models in supporting HISI implementation, evaluation, and practices—for instance, the decentralization of a telemedicine infrastructure, the innovative application of e-technology for nurses, and the evaluation of a fuzzy ontology-based medical information system. Finally, Section IV, which includes Chapter XVII through Chapter XX, concludes the volume with a gleam of HISI policy and knowledge transfer processes.

Many young researchers neglect theory building when performing a literature review, and the majority of new researchers fail to appreciate the necessity of closing the "gaps" that are currently challenging the growth of an emerging field. In relation to identifying "gaps" and HISI theoretical development, Chapter I of this volume illustrates how an important "gap" in the HISI area can be used to generate a new perspective in HISI research. In "Designing a M-Health Framework for Conceptualizing Mobile Health," Olla and Tan adopt a structured and discipline-based theoretical approach to breaking down and compartmentalizing the mobile health (M-Health) systems into principal dimensions, based on content analysis of the extant literature. As noted, these dimensions include communication infrastructure, application purpose, device type, data display and application domain. Communication infrastructure refers to the mobile telecommunication technologies and networks. Application purpose identifies the goal and objectives for the application of a M-Health system, such as e-prescription, clinical data exchange, decision support, or various other purposes. Device type relates to the type of device being used, such as tablet PCs, portable data assistants (PDAs), sensors, or other devices. Data display describes how the data will be presented and transmitted to the user, for example, through a series of images, emails, and/or textual data. Application domain categorizes the domain of mobile technology application, and, more specifically, the defined area, in which the m-health system will be implemented, such as rural community health, wireless home healthcare, or some other domain. Altogether, the M-Health Reference Model serves as a guide to healthcare stakeholders and m-health system implementers in identifying and understanding the technological infrastructure, business requirements, and operational needs of the m-health systems.

Although information and communications technology (ICT) is being used in the United Kingdoms National Health Services (NHS) to improve medical delivery, it has not been sufficiently tested and applied to improve our understanding of the factors motivating health organizational behavioral changes in terms of accepting HISI applications and use. In Osbourne-Clarke's Chapter II, "Factors Motivating the Acceptance of New Information and Communication Technologies in the UK Healthcare," three popular theoretical models, namely, the technology acceptance model (TAM), Rogers' diffusion of innovation theory (IDT), and the Triandis theory of interpersonal behavior (TIB), were contrasted and integrated as a means of understanding effective ways that technology can be employed to support telemedicine initiatives. ICT—as a basis for telemedicine to reduce existing communication barriers and initiate new forms of information exchange between medical professionals and patients—is conceptualized and evaluated. An overview of the UK healthcare system and its problems of communication between hospital specialists and general practitioners, as well as the difficulties for healthcare professionals, particularly general practitioners, to see patients outside normal working hours, are highlighted. The authors demonstrate how an integrated theoretical approach to relate and combine existing theories could best be used to explain ICT acceptance and adoption behavior. This particular contribution offers the readers an integrated theoretical perspective to explain the impact of key organizational factors for overcoming commonly encountered resistance to telemedicine initiatives.

With Chapter III, "An Overview of HIPAA-Compliant Access Control Model," Cheng and Hung focus on the growing demands of Web-based healthcare applications and the need for HIPAA privacy rules to be standardized in Web services. As no comprehensive solutions to the various privacy issues have been defined in this area, they propose a vocabulary-based Web privacy policy framework with role-based access control (RBAC) and privacy extensions. Accordingly, they argue that the proposed framework is HIPAA-compliance. Again, this contribution aids the HISI research and practice community in understanding how difficult HISI policy can be formulated.

Theories, models, and organizational frameworks provide us with starting points to ask beneficial questions. Essentially, these models and taxonomies serve as guideposts to researchers in identifying some of the missing knowledge "gaps", thus justifying further research and exploration. Furthermore, these foundational works assist researchers in explaining some unexplained but observed phenomena, as well as contribute to our understanding of various HISI domains' behaviors in the real-world systems. Theories are also often used as the basis for crafting various testable hypotheses. Yet, researchers must also rely heavily on proven methodologies to provide the correct answers for questions they have ventured to ask. Such methodologies are also scientifically accepted means of collecting data to discover new knowledge or verify established knowledge, and will, in turn, then become adaptable approaches for others to duplicate claims of what have been previously found. This brings us to Section II: HISI Methodological Approaches.

Here, our attention shifts from a general focus on HISI theory development, as presented in Section I, to a practical means of using powerful statistical modeling to ground theory in empirical datasets. Specifically, Dr. Christopher Reddick concentrates on the use of secondary analysis in Chapter IV on "The Internet and Managing Boomers and Seniors Health." His work provides valuable insights into an emerging and important HISI topic, that is, trends of Internet use for e-health information retrieval among the elderly versus the baby boomers. Accordingly, the author notes that, "For baby boomers, the Internet has become a major source of health information, second only to their family doctor." Whereas seniors probably have the greatest need for health information, the author claims that they do not use the Internet as their primary source of information nearly as extensively as the baby boomers. In short, the Kaiser Family Foundation's e-Health and the Elderly public opinion dataset of online health information access by boomers and seniors was analyzed to show that boomers marginally use online health information more than seniors for the management of their personal health. Moreover, those who are more aware, and have positive feelings towards online health information (for both boomers and seniors), will use the Internet more actively to manage their health. In essence, if people feel more at ease with, and have a better attitude towards using the Internet for e-health information retrieval, they would more likely use it to control their personal health, or do so on someone else's behalf. This partially answers a very important research question that has been asked in many past e-health conferences: "Has online health information actually helped some people manage their health more effectively?"

Next, even more complex statistical modeling using neural networks (NNs) methodology has been applied to discover "knowledge" in empirical healthcare datasets. Through the trauma audit and research network (TARN), Chesney et. al. in Chapter V on "Data Mining Medical Information: Should Artificial Neural Networks Be Used to Analyze Trauma and Audit Data?" formally advocate the use of an innovative data mining approach in creating an artificial neural network (ANN) model. This model would be employed for the analysis of accumulated trauma data, as compared to traditional logistic regression analysis. The authors show how their obtained results from the ANN model with "the output set to be the probability that a patient will die" differed from those using traditional logistic regression analysis. Ten years of TARN (a network designed to provide effective feedback and accurate classification of care for injured patients) data have been analyzed. Essentially, the ANN approach uses a layered system of key inputs, the weighing of factors for classification probability calculations, and an adjusted outcome neural network analysis. In this sense, ANN modeling begins with the system recording injury details such as demographics, the mechanism of the injury, various measurements of the injury's severity, initial and subsequent management interventions, and the probable outcome of the treatment. Such records are then analyzed to accurately discriminate between those patients who are expected to survive and those who are predicted to die. Their results show that both ANNs and traditional analytic approaches achieve roughly the same predictive accuracy, although ANNs model has been found to be more complex to interpret than the logistic regression model. In other words, the authors manage to show how novel forms of sophisticated statistical modeling can be applied as tools to analyze equally complex HISI datasets, although their findings further suggest the usefulness of applying both traditional and non-traditional analysis techniques together, as well as including as many factors in the analysis as possible.

Steven Walczak and colleagues in Chapter VI on "Diagnostic Cost Reduction Using Artificial Neural Networks: The Case of Pulmonary Embolism" demonstrate the robustness of automated intelligence in improving diagnostic capabilities when predicting the likelihood of pulmonary embolism (PE) in a surgical patient population. Accordingly, they claim that the illness—PE—which may have mortality rates as high as 10 percent, is one of the most difficult and costly to diagnose. Fortunately, the complexity of identifying patients at risk for PE can be overcome with the use of intelligent tools, such as nonparametric Neural Networks. According to the authors, superior positive prediction can be achieved with the NN modeling technique. Thus, this contribution to HISI methodology advances the science of prognosis, a complex task for any clinician to handle, with the consequences impacting significantly on the patients.

In the remaining few chapters in this section, we move from statistical and analytic methods to interweaving among survey research, interviews (and triangulation), and the more qualitative case methodology. In Chapter VII, Andersen and Balas, on "A Survey on Computerization of Primary Care in the United States," discuss the use of a survey-based approach to assess information technology (IT) usage among primary care physicians. As these physicians represent a major stakeholder group in the US healthcare system, insights into the adoption and diffusion patterns of IT among them is essential to enhance our knowledge of how IT is being deployed. With increased productivity and improved quality being the main objectives for using and deploying IT in healthcare delivery, many questions arise that require further research. These include what types of IT physicians are using, what their perceived benefits are, and what the major barriers to IT acceptance could be. An interesting—but puzzling—result the authors note was that a high number of physicians did not indicate any interest at all in the types of IT applications being surveyed. Overall, their results reveal that perceived benefits and barriers are important predictors of IT implementation. Their study has significant implications for developing strategies, as well as interfaces, for incorporating IT applications into real-world healthcare settings.

In Chapter VIII, Dana Schwieger, Arlyn Melcher, C. Raganathan and H. Joseph Wen apply a "Case Study" approach, conducted over a ten-month period within the domain of a modified adaptive structuration theory (AST) model, to document the impact of advanced IT and HISI adoption within a medical organization setting. AST, which is rapidly becoming an important theoretical paradigm for comprehending such evaluations, was modified to illustrate the changing interrelationships among the variables affecting the adoption and application of the HISI technology studied. Specifically, the case illustrates the complex interactions between medical billing technology and organizational processes. As the organization attempts to install and implement the new system, the researchers find that in order for the organization to maintain daily operations, several aspects of the organization, technology, and operations would have to be modified and adapted. Then, as the system integrates slowly into operations and the organization's needs evolved through the adaptation process, the researchers, in turn, find that different iterations of the model could emphasize different structures. The case also illustrates that the capacity to manage HISI technologies is often dependent on the organization's abilities to prioritize its needs and focus its energies on a critical structure, while temporarily disregarding others until the primary healthcare processes are under control.

A second survey-based contribution is provided in Chapter IX, "Understanding of Physicians' Acceptance of Computerized Physician Order Entry," a contribution by Liang and colleagues. Computerized physician order entry (CPOE) holds the potential to reduce medical errors, to improve care quality, and to cut healthcare costs. Based on a series of hypotheses generated by the technology acceptance model (TAM), these authors attempt to evaluate physician user acceptance of CPOE in a large general hospital setting in China. Items in the questionnaire are adapted from previous research and designed to measure physicians' perceptions of CPOE. Under the condition of high CPOE experience, the authors find perceived ease of use having no effect on attitude; under the condition of low CPOE experience, however, perceived ease of use has been shown to positively affect attitude. In other words, as physician users become more experienced with CPOE, the issue of usability becomes less important. Yet, this result does not diminish the significance of the need for designers to pay attention to the usability factor. Rather, it actually proves the need for designers to pay special attention to the usability factor, as it positively affects the attitudes of those with low CPOE experience.

In Chapter X, we revert back to the qualitative approach of using a "case study" methodology. Wiggins, Beachboard, Trimmer, and Pumphrey contribute an interesting perspective on IT governance from a rural healthcare perspective. They used a "single-site" case study in their piece, "Entrepreneurial IT Governance: Electronic Medical Records (EMR) in Rural Healthcare," to document the implementation of an EMR in a rural family practice residency program. The residency program, which trains primary care physicians and provides primary care services to rural communities, has initially been aimed to enhance the practice's clinical research capabilities. But this simple goal eventually expands into a much larger goal of extending the system throughout rural clinics and providers in the region. The authors argue that organizations aiming for a successful adoption of IT as a means of improving healthcare in the rural setting should take an innovative, relationship-oriented approach.

The penultimate chapter for this section, Chapter XI, once again features the use of an integrated survey-interview approach, including stakeholder questionnaires and twelve key informant interviews, combined with an extensive literature review in "Telehealth Organizational Implementation Guidelines Issues: A Canadian Perspective." Contributed by Maryan Yeo and Penny A. Jennett to develop theoretically sound and empirically based perspectives, their research uses a triangulation of common methodologies. Results of their study are categorized into the four major themes of organizational readiness, accountability, quality assurance, and continuity. The authors point out that a vast number of their findings relate mostly to the former two themes, whereas the latter two themes have gained only scattered attention. The findings and recommendations, useful in the evolution of telehealth services and their successful management, lead us naturally to the final chapter in this section, a transition to Section III's contributions on HISI implementation, evaluation and practices.

Chapter XII entitled, "Computer Usage by U.S. Group Medical Practices 1994 vs. 2003 and Type of Usage Comparison to IT Practices in Taiwan," contributed by Sobol and Prater, serves as the transitional chapter. The researchers conduct a follow-up of their 1994 study of group medical practices using mail survey of IT use in private group medical practices. Issues they want to address include in-house expertise versus outsourcing, and the use of e-billing systems in these practices; this, in turn, sheds new light on how to reduce the increasing amount of time physicians spend on business administration. Their work addresses the "gap" in previous research, which tended to focus mainly on hospitals and health maintenance organizations (HMOs) but not private physician practices. Accordingly, the authors report on achieving a "longitudinal" picture of these private group practices' IT services adoption patterns. Results of their study provide insights into key issues and challenges faced by these practices, including the types of IT applications used, the different types of savings arising from IT adoption, the percentage of time spent by physicians on business administration, and the different sources of information these physicians relied upon to develop the business aspects of their practice. This transits us to Section III, which focuses on HISI implementation, evaluation, and practices.

In this section, we begin with Chapter XIII, a contribution from Apostolakis, Valsamos, and Varlamis. In "Decentralization of the Greek National Telemedicine System," these authors demonstrate a practical implementation of a Greek telemedicine system at a national level by recording and analyzing the shortcomings and difficulties of the existing Greek Telemedicine system. They suggest upgrading the

Regional Telemedicine Centers' role to become the cornerstone of the new system. By highlighting the necessary actions for a smooth transition to a new system at the technical, operational, and organizational levels, their analysis uncovers the shortcomings and inefficiencies in the usage of Telemedicine Centers in the National Health System, and dictates the development of the Regional Telemedicine Centers (RTCs). The binding of the new RTCs with the existing telemedicine system could then be performed with minimum cost by presuming recording and reusing existing infrastructure, training of personnel, and smoothly transiting to the new telemedicine structure. Their shared experience of a HISI implementation model provides insights to future HISI practices.

The remaining chapters in Section III incorporate more HISI evaluation and practices. The empirical study covered in Chapter XIV by Davis and Thakkar uses a two-phase approach to identify the status of Electronic health records systems (EHR) in U.S. hospitals. In "Perceived Level of Benefits and Risks of Core Functionalities of an EHR System," they report on interviewing seven healthcare and information systems professionals from three hospitals to develop a sound instrument to identify and draw relevant measures from the extant literature. They attempt to address the following question: If, with the use of "core" functionality in an EHR system, does a significant relationship exist between perceived levels of benefit and risk? In their study, "core" functionality was defined as "health information, results management, order entry/management, decision support, electronic communication, patient support, administrative processes, reporting, and population health management functionalities of an EHR system." Moreover, they want to detect any relationship between the status of the EHR system and the size of hospital. Their results show a significant positive correlation between perceived benefits and risks in all of the eight core functionalities, but no significant relationship between status of EHR system and the size of hospital. They conclude that each of these eight core functionalities might be adopted by hospitals either individually or as an entire EHR system. In a manner similar to the preceding contributions, the usefulness of conducting appropriately managed surveys (as well as interviews) for exploring HISI practices is clearly documented in this study.

In Chapter XV, "Using Pocket PCs for Nurses Shift Reports and Patient Care," Chang, Lutes, Braswell, and Nielsen evaluate the use of an emerging IT solution to overcome inefficiencies in providing quality nursing care, specifically in hospitals supported by paper-based systems. In their contribution, the emerging IT solution comprises using Pocket PCs and a desktop PC interfaced to a hospital's mainframe system to manage nursing care inefficiencies. This system has been introduced and evaluated on nurses working in traditional paper-based hospital systems. The goal is to apply mobile IT, allowing nurses easier access to patient information. The authors describe the development of the prototype and report the results of a pilot test, comparing the time spent in taking and giving shift reports before and after the study, as well as nurses' perceptions of the mobile IT system. In the end, nurses appeared to have provided strong verbal support for the use of the system. With the deployment of such a system, the key question of returns on investments (ROI) is left to the readers. This study contributes to our understanding of the potential of mobile technology, integrated with a hospital's mainframe system, and how and what such a system could impact on the efficiency of communications in nursing shift reports, and in accessing information relevant to patient care.

In Chapter XVI, "Evaluation of a Fuzzy Ontology-based Medical Information System," Dr. Dave Parry emphasizes evidence-based medicine (EBM) to demonstrate how appropriate information should be made available to clinicians at the point of care. Electronic sources of information may fulfill this need, but require a high level of skill to use successfully. David Parry concentrates on the diffusion of e-technology, and describes the rationale behind, and initial testing of, a system to allow collaborative search and ontology construction for professional groups in the health sector. The approach, which is based on the use of a browser linked to a fuzzy ontology rooted in the National Library of Medicine (NLM) unified medical language system (UMLS), is seen to provide high quality information for professionals in making future EBM decisions. This concludes Section III and puts us into the final section of this volume, Section IV on HISI Policies and Knowledge Transfer Processes.

Given the significance of HISI research and practice, Part IV concludes the volume with an attempt to illustrate how these two components can be linked. A gleam of HISI policy and knowledge dissemination and transfers is provided through the chapters in this section. Chapter XVII highlights the current alternative paradigms to e-health pedagogy; Chapter XVIII takes a novel approach to examining healthcare information technology (HIT) usage and user satisfaction in healthcare organizations; and Chapter XIX reviews the competitive forces challenging e-health. Finally, Chapter XX provides a methodology for translating theory into best practices in the area of healthcare technology management, within the setting of a Canadian teaching hospital.

In Chapter XVII, "Applying Personal Health Informatics to Create Effective Patient-Centered E-Health," Wilson reviews and compares the current alternative paradigms to e-health pedagogy. Adopting a personal health informatics (PHI) perspective, he integrates three previously held paradigms—namely, the e-commerce paradigm, the personal health record paradigm, and the consumer health informatics paradigm. In this light, he attempts to develop a conceptual model of a new paradigm, the PHI. This paradigm incorporates the significant features of previous paradigms by integrating multiple perspectives of informatics, both personal and healthcare. The significance of this work lies in the model for enhancing knowledge dissemination in e-health design, development, and management. Overall, this work helps advance our contemporary understanding of the various health informatics issues, and points out future directions for HISI policy and knowledge transfer process, in particular, the design and development of pedagogy encompassing e-health.

In Chapter XVIII, Hikmet and Bhattacherjee, in their contribution of "The Impact of Professional Certifications on Healthcare Information Technology Use," take a novel approach to examine HIT usage and user satisfaction in healthcare organizations. The authors examine the effect of professional certifications, such as that of the Joint Commission of Accreditation of Healthcare Organizations (JCAHO), in motivating health information technology (HIT) use among healthcare administrators. Their study examines only two of several organizational factors, namely professional certifications and facility type (size). Their survey-based approach concludes that these types of certifications do, indeed, enhance HIT usage and user satisfaction. Their study also raises noteworthy questions about the effect of external entities and factors on HIT use. Since HIT usage tends to be positively correlated with user satisfaction, this divergence of effects is theoretically perplexing and worthy of further research.

In Chapter XIX, Wickramasinghe, Misra, Jenkins, and Vogel advocate the use of a "Competitive Forces" framework to provide a unified system for understanding various e-health initiatives, as well as their relative strengths and deficiencies in improving access, quality, and value of healthcare services. They note that superior access, quality, and value of healthcare services have become national priorities for healthcare owing to the challenge of controlling exponentially increasing costs of healthcare expenditure. Their proposed evaluation system is developed on the basis of three key components: (a) an understanding of how e-health can modify the interactions between the various stakeholders; (b) an understanding of the competitive forces facing e-health organizations and the role of the Internet in modifying these forces; and (c) the introduction of a framework that serves to identify the key forces facing e-health. This chapter also provides some suggestions of how any health organization can structure itself to be e-health "ready".

To conclude this volume, Chapter XX, contributed by Eisler, Tan, and Sheps in "From Theory to Practice: Healthcare Technology Management (HCTM) Conceptualization, Measures, and Practices" shows how the different aspects of HISI research, practice, policy formulation and knowledge transfers could be integrated. Their work illustrates how theory-based research drives the development of a sound measuring instrument, which can, in turn, be applied to improve HCTM practice in the field; in essence, the entire process of HISI knowledge transfers from the laboratory to the field. Using a triangulation method—combining expert panel review, survey, and cross-validation of their research findings with study results from an independent external source—they show that the development of a valid HCTM instrument could be used to guide policy formulation, dictate future HISI research and practice, and provide a model for structuring HISI education and knowledge diffusion. In this context, the instrument they develop to measure HCTM practice entails key performance indicators that differentiate among high and low performing health organizations.

Owing to the rapid diffusion of digital library capabilities and the proliferation of Internet-based data exchanges in this age of increased globalization, we are witnessing an explosion of knowledge in HISI. Who would have imagined just a decade ago that the HISI field would have attracted researchers and practitioners from so many different walks of life? The HISI advanced series represent the cross-pollination of ideas from trained experts across a myriad of disciplines. This volume, in and of itself, is the beginning of an accumulation of contributions that is germinating an emergent body of HISI literature, so that future HISI research and practice may be informed. Contributors are primarily from researchers and practitioners of many different walks of life, with expertise in the area of healthcare computing, industrial processes and biomedical engineering, nursing informatics, health information sciences, management information systems, operations research, applied systems sciences, digital networks, web security standards and services, mobile health care, wireless networks and sensor networks, e-medicine, as well as e-home healthcare delivery systems.

This entire discussion brings me back to the central question we hinted in the beginning of this Preface—What would differentiate HISI from the other disciplines? Consider the question of how a discipline emerges to evolve a network of inter-related researchers and practitioners. If we sincerely wish to seek the answers, we must ask ourselves another follow-up question—what makes an emerging discipline attractive and appealing enough to gain the attention of new (and even established) researchers and students from other well-rooted and more traditionally-recognized disciplines? Soon, we will realize that what defines a discipline is nothing more than the accumulation of specific theories and practices that are relevant and applicable to the challenges of that discipline, and not just to any discipline. Indubitably, a critical mass of researchers and a substantial body of identifiable research literature must also exist for a discipline to thrive. Since numerous theories can be applied across multiple disciplines, each new and evolving discipline will be defined by its continuous drawing of theoretical concepts from other more established disciplines, as well as the growing number of researchers resolving "gaps" encountered within the discipline to give it an identity of its own. Over the years, therefore, if a discipline is to be increasingly recognized, it must germinate its own roots and bodies of literature in the form of accepted theories, frameworks, and models, alongside conclusions of identifiable, discipline-specific "gaps" in knowledge and practices. This is why theory-based, methodologically rigorous research in HISI is critical to advancing the field; this volume is a call for researchers to come forward and contribute to the building of the HISI discipline through the conduct of both basic and applied HISI research.

Altogether, the primary aim of this first HISI Advances Series volume is, therefore, to educate new researchers, practitioners, and interested students on the significance of research and best practices in carving out the HISI space. A secondary aim is to showcase how both HISI basic and applied research can contribute to real-world HISI practices. This understanding will not only enable us to better manage the future of HISI applications, but also to better appreciate how specific current HISI challenges and evolving HISI practices could, in and of themselves, beneficially impact individuals, groups, organizations, the economy, and society on an even greater scale.

Section I

HISI Theoretical Development

Chapter I

Designing a M-Health Framework for Conceptualizing Mobile Health Systems

Phillip Olla, Madonna University, USA

Joseph Tan, Wayne State University, USA

Abstract

The reference model presented in this chapter encourages the breakdown of m-health systems into the following five key dimensions: communication infrastructure: this is a description of the mobile telecommunication technologies and networks; device type: this relates to the type of device being used such as PDA, sensor, or tablet PC; data display: describes how the data will be displayed to the user and transmitted such as images, e-mail and textual data; application purpose: identification of the objective for the m-health system; application domain: definition of the area that the system will be implemented. Healthcare stakeholders and system implementer can use the reference model presented in this chapter to understand the security implications of the proposed system, identify the technological infrastructure, business requirements and operational needs of the m-health systems being implemented. A reference model to encapsulate the emerging m-health field is needed for cumulative progress in this field. Currently, the m-health field is disjointed and it is often unclear what constitutes an m-health system. In the future, m-health applications will take advantage of technological advances such as device miniaturizations, device convergence, high-speed mobile networks, and improved medical sensors. This will lead to the increased diffusion of clinical m-health systems requiring better understanding of the components, which constitute the m-health system.

Introduction

M-health is defined as "mobile computing, medical sensor, and communications technologies for healthcare" (Istepanian & Zhang, 2004). The first occurrence of the terminology 'M-Health' in the literature was in the "Unwired e-med" special issue on wireless telemedicine systems (Istepanian & Laxminaryan, 2000). Since then, there has been an increase use of the term, encapsulating various types of healthcare systems. The use of the m-health terminology relates to applications and systems such as telemedicine (Istepanian & Wang, 2003), telehealth (Istepanian & Lacal, 2003) and biomedical sensing system (Budinger, 2003). Until now, there has been considerable confusion and overlap with the use of these terms are (Tulu & Chatterjee, 2005).

The rapid advances in information communication technology (ICT) (Godoe, 2000), nanotechnology, bio monitoring (Budinger, 2003) mobile networks (Olla, 2005a), pervasive computing (Akyildiz & Rudin, 2001) , wearable systems , and drug delivery approaches (Grayson, et al., 2004) are transforming the healthcare sector. The insurgence of innovative technology into the healthcare practice is not only blurring the boundaries of the various technologies and fields, but is also causing a paradigm shift that is blurring the boundaries between public health, acute care, and preventative health (Hatcher & Heetebry, 2004). These developments have not only had a significant impact on current e-health and telemedical systems (Istepanian & Zhang, 2004), but they are also leading to the creation of a new generation of m-health systems with convergence of devices, technologies and networks at the forefront of the innovation.

This chapter proposes the use of a five dimensional reference models to assist system implementers and business stakeholders in understanding the various components of an m-health system. The approach used in this chapter focuses on identifying different dimensions of a mobile healthcare delivery system (MHDS) (Wickramas-inghe & Misra, 2005) which can then be used to identify user security requirements for different categories in an organized manner. These dimensions were driven from our literature review (Field, 1996; Bashshur, et al., 2000; Bashshur, 2002; Moore, 2002; Olla & Patel, 2003; Raskovic, Martin, & Jovanov, 2004; Istepanian, et al., 2005; Jovanov, et al., 2005) and the model reflects a combination of various classification schemes proposed in earlier studies to classify telemedicine and tele-health systems

Based on the definition above, m-health is a broad area transcending multiple disciplines and utilizing a broad range of technologies. There are a variety of applications, devices, and communication technologies emerging in the m-health arena, which can be combined to create the m-health system. The dimensions consist of:

1. **Communication infrastructure:** Description of the mobile telecommunication technologies that will be used, such as Bluetooth, wireless local area networks or third generation technologies (Olla, 2005)

2. **Device type:** This relates to the type of device being used to collect the medical data such as personal digital assistance (PDA), sensor, tablet PC (Parmanto, et al., 2005)

3. **Data display:** Describes how the data will be displayed to the user and transmitted such as images, e-mail, textual data and other types of data presentation languages (Tulu & Chatterjee, 2005)

4. **Application purpose:** Identification of the objective for the m-health system (Field, 1996)

5. **Application domain:** Definition of the area that the system will be implemented such as clinical (dermatology, radiology, etc.) or non-clinical (billing, maintenance, etc.) domains (Bashshur, et al., 2000)

Selecting different alternatives in the five dimensions will have implications on the functionality of the system, however the key focus of this discussion will be the emphasis on how the security and integrity of the m-health system is maintained based on the dimension choices.

The rest of the chapter is organized as follows. The Background section gives a brief overview of the evolution of m-health. The next sections provides an overview of existing and new mobile technologies suitable for the healthcare sector. Following is the section that introduces the five dimensions of the m-health reference model. The penultimate section uses the reference model to decompose a real-life mobile health delivery system to illustrate the security concerns. This is followed by the conclusion.

Background of M-Health

The phenomenon to provide care remotely using ICT can be placed into a number of areas such as m-health, telemedicine, e-health, but as summed up by Bashur, the president emeritus of the American Telemedicine Association, the terminology is not the important aspect. "It does not really matter what we call it or where we draw boundaries. …collective and collaborative efforts from various fields of science, including what we call now telemedicine is necessary" (Bashshur, 2002). Emphasis on the various components and objectives of the various types of systems should be the priority, as this will increase the chances of implementing efficient and effective systems, generating viable business models, and creating secure systems that meet the needs of the stakeholders (Olla & Patel, 2003). Over the evolution of telemedicine, new terminologies have been created as new health applications and delivery options became available and the application areas extended to most healthcare domains. Confusion and identification of what falls under telemedicine and what falls under tele-health or e-health became more complicated as the field advanced. New concepts such as pervasive health and m-health are also adding to this confusion. Before understanding the scope and components of m-health, it is important to briefly mention the history of telemedicine and the advancements of mobile networks, which are collectively the foundation of m-health. The evolution and growth of telemedicine is highly correlated with ICT advancements and software development. Telemedicine advancements can be categorized into three eras (Bashshur, et al., 2000; Tulu & Chatterjee, 2005).

The *first era* of telemedicine solely focused on the medical care as the only function of telemedicine. This era can be named as telecommunications era of the 1970s. The applications in this era were dependent on broadcast and television technologies in which telemedicine application were not integrated with any other clinical data. The *second era* of telemedicine was a result of digitalization in telecommunications and it grew during the 1990s. The transmission of data was supported by various communication mediums ranging from telephone lines to integrated service digital network (ISDN) lines. During this period, there were a high costs attached to the communication mediums that provided higher bandwidth. The bandwidth issue became a significant bottleneck for telemedicine in this era. Resolving the bandwidth constraints has been a critical research challenge for the past decade, with new approaches and opportunities created by the Internet revolution; now more complex and ubiquitous networks are supporting the telemedicine. The *third era* of telemedicine was supported by the networking technology that was cheaper and accessible to an increasing user population. The improved speed and quality offered by Internet2 is providing new opportunities in telemedicine. In this new era of telemedicine, the focus shifted from a technology assessment to a deeper appreciation of the functional relationships between telemedicine technology and the outcomes of cost, quality, and access.

This chapter proposes a *fourth era* which is characterized by the use of Internet protocol (IP) technologies, ubiquitous networks and mobile/wireless networking capabilities and can be observed by the proliferation of m-health applications that perform both clinical and non-clinical functions. Since, the proliferation of mobile networks telemedicine has attracted a lot more interest from both academic researchers and industry (Tachakra, et al., 2003). This has resulted in many mobile/wireless telemedicine applications being developed and implemented (Istepanian & Laxminaryan, 2000; Pattichis, et al., 2002; Budinger, 2003; Istepanian & Lacal, 2003; Jovanov, et al., 2003; Webb, 2004). Critical healthcare information regularly travels with patients and clinicians and therefore the need for information to become securely and accurately available over mobile telecommunication networks is key to reliable patient care and reliable medical systems.

Health organizations are required by the Health Insurance Portability and Accountability Act of 1996 (HIPAA) to maintain the privacy of protected health information and to provide individuals with notice of its legal duties and privacy policies with respect to this information (HIPPA, 2005). Specifically, the law requires that:

- Any medical information that identifies a person be kept private
- Notice of legal duties and privacy practices with respect to protected health information be made available
- The organization abide by the terms of their notices currently in effect

HIPAA also requires that:

- Computers and data containing protected health information (PHI) are protected from compromise or loss
- Audit trails of access to PHI are kept
- Electronic transmissions of PHI are authenticated and protected from observation or change

Failure to comply with these requirements (for both HIPAA privacy and security) can result in civil and criminal penalties ranging from $100 to $250,000, and up to 10 years in jail. Medical information has always been considered sensitive, and never more so than now due to the security issues created by mobility. Many countries have imposed strict regulations with heavy penalties to ensure the confidentiality and authorized distribution of personal medical information. Following the lead of European Union Directive 95/46/EC, that protects both medical and financial personal information, the United States and Canada passed important legislation (HIPAA and PIPED, respectively) that imposes substantial penalties, both civil and criminal, for negligent or intentional exposure of personal medical information to unauthorized parties.

The telecommunication industry has progressed significantly over the last decade. There has been significant innovation in digital mobile technologies. The mobile telecommunication industry has advances through three generations of systems and is currently on the verge of designing the fourth generation of systems (Olla, 2005b). The recent developments in digital mobile technologies are reflected in the fast growing commercial domain of mobile tele-medical services (Istepanian, et al., 2005). Specific examples include mobile ECG transmissions; video images and tele-radiology; wireless ambulance services to predict emergency and stroke morbidity; and other integrated mobile tele-medical monitoring systems (Warren, 2003; Istepanian & Zhang, 2004). There is no doubt that mobile networks can introduce additional security concerns to the healthcare sector.

Implementing a mobile trust model will ensure that a mobile transaction safely navigates multiple technologies and devices without compromising the data or the healthcare systems. M-health transactions can be made secure by adopting practices that extend beyond the security of the wireless network used and implementing a trusted model for secure end-to-end mobile transactions. The mobile trust model proposed by Wickramasinghe (2005) utilizes both technology and adequate operational practices to achieve a secure end-to-end mobile transaction. The first level highlights the application of technologies to secure elements of a mobile transaction. The next level of the model shows the operational policies and procedures needed to complement technologies used. No additional activity is proposed for the mobile network infrastructure since this element is not within the control of the provider or the hospital.

The next section will discuss the mobile network technologies and infrastructure, this is a key component of any m-health system; the network infrastructure acts as a channel for data transmission and is subject to the same vulnerabilities, such as sniffing, as in the case of fixed network transaction. The mobile networks discussed in the next section are creating the growth and increased adoption of m-health applications in the healthcare sector.

Mobile Healthcare Delivery System Networks

The implementation of an m-health application in the healthcare environment leads to the creation of a mobile healthcare delivery system (MHDS); an MHDS can be defined as the carrying out of healthcare-related activities using mobile devices such as a wireless tablet computer, personal digital assistant (PDA), or a wireless-enabled computer. An activity occurs when an authorized healthcare personnel accesses the clinical or administrative systems of a healthcare institution using a mobile device (Wickramasinghe & Misra, 2005). The transaction is said to be complete when medical personnel decide to access medical records (patient or administrative) via a mobile network to either browse or update the record.

Over the past decade there has been an increase in the use of new mobile technologies in healthcare such as Bluetooth, and wireless local area networks (WLAN) that

Table 1. Comparison of mobile networks based on range and speed (Copyright Authors, used with permission)

Networks	Speed	Range and Coverage	Main Issues for M-Health
2nd Generation GSM	9.6 kilobits per second (KBPS)	World wide coverage, dependent on network operators roaming agreements.	Bandwidth limitation, Interference.
High Speed Circuit Switched Data (HSCSD)	Between 28.8 KBPS and 57.6 KBPS.	Not global, only supported by service providers network.	Not widely available, scarcity of devices.
General Packet Radio Service (GPRS)	171.2 KBPS	Not global, only supported by service providers network.	Not widely available.
EDGE	384 KBPS	Not global, only supported by service providers network.	Not widely available, scarcity of devices
UMTS	144 KBPS - 2 MBPS depending on mobility	When fully implemented should offer interoperability between networks, global coverage.	Device battery life, operational costs.
Wireless Local Area	54 MBPS	30–50 m indoors and 100–500 m outdoors. Must be in the vicinity of hot spot.	Privacy, security.
Personal Area Networks – Bluetooth	400 KBPS symmetrically 150 -700 KBPS asymmetrically	10 – 100m	Privacy, security, low bandwidth.
Personal Area Networks – Zigbee	20 kb/s – 250 KBPS depending on band	30m	Security, privacy, low bandwidth.
WiMAX	Up to 70MBPS	Approx. 40m from base station.	Currently no devices and networks cards.
RFID	100 KBPS	1 m Non line-of-sight and contact less transfer of data between a tag and Reader.	Security, privacy.
Satellite Networks	400 to 512 KBPS new satellites have potential of 155MBPS.	Global coverage.	Data costs, shortage of devices with roaming capabilities. Bandwidth limitations.

use different protocols from the standard digital mobile technologies such as 2G, 2.5 and 3G technologies. A summary of these technologies are presented below, and a précis of the speeds and range is presented in Table 1.

These mobile networks are being deployed to allow physicians and nurses easy access to patient records while on rounds, to add observations to the central databases and to check on medications, among a growing number of other functions. The ease of access that wireless networks offer is matched by the security and privacy challenges presented by the networks. This serious issue requires further investigation and research to identify the real threats for the various types of networks in the healthcare domain.

Second generation systems (2G /2.5G): The second-generation cellular systems (2G) were the first to apply digital transmission technologies such as time division multiple access (TDMA) for voice and data communication. The data transfer rate was on the order of tens of kbits/s. Other examples of technologies in 2G systems include frequency division multiple access (FDMA) and code division multiple access (CDMA).

The 2G networks deliver high quality and secure mobile voice and basic data services such as fax and text messaging, along with full roaming capabilities across the world. Second Generation technology is in use by more than 10% of the world's population and it is estimated that 1.3 billion customers across more than 200 countries and territories around the world use this technology (GSM_Home, 2005). The later advanced technological applications are called 2.5G technologies and include networks such as general packet radio service (GPRS) and EDGE. GPRS-enabled networks provides functionality such as: 'always-on', higher capacity, Internet-based content and packet-based data services enabling services such as colour Internet browsing, e-mail on the move, visual communications, multimedia messages and location-based services. Another complimentary 2.5G service is enhanced data rates for GSM evolution (EDGE) which offers similar capabilities to the GPRS network.

Third generation systems (3G): The most promising period is the advent of 3G networks which are also referred to as the universal mobile telecommunications systems (UMTS). A significant feature of 3G technology is its ability to unify existing cellular standards, such as code-division multiple-access (CDMA), global system for mobile communications (GSM_Home, 2005), and time-division multiple-access (TDMA), under one umbrella (IEEE special issue). Over 85% of the world's network operators have chosen 3G as the underlying technology platform to deliver their third generation services (GSM-Information). Efforts are underway to integrate the many diverse mobile environments in addition to blurring the distinction between the fixed and mobile networks. The continual roll out of advanced wireless communication and mobile network technologies will be the major driving force for future developments in m-health systems (Istepanian & Zhang, 2004). Currently, the GSM version of 3G alone saw the addition of more than 13.5 million users, representing an annual growth rate of more than 500% in 2004. As of December 2004, 60 operators in 30 countries were offering 3GSM services. The global 3GSM customer base is approaching 20 million and has already been commercially launched in Africa, the Americas, Asia Pacific, Europe, and the Middle East (GSM_Home, 2005), thus making this technology ideal for developing affordable global m-health systems.

Fourth generation (4G): The benefits of the 4th generation network technology include: (Qiu, Zhu, Zhang, 2002; Istepanian, et al., 2005; Olla, 2005a;) voice-data integration, support for mobile and fixed networking, enhanced services through the use of simple networks with intelligent terminal devices. 4G also incorporates a flexible method of payment for network connectivity that will support a large number of network operators in a highly competitive environment. Over the last decade, the Internet has been dominated by non-real-time, person-to machine communications (UMTS-Forum-Report14, 2002). The current developments in progress will incorporate real-time person-to-person communications, including high-quality voice and video telecommunications along with extensive use of machine-to-machine interactions to simplify and enhance the user experience.

Currently, the Internet is used solely to interconnect computer networks. IP compatibility is being added to many types of devices such as set-top boxes to automotive and home electronics. The large-scale deployment of IP-based networks will reduce the acquisition costs of the associated devices. The future vision is to integrate mobile voice communications and Internet technologies, bringing the control and multiplicity of Internet application services to mobile users (Olla, 2005b). 4G advances will provide both mobile patients and citizens the choices that will fit their lifestyle and make it easier for them to interactively get the medical attention and advice they need, when and where it is required and how they want it regardless of any geographical barriers or mobility constraints.

Worldwide interoperability for microwave access (WiMAX): WiMAX is considered to be the next generation of wireless fidelity (WiFi/Wireless networking technology that will connect you to the Internet at faster speeds and from much longer ranges than current wireless technology allows (http://wimaxxed.com/). WiMax has been undergoing testing and is expected to launch commercially by 2007. Research firm Allied Business Research predicts that by 2009, sales of WiMax accessories will top $1 billion (Taylor & Kendall, 2005) and Strategy Analytics predicts a market of more than 20 million WiMAX subscriber terminals and base stations per year in 2009 (ABI-Website, 2005).

The technology holds a lot of potential for m-health applications, with the capabilities of providing data rates of up to 70 mbps over distances of up to 50 km. The benefits to both developing and developed nations are immense. There has been a gradual increase in popularity of this technology. Intel recently announced plans to mass produce and release processors aimed to power WiMax-enabled devices (WiMax, 2005). Other technology organizations investing to further the advancement of this technology include Qwest, British Telecom, Siemens and Texas Instruments. They aim to get the prices of the devices powered by WiMax to affordable levels so that the public can adopt them in large numbers, making it the next global wireless standard. There are already Internet service providers in metropolitan areas offering pre-WiMAX service to enterprises in a number of cities including New York, Boston and Los Angeles (WiMax, 2005).

Wireless local area networks: Wireless local area networks (WLAN) use radio or infrared waves and spread spectrum technology to enable communication between devices in a limited area. WLAN allows users to access a data network at high speeds of up to 54 Mb/s as long as users are located within a relatively short range (typically 30-50 m indoors and 100-500 m outdoors) of a WLAN base station (or antenna). Devices may roam freely within the coverage areas created by wireless "access points," the receivers and transmitters connected to the enterprise network. WLANs are a good solution for healthcare today, plus they are significantly less expensive to operate than wireless WAN solutions such as 3G (Daou-Systems, 2001).

Personal area networks: A wireless personal area network (WPAN) (IBM-Research; Istepanian, Robert & Zhang, 2004) is the interconnection of information technology devices within the range of an individual person, typically within a range of 10 meters. For example, a person traveling with a laptop, a personal digital assistant (PDA), and a portable printer could wirelessly interconnect all the devices, using some form of wireless technology. WPANs are defined by IEEE standard 802.15 (IEEE-Working-Group). The most relevant enabling technologies for m-health systems are Bluetooth (Bluetooth-home) and ZigBee (ZigBee-Alliance). *ZigBee* is a set of high-level communication protocols designed to use small, low power digital radios based on the IEEE 802.15.4 standard for wireless personal area networks. ZigBee is aimed at applications with low data rates and low power consumption. ZigBee's current focus is to define a general-purpose, inexpensive self-organizing network that can be shared by industrial controls, medical devices, smoke and intruder alarms, building automation and home automation. The network is designed to use very small amounts of power, so that individual devices might run for a year or two with a single alkaline battery which is ideal for use in small medical devices and sensors. The Bluetooth specification was first developed by Ericsson, and later formalized by the Bluetooth Special Interest Group established by Sony Ericsson, IBM, Intel, Toshiba and Nokia, and later joined by many other companies. A Bluetooth WPAN is also called a *piconet*, and is composed of up to eight active devices in a master-slave relationship. A piconet typically has a range of 10 meters, although ranges of up to 100 meters can be reached under ideal circumstances. Implementations with Bluetooth versions 1.1 and 1.2 reach speeds of 723.1 kbit/s. Version 2.0 implementations feature *Bluetooth enhanced data rate (EDR)*, and thus reach 2.1 Mbit/s (Bluetooth-home; encyclopedia).

Radio frequency identification (RFID): RFID systems consist of two key elements: a 'tag' and a reader/writer unit capable of transferring data to and from the tag. An antennae linked to each element allows power to be transferred between the reader/writer and remotely sited tag through inductive coupling. Since this is a bi-directional process, modulation of the tag antenna will be 'reflected' back to the reader's/writer's antenna, allowing data to be transferred in both directions. Some of the advantages of RFID that makes this technology appealing to the healthcare sector are:

- No line-of-sight required between tag and reader
- Non-contact transfer of data between a tag and reader
- Tags are passive, which means no power source is required for the tag component
- Data transfer range of up to 1 meter is possible
- Rapid data transfer rates of up to 100 Kbits/sec.

The use of RFID in the healthcare environment is set to rise and is currently being used for drug tracking. RFID technology is expected to decrease counterfeit medicines and make obtaining drugs all the more difficult for addicts (Weil, 2005). There are also applications that allow tagging of patients, beds, and expensive hospital equipment.

Satellite technologies: Satellite broadband uses a satellite to connect customers to the Internet. Two-way satellite broadband uses a satellite link to both send and receive data. Typical download speeds are 400 to 512 kbps, while upload speeds on two-way services are typically 64 to 128 kbps. Various organizations (Imrasat-Swift, 2000) have been investigating the development of an ultra-high-data-rate Internet test satellite for use for making a high-speed Internet society a reality (JAXA, 2005). Satellite-based telemedicine service will allow a real-time transmission of electronic medical records and medical information anywhere on earth. This will make it possible for doctors to diagnose emergency patients even from remote areas and also will increase the chances of saving lives by receiving early information as ambulance data rates of 155mbps are expected. One considerable drawback associated with using this technology is cost (Olla, 2004).

This section has summarized the various mobile network technologies that are being used in the healthcare sector. The mobile technologies described above have a significant impact on the ability to deploy m-healthcare application and systems; however, there are combinations of other important factors described in the next section. The next section will present a five-layered model that uses mobile network technologies along with device type, data display, application purpose and application domain to categorize m-health systems.

The M-Health Reference Model

The financial cost of delivering quality healthcare is increasing exponentially not only in North America but also world wide. To satisfy increasing healthcare challenges, organizations in the healthcare sector are investing in innovative technological solutions to meet these higher expectations placed on practice management

Figure 1.   M-Health reference model for identifying components of healthcare delivery systems (Copyright Authors, used with permission)

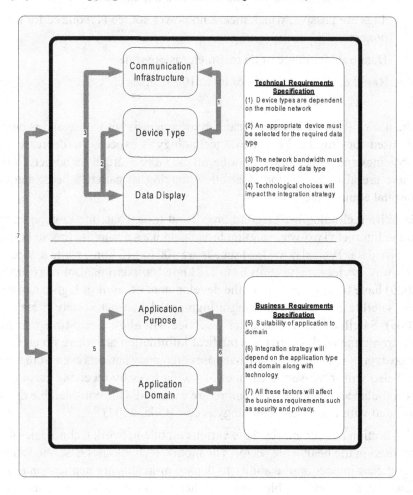

(Wickramasinghe & Silvers, 2002; Wickramasinghe & Misra, 2005). The evolution of m-health solutions such as the use of wireless networks to access patient records and other healthcare services such as billing and prescription are becoming popular especially in the U.S. and Canada (Goldberg & Wickramasinghe, 2002) and in many European countries (Sorby, 2002). However, these wireless solutions also bring with them their own challenges, security being one of the most important issues in m-health. This is because m-health systems transmit highly sensitive information, such as patient data over cyberspace, and there is a need for high-level end-to-end security, confidentiality and privacy.

This section presents a reference model to describe each m-health system to address the security challenges. Specifically, we present a reference model and show how our model can facilitate a higher level of end-to-end security in a wireless or mobile healthcare environment. Despite the advancements of wireless technologies, the use of wireless security in healthcare is in its infancy and a robust mobile healthcare model needs to be developed to allow further innovation of m-health applications and services to fulfill the growing needs of the healthcare sector.

This section presents a reference model that can be utilized to classify m-health systems by identifying the system components for a specific m-health system. As previously indicated, the approach used to develop the reference model concentrated on identifying different dimensions of a mobile healthcare delivery system (MHDS), which provides the capability to identify user security requirements for different categories in an organized manner. The reference model was formulated by reviewing the literature and the model reflects an amalgamation of various classification schemes proposed by previous experts to categorize telemedicine and tele-health systems. The following sub sections will provide a description of these five domains for the m-health reference model illustrated in Figure 1. These domains include communication infrastructure, device type, data display, application purpose, and application domain.

Mobile Communication Infrastructure

The first dimension defines the mobile infrastructure used to transmit, encode and receive the data. There are numerous wireless infrastructures available for healthcare providers to choose from. Examples of networks that provide personal area networks include Bluetooth and Zigbee. Mobile networks that provide connectivity within buildings include wireless local area networks (WLAN); these use different protocols from the standard digital mobile technologies such as 2G, 2.5 and 3G technologies which provide wide-area connectivity. A summary of these technologies was provided in a previous section.

Device Type

The second section is referred to as 'Device Type'. Due to the advances in medical sensor technologies and handheld computers, m-health has the potential to deliver services beyond the scope of mobile telemedicine discussed in the previous section. The integration of medical sensors with ICT allows physicians to diagnose, monitor, and treat patients remotely without compromising standards of care. Advances of new materials and signal processing research is allowing the design of smart medical sensors, which utilize the real-time data recording, and processing of multi-physiological signals.

There is a multiplicity of sensors commercially available on the market such as piezo-electrical materials for pressure measurements, infrared sensors for body temperature estimation, and optoelectronic sensors monitoring heart rate and blood pressure. These sensors are being embedded into wearable items and accessories such as sunglasses and rings that can easily be carried. With the continual improvements to the sensors and the miniaturization of computing devices, these wearable devices for the monitoring, diagnosis, and treatment of illnesses are becoming more readily available. Hitachi has developed a wristwatch, which can measure the wearer's health conditions such as pulse, moves, and body temperature. The monitoring wristwatch can send the data wirelessly via the Internet to remote monitoring services. Hitachi aims to commercially launch the wireless wristwatch within 3 years (Nikkei-Business-Publications, 2005), targeting the healthcare service industry for elderly people. The benefit of wearable sensors for physiological data collection is that they can be used to monitor human health constantly without unsettling the patients' day-to-day activities. Examples include rings, vests, and watches (IBM-Research 2004), wearable intelligent sensors and systems for e-medicine (Winters & Wang, 2003). Wireless communication such as WAN is used for transmitting information and accessing healthcare databases wherever appropriate to allow free movement of the user (Jovanov, et al., 2005).

Personal digital assistants (PDA) have been popular among healthcare practitioners in the last few years. PDA penetration among physicians is at 25%, much higher than the 4% penetration for the general population (Forrester, 2001; Harris-Interactive, 2001; Fischer, et al., 2003; Parmanto, et al., 2005). Studies have shown that the integration of PDAs into clinical practice has led to decreased medication error rates (Grasso, et al, 2002) and the improvement in physicians' adherence to a clinical practice guidelines (Shiffman, 1999; 2000).

Although the PDA has great potential in supporting evidence-based medicine, there are some considerable drawbacks (Parmanto, et al., 2005). The small screen is a poor match for information resources designed for full-size desktop computers. Presenting vast amounts of information in the limited space of the PDA display is a significant technical barrier to the realization of the PDA's potential (Larkin, 2001; Peterson, 2002; Fischer, et al., 2003). Other technical PDA drawbacks include low resolution, limited memory, slow processor, and problematic data input. An alternative for the PDA is a tablet PC. These are being adopted in the healthcare sector for information capture at the patient's bedside.

Data Display

This key dimension describes how the information from the m-health application is to be processed and transmitted. The chosen delivery options can have an important effect on the final quality of the telemedicine event and the outcome. Delivery options in telemedicine can be categorized under two main groups according to Tulu and Chatterjee (2005): (1) synchronous and (2) asynchronous. Information transactions that occur between two or more participants simultaneously are called synchronous communications. In asynchronous communications, these transactions occur at different points in time. The data displays for both synchronous and asynchronous presentations can be grouped into the following categories: text, data, video, and multimedia (combination).

Application Purpose

The fourth dimension is the application purpose. This domain describes the intended use of the application. Field (1996) categorized this field   into two main groups: clinical and non-clinical systems.

The *Committee on Evaluating Clinical Applications of Telemedicine in 1996 grouped* Clinical applications into five categories (Committee, 1996):

1.   Initial urgent evaluation
2.   Supervision of primary care
3.   Provision of specialty care
4.   Consultation
5.   Monitoring

Due to the rapid advances made in the m-health field, three additional categories were added by Tulu and Samir (2005):

6.   Use of remote information and decision analysis resources to support or guide care for specific patients
7.   Diagnostic
8.   Treatment (surgical and non-surgical)

 In addition to these groups, two additional categories have been added by the authors to reflect the future trends of m-health systems:

9.   Drug delivery
10. Patient identification

The use of m-health systems for non-clinical purpose includes medical education, and administrative duties that do not involve decisions about care for particular patients. Some examples of m-health non- clinical applications include:

1.   Mobile access to the latest drug reference database
2.   Bedside access to patient records: Increase efficiency by reducing demand for paper records
3.   ePrescribing: Mobile prescription writing and verification of drug interactions
4.   Prescription formulary reference: Electronically identify most economic pharmaceuticals for a patient
5.   Electronic billing for in-home healthcare workers
6.   Patient/drug verification: Scan patient and drug bar codes to help ensure the appropriate medicine is being administered to the correct patient
7.   Delivery applications: Healthcare supply delivery, tracking and billing
8.   Patient encounter data capture

Application Area

The final dimension is called application area. This dimension described to the medical field which is implementing the m-health technology. The application area can also be sub-divided into clinical and non-clinical use. Clinical use relates to medical departments such as emergency, ophthalmology, paediatrician, and surgery. Non-clinical use relates to areas maintenance such as, charge capture, billing, and administration. The importance of this domain is to highlight the differences in the environments and to identify procedures that are specific to a particular healthcare domain.

In summary, the reference model highlights some of the important elements of an m-health system. It is important to understand all of the dimensions of the reference model for each mobile healthcare system. Using the above dimensions to describe an application will allow an m-health system to be broken down into meaningful components.

The next section presents a case, which features the use of an m-health application that uses a PDA to collect private medical data in remote African communities. The case in the next section illustrates how the reference model can be used to derive the components of an m-health system; this allows issues such as security, privacy, hosting requirements, interference of devices, and integration to be investigated simultaneously.

Overview of Blood Donor Recruitment (BDR) Project

As an increased number of healthcare industry professionals adopt mobile-enabled handheld devices to collect, store, and retrieve critical medical information, the need for security has become a top-priority IT challenge. These mobile benefits come with immense corporate and regulatory risk. PDA devices left unsecured while electronic health information is being hotsynced to a PC can become a primary source for the intentional malicious interception of confidential information. Furthermore, the recent adoption of the Patient Privacy and Federal Health Insurance Portability and Accountability Act (HIPPA) are strong reasons not to have protected health information on any unsecured devices, especially a PDA. This section will provide an example of how the reference model described in the previous sections can be used to describe a project initiated by the Red Cross.

The medical informatics data analyst/IT manager of the Uganda Red Cross Society identified a potential weakness in the use of mobile devices in the community health field. One of the authors was consulted to assist in developing a model that addressed data security to ensure the main IT security goals: confidentiality, integrity, and availability are achieved. Mobile devices were used in blood donor recruitment (BDR) activities to register blood donors' details. The medical history is stored for blood screening purposes. The data is very confidential because some of the blood donors' results are positive for HIV, hepatitis or syphilis. The system specifications are as follows:

Palm M125 with the following software:

- Palm Desktop software for Windows v. 4.0
- Pendragon form 3.2
- Pendragon Distribution Tollkit 2.0
- Window Xp on the PC
- Microsoft Access 2000

The volume of data is about 10mb records on the PDA.

This information is transferred to the computer server by either wired synchronization (HotSynced) or wireless network. The hotsync option requires the user to be in the confines of the hospital or office because it involves the use of the wired cradle. The other alternative, which is being considered, is the use of a wireless network such as WiFi or GSM to transfer the data to the computer. Once the data is stored on the computer it is manipulated using various software tools.

Table 2a. Using the reference model to describe the blood donor system using a cradle solution (Copyright Authors, used with permission)

System	Purpose	Data	Network	Device	Application Area
Blood Donor Recruitment (BDR)	Blood donor data capture and transfer	Textual data	Fixed cable	Palm PDA	Rural community health
Security Model					
•Data sent from the PDA and to the PDA must be secured with encryption.					
•User and server authentication must be in place.					
•Access to data in the server from a computer or PDA different from where the server runs must be secured with encryption and user / server authentication.					
•Advances authentication methods such as biometrics will provide added security features.					

Using the m-health reference model described in the previous section, the BDR system was broken down into the various components as highlighted in Table 2a and 2b. The following general recommendations were suggested to the client.

1. Upgrade memory on mobile device
2. Formulate an enforceable end-to-end security policy
3. Evaluate encryption software that can run both on the PDA and the PC
4. Implement a solution that ensures captured data on the PDA can be encrypted before being hotsynced on the PC
5. Try out software prior to purchase

There are various software solutions that can be used to secure the health system described above, which vary by encryption method, price, and device compatibility, however there is no single solution to securing a system. It is important that each scenario is addressed differently irrespective of how similar they seem.

A software solution that would fulfill the requirements for the scenario described in Table 2a and 2b, the PDASecure™ by Trust Digital software, provides six different selectable encryption algorithms. Additional protection features includes strong password protection to prevent unauthorized synchronizing or beaming of data, unauthorized deletion of files due to viruses or malicious code, and a user requirement to authenticate themselves to devices before data can be decrypted. IT administrators can control who can access data and networks with wireless handheld devices, encrypt 100% of the data, and password-protect devices so that they are useless if stolen or compromised.

Table 2b. Using the reference model to describe the blood donor system using a wireless solution (Copyright Authors, used with permission)

System	Purpose	Data	Network	Device	Application Area
Blood Donor Recruitment (BDR)	Blood donor data capture and transfer	Textual data	WIFI/ GPRS	Palm PDA	Rural community health
Security Model •Data sent to/ from the PDA must be secured with encryption. •User and server authentication must be in place. •No data storage in network operator environment (GPRS/UMTS Operator) •WiFi network must be secured.					

Using mobile networks allows data to travel over the open air when the data transmission is wireless and there is a possibility of interception of the radio transmission as well as unauthorized access of the hospital system. Poorly designed WiFi local area networks can be leaky and accessible beyond the intended boundary of use. If an unauthorized access of any kind occurs, it cannot only lead to the loss of the patient's privacy but could also lead to other potential consequences.

In Table 2a, the wireless network is not used and the mobile device must be co-located with the computer system and server to transfer and copy data. This option also presents a different set of security problems. Due to the storage capacities of the mobile devices and the growing trend of today's mobile workforce, every port, external disk drive, or JumpDrive can become a security risk. In the corporate environment, IT experts have turned to soldering and gluing USB ports to prevent intrusion, or have installed titanium chastity belts around computers. USB ports and PDA cradles can be used for a variety of functions from input devices as inconspicuous as iPODs which are now capable of not only downloading more than 30 gigabits of data.

In summary, using the reference model presented in this chapter to decompose Red Cross blood donor system ensured that the security issues were identified and appropriately addressed; the model was also valuable for discovering technical specifications of the system and understanding what upgrades were required to reduce the vulnerabilities of the system. In the future, this model can be improved by the creation of a set of guidelines and standards that are appropriate for a particular type of m-health system. This will be valuable for governments and private vendors implementing innovative healthcare systems. The model also aids the healthcare stakeholders to identify the technological infrastructure, business requirements and operational needs for the different types of m-health systems.

Conclusion

In the clinical domain, considerable leaps in the fields of biomedical telemetry, nanotechnology, ICT, and drug deliver techniques will encourage m-health applications to evolve rapidly over the next decade. These new m-health applications will take advantage of technological advances such as device miniaturizations, device convergence, high-speed mobile networks, reduction in power consumption and improved medical sensors. This will lead to the increased diffusion of clinical m-health systems and this will impact reshaping the healthcare sector.

The non-clinical use of m-health enterprise systems will also see an increased rate of adoption due to the potential benefits of the mobile solutions. Potential quality improvements may be achieved by implementing platforms that contain functionality that allows organizations to: perform clinical results viewing, e-prescribing, medication administration, and specimen collection, charge capture and physician dictation capture. These systems help reduce errors by making the patient's medical record and appropriate medical knowledge available at the point of care and the point of decision.

The reference model presented in this chapter aids the breakdown of m-health systems into the following five key dimensions: communication infrastructure: this dimension describes mobile telecommunication technologies and networks; device type: this relates to the type of device being used such as PDA, sensor, and tablet PC; data display: describes how the data will be displayed to the user and transmitted such as images, e-mail and textual data; application purpose: identification of the objective for the m-health system; application domain: definition of the area that the system will be implemented.

The reference model described in this chapter encapsulates the emerging m-health field and is needed to assist in clarifying the rapid progress in this field. Currently, the m-health field is disjointed and it is often unclear what component constitutes an m-health system. This is addressed by the reference model. Further work is needed to identify the appropriate standards and guidelines for implementing the various types of m-health systems. This would benefit vendors and system implementer by allowing them to understand the various conditions that may apply to a system that uses specific set of the m-health reference model variables. The reference model would also benefit from further work that defines how the choice of dimensions can impact the business models and security policy for the implementation of the system.

References

ABI-Website. (2005). WIFI - WIMAX. *http://www.abiresearch.com/category/Wi-Fi_WiMAX.*

Akyildiz, I., & Rudin, H. (2001). Pervasive computing. *Computer Networks-The International Journal of Computer and Telecommunications Networking, 35*(4), 371.

Bashshur, R. (2002). Telemedicine and healthcare. *Telemedicine Journal and e-Health, 8,* 5-12.

Bashshur, R., Reardon, T., & Shannon, G. (2000). Telemedicine: A new healthcare delivery system. *Annual Review of Public Health, 21,* 613-637.

Bluetooth-home. http://www.bluetooth.org/.

Budinger, T. (2003). Biomonitoring with wireless communications. *Annu. Rev. Biomed Eng, 5,* 412.

Committee. (1996). *Committee on evaluating clinical applications of telemedicine, temeledicine: A guide to assessing telecommunications in healthcare.*

Daou-Systems. (2001). *Going mobile: From e-health to m-health.* http://www.daou.com/emerging/pdf/mHealth_White_Paper_April_2001.PDF.

Encyclopedia. http://en.wikipedia.org/wiki.

Field, M. (1996). *Telemedicine: A guide to assessing telecommunications in health-care.* Paper presented at the National Academy Press. Washington, D.C.

Fischer, S., Stewart, T. E., Mehta, S., Wax, R., & Lapinsky, S. E. (2003). Review Paper & bull; Handheld computing in medicine. *Journal -American Medical Informatics Association, 10*(2), 139-149.

Forrester, T. (2001). *Doctors connect with handhelds.*

Godoe, H. (2000). Innovation regimes, R&D and radical innovations in telecom-munications. *Research Policy, 29*(9), 1033-1046.

Goldberg, S., & Wickramasinghe, N. (2002). *Mobilizing healthcare. Proceedings of the 5th ICECR Conference.* Montreal.

Grasso, B. C., Genest, R., Yung, K., & Arnold, C. (2002). Reducing errors in discharge medication lists by using personal digital assistants. *Psychiatric Services, 53*(10), 1325-1326.

Grayson, A. C. R., Shawgo, R. S., Johnson, A. M., Flynn, N. T., Li, Y., Cima, M. J., et al. (2004). A BioMEMS review: MEMS technology for physiologically integrated devices (Invited paper). *Proceedings of the IEEE, 92*(1), 6-21. GSM_Home. (2005). http://www.gsmworld.com/index.shtml.

GSM-Information. (2004). http://www.gsmworld.com/index.shtml.

Harris-Interactive. (2001). Physicians' use of handheld personal computing devices increases from 15% in 1999 to 26% in 2001. *Harris Interactive Healthcare News, 1*(25).

Hatcher, M., & Heetebry, I. (2004). Information technology in the future of health-care. *Journal of Medical Systems Issue, 28*(6), 673-688.

HIPPA. (2005). United States Department of Health and Human Services, Office for Civil Rights, Health Insurance Portability and Accountability Act of 1996 Fact Sheets. Retrieved September 30, 2005, from www.hhs.gov/ocr/hipaa/.

IBM-Research. http://www.research.ibm.com/topics/popups/smart/mobile/html/phow.html).

IEEE-Working-Group. http://www.ieee802.org/15/. *IEEE 802.15 Working Group for WPAN [Online]*.

Imrasat-Swift64. (2000). *Inmarsat announces availability of the 64kbit/S mobile office in the sky.* http://www.inmarsat.com/swift64/press_1.htm.

Istepanian, R., & Laxminaryan, S. (2000). UNWIRED, the next generation of wireless and internetable telemedicine systems-editorial paper. *IEEE Trans. Inform. Technol. Biomed., 4*(189-194).

Istepanian, R. S. H., Laxminarayan, S., & Pattichis, C. S. (2006). *M-health: Emerging mobile health systems.* Topics in biomedical engineering international book series. New York: Springer.

Istepanian, R., & Zhang, Y. (2004). Guest editorial introduction to the special section on m-health: Beyond seamless mobility and global wireless healthcare connectivity. *Ieee Transactions On Information Technology In Biomedicine, 8*(4).

Istepanian, R., & Lacal, J. (2003). M-health systems: Future directions. *Proceedings of the 25th Annual International Conference IEEE Engineering Medicine and Biology.* Cancun, Mexico.

Istepanian, R., & Wang, H. (Eds.). (2003). Telemedicine in the UK, in *European Telemedicine Glossary of Concepts, Standards Technologies.* Brussels, Belgium: European Commission Information Society Directorate-General.

J. M. Winters, J., Y. W., and J. M. Winters. (2003). Wearable sensors and telereha-bilitation: Integrating intelligent telerehabilitation assistants with a model for optimizing home therapy. *EEE Eng. Med. Biol. Mag, 1*(22), 56-65.

JAXA. (2005). *Aerospace exploration agency.*

Jovanov, E., Lords, A., Raskovic, D., Cox, P., Adhami, R., & Andrasik, F. (2003). Stress monitoring using a distributed wireless intelligent sensor system. *IEEE Eng. Med. Biol. Mag., 22*(3), 49-55.

Jovanov, E., Milenkovic, A., Otto, C., & Groen, P. (2005). A wireless body area network of intelligent motion sensors for computer assisted physical rehabilitation. *Journal of NeuroEngineering and Rehabilitation, 2*(6).

Larkin, M. (2001). Can handheld computers improve the quality of care?. *Lancet, 358*(9291), 1438.

Moore, S. (2002). Extending healthcare's reach: Telemedicine can help spread medical expertise around the globe. *IEEE Spectrum, 39*(66-71).

New-scientist. (2005). Future trends, convergence is. *NewScientist, 12,* 53.

Nikkei-Business-Publications. (2005). Hitachi's wireless health monitoring wristwatch. *http://techon.nikkeibp.co.jp/english/NEWS_EN/20050526/105103/ ?ST=english.*

Olla, P. (2004). A convergent mobile infrastructure: Competition or co-operation. *Journal of Computing and Information Technology: Special Issue on Information Systems: Healthcare and Mobile Computing, 12*(4), 309-322.

Olla, P. (2005a). Evolution of GSM network technology. In: M. Pagani (Ed.), *Encyclopaedia of multimedia technology and networking.* Hershey, PA: Idea Group Publishing.

Olla, P. (2005b). Incorporating commercial space technology into mobile services: Developing innovative business models. In: M. Pagani (Ed.), *Mobile and wireless systems beyond 3G: Managing new business opportunities.* IRM Press.

Olla, P., & Patel, N. (2003). Framework for delivering secure mobile location information. *International Journal of Mobile Communications, 1*(3), 289-300.

Parmanto, B., Saptono, A., Ferrydiansyah, R., & Sugiantara, W. (2005). Transcoding biomedical information resources for mobile handhelds. *Proceedings of the 38th Hawaii International Conference on System Sciences.* Hawaii.

Pattichis, C., Kyriacou, E., Voskarides, S., Pattichis, M., Istepanian, R., & Schizas, C. (2002). Wireless telemedicine systems: An overview. *IEEE Antennas Propagat. Mag., 44*(2), 143-153.

Peterson, M. (2002). The right information at the point of care library delivery via hand-held computers. *Proceeding of the EAHIL Conference of Health and Medical Libraries.* Cologne.

Qiu, R., & Zhang, Y. (2002). Third-generation and beyond (3.5G) wireless networks and its applications. *IEEE International Symposium on Circuits and Systems (ISCS).* Scottsdale, Arizona.

Raskovic, D., & Jovanov, E. (2004). Medical monitoring applications for wearable computing. *Comput. J, 47*(4), 495-504.

Shiffman, R. (1999). User satisfaction and frustration with a handheld, pen-based guideline implementation system for asthma. *Proceedings of the AMIA Symposium.*

Shiffman, R. (2000). A guideline implementation system using handheld computers for office management of asthma: Effects on adherence and patient outcomes. *Pediatrics, 105*(4), 767-773.

Sorby, I. (2002). Characterising cooperation in the ward—a framework for producing requirements to mobile electronic healthcare records. *Proceedings of the 2nd Hospital of the Future Conferenc.* Chicago, IL.

Tachakra, S., Wang, X., Istepanian, R., & Song, Y. (2003). Mobile e-health: The unwired evolution of telemedicine mobile. *Telemedicine Journal and e-Health, 9*(3).

Taylor, C., & Kendall, P. (2005). *Strategy analytics: WiMAX 3G killer or fixed broadband wireless standard?*.

Tulu, B., & Chatterjee, S. (2005). A taxonomy of telemedicine efforts with respect to applications, infrastructure, delivery tools, type of setting and purpose. *Proceedings of the 38th Hawaii International Conference on System Sciences.* Hawaii.

UMTS-Forum-Report14. (2002). *Support of third-generation services using UMTS in a converging network environment.* http://www.umts-forum.org/servlet/dycon/ztumts/umts/Live/en/umts/Resources_Reports_index: **UMTS.**

Warren, S. (2003). Beyond telemedicine: Infrastructures for intelligent home care technology. *Pre-ICADI Workshop Technology for Aging, Disability, and Independence.* London, UK.

Webb, C. (2004). Chip shots. *IEEE Spectr, 41*(10), 48-53.

Weil, N. (2005). Companies announce RFID drug-tracking project: Unisys and SupplyScape plan to track Oxycontin through the supply chain. *Cpmputerworld Magazine.*

Wickramasinghe, N., & Misra, S. (2005). A wireless trust model for healthcare. *International Journal of Electronic Healthcare, 1*(1).

Wickramasinghe, N., & Silvers, J. (2002). IS/IT the prescription to enable medical group practices attain their goals. *Healthcare Management Science.*

WiMax. (2005). http://wimaxxed.com.

ZigBee-Alliance. http://www.zigbee.org/.

Chapter II

Factors Motivating the Acceptance of New Information and Communication Technologies in UK Healthcare:
A Test of Three Models

Janice A. Osbourne, Brunel University, UK

Malcolm Clarke, Brunel University, UK

Abstract

This paper discusses the use of three published models, the technology acceptance model (TAM), Rogers diffusion of innovation theory (IDT), and the Triandis theory of interpersonal behaviour (TIB), and attempts to bring them together in an integrated model to better predict the adoption of new information and communication tech-

nologies by a cohort of health professionals within UK primary care in an attempt
to aid implementers in bringing technology in at an organizational level.

Introduction

Over the last 25 years, public healthcare delivery has been undergoing continuing changes. This has included the use of new information and communication technologies in a bid to improve services to patients, speed up waiting times, and addressing structural problems in the National Health Service (NHS). These changes have been largely driven by technical competence on the medical side but not matched sufficiently in technical organizational improvements. This chapter discusses the use of three published models, the technology acceptance model (TAM), Rogers diffusion of innovation theory (IDT), and the Triandis Theory of Interpersonal behaviour (TIB), and attempts to bring them together to assist in the political decision to bring technology in at the organization level too.

Public Healthcare in the UK: An Overview

Within the United Kingdom, there exists a plethora of organizations and bodies providing the majority of healthcare in the UK including general practitioners to accidents and emergency departments, and dentistry. These organizations all fall under the National Health Service (NHS), the publicly funded healthcare system of each part of the UK, which in theory is managed by the Department of Health. Services provided under this organization are characterised by free service to all citizens and is divided into two levels of care, primary and secondary.

In the United Kingdom, a patient must first see their own doctor (referred to as the GP) located in close proximity to the patient's home. GP's are the first point of contact for users in the UK. This level of service provided is known as primary care. At present, 90% of all health and social care contacts with the NHS are through primary healthcare (NHS, 2001). Primary healthcare is provided through a combination of general practitioners and community medical workers. Services such as district nursing and child health monitoring are provided by community medical workers. If specialist help is required by a patient, he or she will be referred to a hospital or a consultant by their GPs. This is referred to as secondary care, as self-referral is not allowed and the clinical condition presenting normally cannot be dealt with by a primary care specialist and so is dealt with at this level.

One major problem in the NHS is that of communication between hospital specialists and general practitioners particularly in inner city areas. The written communication between GPs and consultants have been highlighted as being of poor quality (Rowland, 1992) and often having poor educational value (AGHTA, 1996). This problem has led to problems occurring in the outpatient referral system in terms of delays for hospital appointments, leading to frustration by patients (DOH, 1991).

In addition to this, there have been problems with out of hours GP services (Hallam, 1994), which has led to recommendations being made for more access to the healthcare system through entry points such as NHS Direct (Rogers, Chapple, & Sergison, 1999).

The government, in an effort to modernize the National Health Service and to deal with the numerous structural problems, have emphasized in policy initiatives the vision for connecting health policies with the capabilities of new information and communication technologies, which are able to provide new kinds of service that are more responsive to public needs and speed up access to healthcare. *The Information Strategy for the Modern NHS* (1998-2005) was seen as both visionary and relevant to the needs of the NHS. In the *Information for health* policy document for example, removing distance from healthcare was seen as a goal of the innovative technology Telemedicine.

Opportunities in the field of telemedicine will be seized to remove distance from healthcare, to improve the quality of that care, and to help deliver new and integrated services. GP's will be able to send test readings or images electronically to hospital specialists many miles away and in the same way receive results and advice more quickly (National Health Service Executive, 1998)

One of the major programmes, which the government has initiated, is the National Programme for IT for which an overview is provided.

National Programme for IT (Formerly NPfit)

The National Programme for Information Technology (Npfit) came about in 2002 as a result of the UK government's decision to make an unprecedented investment in information technology as essential to its plans for the National Health Service. This programme has been seen as one of the most expensive information technology programmes in the world with costs estimated to run over £18billion over ten years. (Brennan, 2005).

The programme aims to connect 30,000 general practitioners and 270 acute, community, and mental health trusts to a single, secure, national system to make information available when and where it is needed, including to patients themselves (Hutton, 2004).

In tracing its history, the Npfit programme came about as a result of suggestions made in the Wanless Treasury's report (Wanless, 2002). The report gave reasons as to why previous targets set by the NHS Executive, of all NHS trust having electronic medical reports implemented by 2005, had not been achieved. These reasons included budgets for information technology being used to relieve financial pressures elsewhere instead of locally and an inadequate setting of central information technology (IT) standards.

The Report recommended that the NHS double the proportion of its budget invested in information technology to 4%, to bring it closer into lines with the healthcare in the United States, which has a budget of 6%. They concluded that without a major advance in the effective use of information and communication technology, the health service would find it difficult to deliver the efficient high quality service, which the public will demand. The government's response to this was to allocate £2.3bn for a new national programme for IT (Doh, 2002). The Primary aim of the programme is **for** electronic patient records to be implemented in all acute trusts by the end of 2007. In 2005, the government established an agency, *Connecting for health,* as the single national provider of IT, which would deliver the National programme ensuring the maintenance, development, and effective delivery of the IT products and services delivered by the former NHS information authority.

There are several products that the National Programme plans to deliver, which includes:

- **A National care record system (NCRS):** *Connecting for health* plans to produce holistic records for patients from birth to death gradually, holding a review of the person's health and all his or her health contacts within the National Health Service. This summary patient record called the "spine" will be accessible 24 hours a day, seven days a week by health professionals, whether they work in hospitals, primary care, or community services.

- **Electronic booking:** This programme, *Choose and book*, will allow GPs and other primary care staff to make initial hospital or clinic outpatient appointments at a convenient time, date, and place for the patient. If the patient prefers, he or she can make their appointment later online or through a telephone booking service.

- **Electronic transfer of prescriptions:** This will allow for prescribers to create and transfer prescriptions directly to a patient's community pharmacist and the Prescription Pricing Authority (PPA). It's aim is to reduce reliance on article prescriptions and it is expected to reduce prescription errors and provide better information at the point of prescribing.

- **New National Networking Service (N3):** This will provide the NHS with world-class networking services, including secure broadband connectivity, from every site where NHS services are delivered or managed

Based on the expenditure of this and similar programmes, we deduce that money is available so the choice is between spending the time to do it well, seeing that the government intends to have information technology playing a central part in healthcare within the very near future, or to do it badly on time. This then leads us to look at external models on which to identify factors, which play a part in technology adoption.

Development of Research Model

There have been several theoretical perspectives, which have been used to study the determinants of IT acceptance and adoption across a variety of disciplines including Communications (Rogers, 1995), Sociology (Wejnert, 2002), and Information systems research (Knol & Stroeken, 2001).

Intention-based models and behavioural decision theories have been used to explain usage of information systems (e.g., Agarwal & Prasad, 1997; Davis, 1989) and results further show that behavioural intentions are significantly and positively correlated with actual behaviour. According to these theories, user adoption and usage behaviours are determined by intention to use information technology, which in turn is influenced by beliefs and attitudes about information technology.

Although there are many theories, which can be used to explain intention we have selected three. The technology acceptance model, the theory of interpersonal behaviour, and Rogers innovation and diffusion model. These models will form the basis of our conceptual model.

Technology Acceptance Model (TAM)

The technology acceptance model (TAM, Davis, 1993) is described as the most dominant theoretical model in information technology acceptance (Misiolek, Zakaria, & Zhang) and is an adaptation of the theory of reasoned action (TRA, Fishbein & Ajzen, 1980). The TAM's goal is to provide an explanation of the determinants of computer acceptance that is generally capable of explaining user behaviour across a broad range of end-user computing technologies and user populations (Davis, Bagozzi, & Warshaw, 1989).

The TAM identifies two beliefs perceived usefulness and perceived ease of use, as being of primary importance for computer acceptance behaviour. The model posts that a users adoption of an information system is determined by behavioural intention, which is determined by the user's belief about the system, similar to the TRA. The model differs from the TRA in that behavioural intention is viewed as being determined by the individual's attitude and perceived usefulness. The TAM does not however include the subjective norms of the TRA as it was not found to be significant (Davis, 1989).

The Triandis Theory of Interpersonal Behaviour

The Triandis model (Triandis, 1980, see Figure 1) explains individuals' behaviour in terms of what they have always done (habit), by what they think they should do (social norms) and by the consequences, they associate with a behaviour (perceived consequences). The model also contains aspects that are directly related to the individual, for example attitudes, genetic factors, intention, and behaviour and others that are related to the individual's environment, for example culture, facilitating conditions, and social situations.

Rogers Innovation and Diffusion Theory

The innovation and diffusion theory proposes that an innovation is an idea or practice perceived as new by an individual, group, or organization (Rogers, 1995). Diffusion is described as the process by which an innovation spreads. The individuals' decision to accept or reject an innovation occurs in the following stages, awareness

Figure 1. Triandis Theory of Interpersonal Behaviour

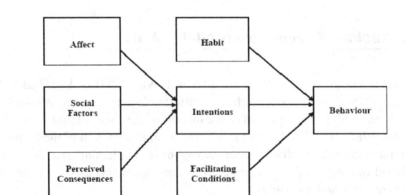

of the innovation, which leads to an attitude being formed towards it based on the individuals perception of the innovation. The decision to adopt or reject is then made, implementation takes place, and the individual confirms his or her decision. The perceived characteristics of an innovation include its relative advantage, compatibility, complexity, trialability, and observability (Rogers, 1995).

Reasons Behind Integration

Previous models described here can contribute to our proposal of an integrated model in a variety of ways, which are:

Incompleteness

Although strong empirical support for the TAM has been established through numerous studies (Karahanna, Straub, & Chervany, 1999; Venkatesh & Davis, 2000; Venkatesh, Morris, Davis, & Davis, 2003), the TAM has had several criticisms levelled at it, including not offering sufficient understanding to provide system designers with information needed for creating and promoting user acceptance of systems (Mathieson, Peacock, & Chin, 2001), and its assumption that its use is volitional, which means that in there are no barriers to prevent an individual from using a technology or a system if he or she chose to do so (Mathieson et al., 2001). There may be situations in which an individual wants to use an IT, but is prevented by lack of time, money, or expertise (Chau & Hu, 2001; Taylor & Todd, 1995). Given the fact that the information and communication technologies, including mobile health technologies (described as computing technology, comprising software, hardware, and communications specifically associated with mobility, Zaslavsky & Tari , 1988) are fairly new to health professionals, the possibility exists that they may choose not to use the technology because they may not have sufficient skills or the ability to use the technology, hence the model would not give a complete picture of factors affecting adoption.

 Because of the uncertain theoretical status of the TAM, Davis (1989) dropped the subjective norm, which has resulted in studies using the TAM seldom including variables related to the social environment. Technology adoption in healthcare is a current hot topic at the moment and we believe that social pressure plays an important role in explaining reasons behind their use.

Similarities Between the Models

Although these theories focus on different determinants to explain consumer behaviour in the adoption of technology, they have similarities:

1. The TAM and the Triandis model are both intention-based models, which assume that attitudes influence intention, which determines behaviour and the actual use of the technology.

2. Perceived ease of use in TAM is related to the complexity construct of the Innovation Diffusion theory in fact the complexity construct is the exact opposite of the Perceived ease of use construct.

3. Perceived consequences in the Triandis model construct is similar to the construct of perceived usefulness (PU) in the TAM and similar to relative advantage in the Innovation Diffusion theory.

We have divided the technology adoption process into three factor areas, those related to the social environment, those related to the technology, and those related to the individual. We find the Triandis model most relevant for factors related to the social environment; for the technology related section we find the attributes from the diffusion of innovation, which concentrates on both the technology and its compatibility and the TAM more suitable; and for those related to the individual, we find the IDT and the Triandis model more suitable. As these models do not give a complete overview on their own, we find it necessary to combine the three to evaluate adoption.

An Integrative Model

Given their complementary nature, a model that integrates the key research constructs from TAM, TIB, and EDT should explain more variance in IT usage intention than either model alone. Such an integrated model is depicted in Figure 3. In this section, we discuss how the assembled model attempts to do the duties assigned to it.

Social Factors

An individual's perception of social pressure to perform or not perform a behaviour affects intention, (Fishbein & Ajzen, 1975). Perception of social pressure refers to an individual's perception of whether individuals close to or important to them think that they should or should not perform a behaviour. Consequently, we view social factors as norms, values, and roles, which influence an individual's intention to adopt medical technology. These values in our context may be conveyed by interaction with patients and peers.

Figure 2. Integrated model

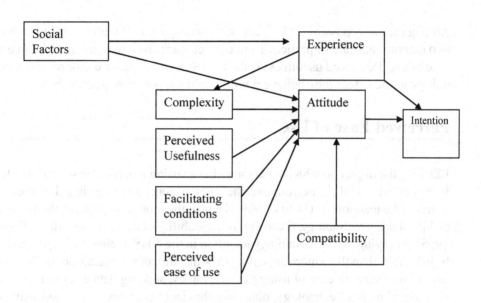

Figure 3. Comparison of the three models

	TAM	TIB	IDT
Variables	Perceived ease of use	Social factors	Relative advantage
	Percieved usefulness	Facilitating conditions	Trialability/ Experience
	Attitude	Perceived consequences	Compatibility
		Genetic Factors	Complexity
		Cultural Factors	Observability

Key:

TAM: Technology acceptance model

TIB: Triandis theory of interpersonal behaviour

IDT: Innovation diffusion theory

There are varying views on physicians being influenced socially. It has been suggested that general medical practitioners are influenced in their decision-making by medical specialists, who are seen as being innovative and creative. (Blumberg, 1999). Such opinion leaders can activate local networks to diffuse an innovation by facilitating transfer of information (Young, Hollands, Ward, & Holman, 2003).

Perceived Usefulness

Among the many possible influences on technology use, Davis (1989) suggests that two determinants are of particular importance: perceived usefulness and perceived ease of use. Perceived usefulness is the tendency of people to use or not use a technology to the extent they believe it will help them perform their job better.

Perceived Ease of Use

PEOU is the degree to which a person believes using a particular system would be free of effort, and if the performance benefits of usage are outweighed by the effort of using the technology (Davis, 1989). Hence, the more complex the innovation of an information technology, the lower the probability of its adoption will be (Rogers, 1995). Applying this to technology adoption in the NHS, technologies perceived to be user friendly will be more appealing to both patients and practitioners. Perceived ease of use refers to ease of using the technology, sending data electronically as in the case of mobile technology, obtaining the data necessary to proceed with consultations as in the case of General Practitioners.

Facilitating Conditions

Facilitating conditions are the objective factors that make a behaviour easy or difficult. In the Triandis model, facilitating conditions are important determinants of behaviour. Even if intentions to perform the behaviour are high, the habits are well established and the physiological arousals are optimal, there may be no action/behaviour if the situation or objective factors do not warrant the behaviour (Triandis, 1980). A simplified explanation of this is that facilitating conditions are important in that individuals with the intention of accomplishing something may be unable to do because their environment prevents the activity from being performed.

Triandis hypothesizes that facilitating conditions directly affect the actual behaviour rather than intentions because he argues that one might have the intention to perform a certain act, but if the environment does not support this behaviour then the act will most likely not be executed. We define facilitating conditions as those factors in an individual's environment that facilitate the act of adopting technology. Empirical investigations have shown that facilitating conditions could also have a significant positive impact on attitude (Chang & Cheung, 2001).

We expect facilitating conditions to have a positive influence on technology adoption.

Perceived Consequences

According to Triandis, each act or behaviour is perceived as having a potential outcome that can be either positive or negative. An individual's choice of behaviour is based on the probability that an action will provoke a specific consequence.

Relative Advantage

Relative advantage is the degree to which an innovation is perceived as better than the idea it supersedes. Physician perceptions of new technologies affect the adoption of innovation in clinical practice. For example, physician perceptions related to teledermatology suggest that this new technology needs to be quick, efficient, reliable, and easily used (Weinstock, Nguyen, & Risica, 2002). If new technologies are too time consuming or complicated, they may not be widely adopted and used. In a study on the perceptions of GPs towards teledermatology, the results reported a preference for reliable, efficient, and easy-to-use technology (Collins, Nicolson, Bowns, & Walters, 2000).

Trialability/Experience

Trialability is the degree to which an innovation may be experimented with a limited basis. The more adopters experiment with a new technology and explore its ramifications, the greater the likelihood that the innovation will be used during early stages of adoption (Agarwal & Prasad, 1997; Natek & Lesjak, 2006).

Intention

Behavioural intention refers to "instructions that people give to themselves to behave in certain ways" (Triandis, 1980) or their motivation regarding the performance of a given behaviour. In our model, intention refers to health professionals' motivation to adopt information technologies.

Attitude

According to Fishbein and Ajzen (1980), "attitude is a learned predisposition to respond in a consistently favorable or unfavorable manner with a given object." Attitude is directly related to behavioural intention and adoption because people will only intend to perform behaviour for which they have positive feelings (Han,

Harkke, Mustonen, Seppanen, & Kallio, 2005; Marino, 2004). We hypothesise that attitude is positively related to the users intention to use new ICTs in healthcare

Compatibility

This construct has not been included in most studies on technology adoption apart from those using the IDT (Cho, 2006). Compatibility refers to the conformity of an innovation in our case new ICTs with the values and beliefs of users and with previously introduced ideas and needs (McCole, 2002). Therefore, the adoption of a new technology depends on its compatibility with existing practices. The importance of technology compatibility with the organization and its tasks has been shown to be a significant factor in successful technology implementations (Cooper & Zmud, 1990).We hypothesise that compatibility is positively related to the user's attitude towards new ICT's in healthcare.

Discussion

The primary objective of this chapter was to compare two of the more dominant technology acceptance and adoption models in IT research, namely the TAM and the IDT as well as a less popular model from the social science, the TIB, then extend these models to an integrated model of IT acceptance and adoption.

On their own these models do not fully evaluate the acceptance of technology by individual, however when integrated the weaknesses of the individual models are totally cancelled out by the strengths of the integrated model.

As described earlier, the TAM assumes that there are no barriers to preventing an individual from using a technology if he or she wished. The IDT and the TIB however feature variables, which can affect adoption by the individual, hence filling one of the gaps of the TAM. The Triandis models which attempts to cover all the major component of the individual and their environments with its 34 variables is somewhat difficult to test by virtue of its complexity hence only the variables relating to our study have selected. The IDT focuses on the process of adoption as well as the, this is complementary with both perceived characteristics of the technology complimenting both the TIB and the TAM

Based on these factors, we believe the integrated model will have better explanatory power of user adoption of technology. However dear readers, as with any cake, the proof is in the eating and as such, we will shortly be conducting an exhaustive study on a cohort of health professionals within a Primary Care Trust given new medical technology as part of a government modernization initiative to see if the model lives up to expectation. We ask that you wait with bated breath!

References

Agarwal, R., & Prasad, J. (1997). The role of innovation characteristics and perceived voluntariness in the acceptance of information technologies. *Decision Sciences, 28*(3), 557-583.

AGHTA. (1996). *Advisory group on health technology assessment. Assessing the effects of health technologies: Principles practice proposals.* London: Department of Health.

Blumberg, R. S. (1999). The leadership of innovation. *Gastroenterology, 116*(4), 787.

Brennan, S. (2005). *The NHS IT project.* Abingdon, UK: Radcliff Medical Press.

Chang, M. K., & Cheung, W. (2001). Determinants of the intention to use Internet/WWW at work: A confirmatory study. *Information & Management, 39*(1), 1-14.

Chau, P. Y. K., & Hu, P. J. H. (2001). Information technology acceptance by individual professionals: A model comparison approach. *Decision Sciences, 32*(4), 699-719.

Cho, V. (2006). A study of the roles of trusts and risks in information-oriented online legal services using an integrated model. *Information and Management 43*(4) 502-520.

Collins, K., Nicolson P., Bowns. I, Walters, S. (2000). *General Practitioners' Perception of Telemedicine in Dermatology: A Psychological Perspective Journal of Telemedicine and Telecare 6*(1), 50-53

Cooper, R., & Zmud, R. (1990). Information technology implementation research: A technological diffusion approach. *Management Science, 36*(2), 123-139.

Davis, F. D. (1989). Perceived usefulness, perceived ease of use, and user acceptance of information technology. *MIS Quarterly, 13*(3), 319-340.

Davis, F. D. (1993). User acceptance of information technology: System characteristics, user perceptions, and behavioural impacts. *International Journal of Man-Machine Studies, 38*(3), 475-487.

Davis, F. D., Bagozzi, R. P., & Warshaw, P. R. (1989). User acceptance of computer technology: A comparison of two theoretical models. *Management Science, 35*(8), 982-1003.

Doh. (2002). *Delivering 21st century IT support for the NHS. National strategic programme.* London: Department of Health.

DOH. (1991). *Research for health: A research and development strategy for the NHS.* London: HMSO.

Fishbein, M., & Ajzen, I. (1975). *Belief, attitude, intention, and behaviour: An introduction to theory and research.* Reading, MA: Addison Wesley.

Fishbein, M., & Ajzen, I. (1980). Predicting and understanding consumer behaviour: Attitude behaviour correspondence. In I. Ajzen, & M. Fishbein (Eds.), *Understanding attitudes and predicting social behaviour* (pp. 149-172). Englewood Cliffs, NJ: Prentice Hall.

Hallam, L. (1994). Primary medical care outside normal working hours: Review of published work. *British Medical Journal, 308*(6923), 249-253.

Han, S., Harkke, V., Mustonen, P., Seppanen, M., & Kallio, M. (2005). Understanding physician acceptance of mobile technology: Insights from two telephone interviews in Finland. *International Journal of Electronic Healthcare, 1*(4), 380-395.

Hutton, J. (2004). *National programme for IT. House of commons official report* London: Department of Health.

Karahanna, E., Straub, D. W., & Chervany, N. L. (1999). Information technology adoption across time: A cross-sectional comparison of pre-adoption and post-adoption beliefs. *MIS Quarterly, 23*(2), 183-213.

Knol, W. H., & Stroeken, J. H. M. (2001). The diffusion and adoption of information technology in saml - and mediums - ed enterprises through IT scenarios. *Technology Analysis, & Strategic Management, 13*(2), 227- 46.

Marino, A. (2004). Innovation technology and application issues in Italian e-healthcare. *International Journal of Electronic Healthcare, 1*(2), 210-220.

Mathieson, K., Peacock, E., & Chin, W. W. (2001). Extending the technology acceptance model: The influence of perceived user resources. *DATA BASE for Advances in Information Systems, 32*(3), 86-112.

McCole, P. (2002). The role of trust for electronic commerce in services. *International Journal of Contemporary Hospitality Management, 14*(2), 81-87.

Misiolek, N., Zakaria, N., & Zhang, P. (2002). *Trust in organizational acceptance of information technology: A conceptual model and preliminary evidence.* Paper presented at the annual meeting of the Decision Sciences Institute, San Diego, CA (November 23-26)

Natek, S., & Lesjak, D. (2006). Trial work: The way to successful information system projects in healthcare. *International Journal of Electronic Healthcare, 2*(3), 223-230.

National Health Service Executive. (1998). *Information for health: An information strategy for the modern NHS 1998-2001.* London: National Health Service Executive.

NHS. (2001). *Building the information core—Implementing the NHS plan.* London: Department of Health, UK Government.

Rogers, A., Chapple, A., & Sergison, M. (1999). If a patient is too costly they tend to get rid of you: The impact of people's perceptions of rationing on the use of primary care. *Healthcare Analysis, 7*(3), 25-237.

Rogers, E. M. (1995). *Diffusion of innovations* (4th ed.). New York: The Free Press.

Rowland, M. (1992). Communications between GP's and specialists. In M. Roland, & A. Coulter (Eds.), *Hospital referrals* (pp. 108-22). Oxford: Oxford University Press.

Taylor, S., & Todd, P. A. (1995). Understanding information technology usage: A test of competing models. *Information Systems Research, 6*(2), 144-176.

Triandis, H. C. (1980).Values, attitudes, and interpersonal behaviour. In M. M. Page (Ed.), *Nebraska symposium on motivation 1979* (pp. 195-295). Lincoln: University of Nebraska Press.

Venkatesh, V., & Davis, F. D. (2000). A theoretical extension of the technology acceptance model: Four longitudinal field studies. *Management Science, 46*(2), 186-205.

Venkatesh, V., Morris, M., Davis, G. B., & Davis, F. D. (2003). User acceptance of information technology: Toward a unified view. *MIS Quarterly, 26*(4), 425-478.

Wanless, D. (2002). *Securing our future health: Taking a long-term view. Final report.* Retrieved September 27, 2005, from http://www.hm-treasury.gov.uk./Consultations_and_Legislation/wanless/consult_wanless_final.cfm

Weinstock, M., Nguyen, F., & Risica, P. (2002). Patient and referring provider satisfaction with teledermatology. *Journl of the American Academy of Dermatology, 47*(1), 68-72.

Wejnert, B. (2002). Integrating models of diffusion of innovations: A conceptual framework. *Annual Review Sociology, 28*(1), 297-326.

Young, J. M., Hollands, M. J., Ward, J., & Holman, C. D. J. (2003). Role for opinion leaders in promoting evidence-based surgery. *Archives of Surgery, 138*, 785-791.

Zaslavsky, A., & Tari, Z. (1988). Mobile computing: Overview and status. *The Australian Computer Journal, 30*(2), 42-52.

This work was previously published in International Journal of Healthcare Information Systems and Informatics, Vol. 1, Issue 4, edited by J. Tan, pp. 29-39, copyright 2006 by IGI Publishing, formerly known as Idea Group Publishing (an imprint of IGI Global).

Chapter III

An Overview of the HIPAA-Compliant Privacy Access Control Model

Vivying S.Y. Cheng, Hong Kong University of Science and Technology, Hong Kong

Patrick C.K. Hung, University of Ontario Institute of Technology (UOIT), Canada

Abstract

The Health Insurance Portability and Accountability Act of 1996 (HIPAA) is a set of rules to be followed by health plans, doctors, hospitals and other healthcare providers in the United States of America. HIPAA privacy rules create national standards to protect individuals' health information; it is therefore necessary to create standardized solutions to tackle the various privacy issues. This chapter focuses on the e-health-care privacy issues based on a prior extension of role-based access control (RBAC) model. We review an access control enforcement model in Web services for tackling HIPAA privacy rules and protecting personal health information (PHI) called the Privacy Access Control Model. First, we discuss related backgrounds of, and privacy requirements in the HIPAA legislation. Next, four privacy-related entities (purposes, recipients, obligations, and retentions) are incorporated into the core RBAC model. The HIPAA rules are then embedded into the extended RBAC model as constraints. Then, we present a vocabulary-independent Web services privacy framework in a layered architecture for supporting healthcare applications.

Introduction

People have been concerned about health information privacy for more than two thousand years. For example, the Hippocratic Oath was written as a guideline of medical ethics for doctors in respect to a patient's health condition, and states:

Whatsoever things I see or hear concerning the life of men, in my attendance on the sick or even apart there from, which ought not to be noised abroad, I will keep silence thereon, counting such things to be sacred secrets.

It is obvious that health information is among the most sensitive and personal information that can be collected and shared. The information that needs to be protected in the healthcare sector is often referred to as personal health information (PHI). PHI includes individually identifiable health information and healthcare to an individual relating to past, present, and future physical and mental health conditions. As more and more physicians, researchers, doctors, and patients are using the Internet to access and gather their PHI, the ease of use and access to confidential information over the Internet create increased threats and vulnerabilities (Jones, Ching, & Winslett, 1995).

The principle of information privacy and disposition requires that "All persons have a fundamental right to privacy, and hence to have control over the collection, storage, access, communication, manipulation and disposition of data about themselves" (IMIA, 2001). Based on this principle, the Health Insurance Portability and Accountability Act (HIPAA) of the U.S. (2005) set a national standard to protect and enhance the right of patients to control how their health information is used and shared. Failure to comply with these legislations may lead to civil and/or criminal penalties and/or imprisonment, as well as the loss of reputation and goodwill when the non-compliance is publicized (University of Miami Ethics Programs, 2005).

To comply with the legislative requirements in the healthcare sector, access control is an essential element for limiting PHI access to legitimate users for legitimate use. The principle of access control focuses and depends on specifying requirements which are preset by the application administrator(s) or data owners. The legislation-compliant requirements can be referred to as the fundamental rules in managing those who have the right to access which PHI in the healthcare setting. In particular, the role-based access control (RBAC) model is described as more suited to healthcare than other access control mechanisms in order to meet the authorization requirements for the security of healthcare information (Ferraiolo, Kuhn, & Chandramouli, 2003; NIST, 2005). However, simply using the RBAC model is not adequate for limiting the purpose of access, storage, and disclosure of PHI.

It is therefore necessary to develop applications that are compliant with the legislation. There has been an increasing amount of discussion recently about a privacy framework in both industry and the research community. Microsoft, for example, will launch an online system called the HealthVault (2007) to manage the users' own health records. HealthVault not only allows users to keep their personal health information, but also allows users to upload the health data such as blood glucose and blood pressure from some HealthVault-compatible devices. The HealthVault Web site allows users to control which information they provide to other services through an opt-in program and therefore won an endorsement from the Patient Privacy Rights Foundation (Hachman, 2007). Nevertheless, it is still a question whether this approach is considered as HIPAA-compliant; especially, the role of this Web site play is still unclear (Hachman, 2007). There is still no comprehensive solution that has been defined and developed yet to tackle the various privacy issues in HIPAA. However, from Microsoft and other companies' approaches, we can argue that the industry also agreed that an access control model is on the right track to dealing with the privacy issues.

The remainder of this chapter is organized as follows: "An Overview of Personal Health Information Privacy Legislations" section discusses the health information privacy legislations (e.g., HIPAA) in the U.S and categorizes the legislations into the privacy principles. Section "A Privacy Access Control Model for e-Healthcare Applications" discusses the extension of a role-based access control model into a privacy access control model for personal health information privacy legislations, whereas section "Implementation in Web Services" is the discussion of implementing the privacy access control model and incorporating into the Web services architecture. Finally, the last section concludes the chapter.

An Overview of Personal Health Information Privacy Legislations

The public has concerns at all times about whether their personal health information (PHI) is secure and if their privacy is protected (Bell Canada, 2005). PHI often contains identifiable and sensitive information such as genetic or demographic data about individuals, for example, name, age, sex, address, phone number, employment status, family composition, and DNA profile. Not only will disclosure of PHI of particular individuals potentially create personal embarrassment, it will also lead to social ostracism (Tan & Hung, 2005). Dire consequences include denial of insurance coverage, loss of job opportunities, and refusal of mortgage financing. The government also can impose civil and criminal penalties and/or imprisonment as well as suffer the loss of reputation and goodwill when the non-compliance of legislation is publicized (University of Miami Ethics Programs, 2005). In order to design a HIPAA-compliant software solution, it is vital to clarify all applicable requirements carefully before implementation. Instead of targeting privacy at an individual level, we start from healthcare legislations to model the fundamental privacy requirements.

Health Insurance Portability and Accountability Act (HIPAA)

The HIPAA regulations are divided into four standards or rules: (1) Privacy, (2) Security, (3) Identifiers, and (4) Transactions and Code Sets. We only focus on the privacy rules in HIPAA. The privacy rules are the most comprehensive, setting standards for how PHI "in any form or medium" should be controlled. The rules aim to ensure that organizations collecting PHI use only the relevant healthcare information and only those who need to access the information for healthcare purposes are able to access it. The privacy rule covers all medical records, both paper and electronic-based.

HIPAA compliance is compulsory in the U.S. Compliance with the privacy rules has been a requirement since April 14, 2003 for most covered entities—healthcare providers, insurers, health plan providers, and clearinghouses that process claims on behalf of healthcare providers. Failure in implementation and maintenance of the compliance by covered entities and their employees may result in severe civil and/or criminal penalties imposed by the Department of Health and Human Services (HIPAA, 2005). The government can impose civil and criminal penalties of as much as $50,000 and/or imprisonment for as long as one year. In addition to these penalties, covered entities may even suffer loss of reputation and goodwill when their non-compliance is publicized. Basically, there are six rights to protect PHI (HIPAA, 2005) as follows:

1. **The right to view and get a copy of patients' own medical records:** This allows patients to access their PHI and related information such as insurance claims.

2. **The right to request the correction of inaccurate health information:** This allows the patients to ask for an update of their PHI if it is incomplete or incorrect.

3. **The right to find out where PHI has been shared for purposes other than care, payment, or healthcare operations:** This allows patients to find out how their PHI is used and shared by healthcare providers or health insurers.

4. **The right to request special restrictions on the use or disclosure of PHI:** This protects patients from their PHI being used or shared for any illegitimate purposes unless their express permission (consent) was given. Even if patients have given permissions, they still have the right to revoke it.

5.   **The right to request PHI to be shared with the patient in a particular way:** This allows the patients to request healthcare providers to send their PHI to a certain address such as their home address or office address.

6.   **The right to file complaints:** This allows the patients to file a complaint to the healthcare providers if their PHI has been used or shared in an illegitimate way, or if the patients were not able to exercise any of the rights.

Legislative Principles for Achieving Healthcare Privacy

We categorize the health information privacy legislations into a set of system design principles and summarize their comparison in Cheng and Hung (2005). These principles serve as a technical guideline for developing e-healthcare Web services applications that are compliant with the privacy legislations.

Principle 1: Data-Level Security Protection Principle

All the legislations require security and safeguards in protecting PHI. The three fundamental requirements—confidentiality, integrity and availability—are usually used in referring to security (Fischer-Hubner, 2001).

•   **Confidentiality:** Prevention of unauthorized or improper disclosure of data. Confidentiality is violated when unauthorized parties are able to read the content of PHI.

•   **Integrity:** Prevention of unauthorized modification of information. This includes the prevention of an unauthorized user modifying the information, and an authorized user modifying the information improperly and maintaining the data consistency. The integrity is violated when the correctness and appropriateness of the content of PHI is modified, destroyed, deleted or disclosed.

•   **Availability:** Prevention of unauthorized withholding of data or resources. The availability is violated when an unauthorized user tries to withhold information from disclosure or the system is brought down or malfunctioned by unauthorized users.

The confidentiality and integrity can mainly be implemented using cryptographic tools from the perspectives of communication security, while the protection of availability is technically much harder to achieve (Fischer-Hubner, 2001). It is, however, necessary to protect security in the privacy applications. Therefore, the implemented system must have to address confidentiality, integrity and availability.

Principle 1.1: *PHI shall be protected by security safeguards in a secure way that data confidentiality, integrity and availability can be achieved.*

In addition to this, all the legislations require the data to be accurate, complete and up-to-date and allow the correction of inaccurate or incomplete information. This can be achieved by allowing legitimate access on PHI for any modification.

Principle 1.2: *PHI needs to be accurate, complete and up-to-date. Correction of inaccurate information should be allowed for maintaining data quality.*

Principle 2: Communication-Level Security Protection Principle

Although the legislations do not explicitly cover the communication security, this is one of the core components for data quality assurances.

Principle 2.1: *PHI shall be transported in a secure way that data confidentiality, data integrity and authentication of users/systems/services are achieved.*

Confidentiality can be achieved by encrypting the messages in the communication channel. Only authorized users are able to decrypt and view the message. Unauthorized users are not able to view the content, even if they eavesdrop on the communication channel. Data integrity assures that unauthorized parties have not modified, altered, or destroyed the data. There should be no changes of message content during the transportation or transmission of data. Authentication is the assurance that the parties involved in a transaction are who they claimed they are. Current technologies such as secure socket layer (SSL), virtual private network (VPN) and IP security (IPSec) are example cryptographic tools developed for maintaining communication security.

Principle 3: Consent Requirement Principle

All the three legislations require that consent has to be given by the owner during the collection, disclosure, use, and retention of PHI. Other legislations also suggested that consent must be informed and voluntary. For example, the European Union Directive on data protection (European Union, 1995) compels European countries to make patient consent the paramount principle in the protection of personal health information (Anderson, 1996). Users must first consent to data collection, use, and storage proposals for any PHI. Consent is an important concept in the legislation requirement and thus we propose this consent requirement principle:

Principle 3.1: *Consent must be given by the owner of PHI for the collection, disclosure, use and retention of his/her PHI.*

In practice, consent is usually obtained by a written acknowledgment of receipt of the notice of privacy practices and handling of restrictions to privacy practices. However, consent is rather an abstract idea in the sense of system design and implementation. We therefore transform this idea into four limitations to specify how the PHI can be released upon the request:

1.   **Limitation on collection:** The purpose of collection needs to be stated in order to review PHI. The collection of PHI shall be limited to which is necessary for the purpose only.

2.   **Limitation on data disclosure:** Legitimate users should be able to make special restrictions on the disclosure of PHI.

3.   **Limitation on use:** The use of PHI shall be identified as legitimate use by the service provider or the owner of PHI.

4.   **Limitation on retention:** PHI shall be retained only as long as the purpose for which it is used.

With these limitations, consent can be viewed as access control policies which can easily be implemented by programming languages and/or database queries. For example, Cheng and Hung (2005) demonstrated the use of role-based access control (RBAC) model with privacy enhancement applied to the HIPAA privacy rules.

In addition to this, we also need to allow the PHI owner to set his/her preference in releasing the PHI and review how the PHI is being released shown in the following principles.

Principle 3.2: *Owner of PHI should be allowed to review their own PHI and how their PHI is collected, used, disclosed and retained.*

Principle 3.3: *Owner of PHI should be allowed to control how much of his/her PHI is released.*

A Privacy Access Control Model for E-Healthcare Applications

Role-based access control (RBAC) model has been widely investigated in various research communities for a period of time (Ferraiolo, Kuhn, & Chandramouli, 2003).

According to the NIST draft standard for RBAC, RBAC has a natural fit with many healthcare applications. In RBAC, permissions are associated with roles, and users are made members of appropriate roles thereby acquiring the roles' permissions. In addition, roles can be granted new permissions, and permissions can be revoked from roles as needed. The significant benefit of deploying RBAC is its flexibility to meet the changing needs of an organization (Osborn, Sandhu,& Munawer, 2000). A general access control rule is specified as follows:

ALLOW [Subject]
to perform [Operation] on [Object]

The core RBAC model element sets and relations are illustrated in Figure 1.

The core RBAC includes sets of five basic entities called users (*USERS*), roles (*ROLES*), objects (*OBJECTS*), operations (*OPS*), and permissions (*PRMS*). The core RBAC also includes a set of subjects (*SUBJECTS*) where each subject may map between a user and an activated subset of roles that are assigned to the user. The description of the six element sets and relations are as follows:

- SUBJECTS is a set of subjects in the system.
- USERS ⊆ SUBJECTS, is a set of human users in the system.
- ROLES is a set of roles that describes the authority and responsibility on a member of a role.
- OBJECTS is a set of objects in the system.
- OPS is a set of operations that can be executed in the system.
- PRMS is a set of permissions that approve a particular operation to one or more objects in the system.
- UA is a many-to-many mapping between users and roles.

Figure 1. A role-based access control (RBAC) model

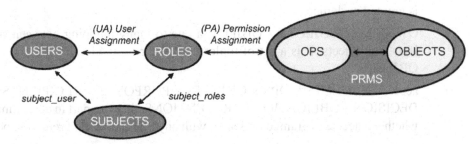

- PA is a many-to-many mapping between permissions and roles.

- assigned_users: (r:ROLES) $\rightarrow$ 2^{USERS}, the mapping of role r onto a set of users. Formally: assigned_users(r) $\subseteq$ { $\forall_{i=1,2,...,n} u_i \in$ USERS $|(u_i, r) \in$ UA}.

- assigned_permissions: (r:ROLES) $\rightarrow$ 2^{PRMS}, the mapping of role r onto a set of permissions. Formally: assigned_permissions(r) $\subseteq$ { $\forall_{i=1,2,...,n} p_i \in$ PRMS$|(p_i, r) \in$ PA}.

- subject_user: (s:SUBJECTS) $\rightarrow$ USERS, the mapping of subject s onto the subject's associated user.

- subject_role: (s:SUBJECTS) $\rightarrow$ 2^{ROLES}, the mapping of subject s onto a set of roles. Formally: subject_role(s) $\subseteq$ { $\forall_{i=1,2,...,n} r_i \in$ ROLES$|$(subject_user(s), r_i) $\in$ UA}.

As discussed in the previous section, the core RBAC model is inadequate for tackling all the privacy requirements for healthcare applications. For example, privacy requirements usually involve access purposes which specify in what condition a user can access an object. A privacy rule may state "doctors may read a patient's PHI for the purposes of treatment." Therefore, we extend the RBAC model with privacy entities, namely *purposes*, *recipients*, *obligations*, and *retentions*, to tackle the privacy rule requirements:

- PURPOSES, is the set of purposes which are used to describe his/her purpose(s) of a request submission.

- RECIPIENTS, is the set of recipients of the result generated by the set of collected object(s) such as analysis reports.

- OBLIGATIONS, is the set of obligations that may be taken after the decision of permission is made. In general, an obligation is opaque and is returned after the permission is granted. The obligations describe what promises a subject must make after gaining the permission.

- RETENTIONS, is the set of retention policies that are to be enforced in the object(s) in effect. Each data custodian may have its own retention policy to enforce the usage of datasets.

- DECISION: {ALLOW,DENY}, a decision for describing whether the access is granted or denied.

- OWNER $\subseteq$ SUBJECTS $\times$ OBJECT, a one-to-many mapping between subjects and objects. It is a set of tuples (s,o) where s $\in$ SUBJECTS and o $\in$ OBJECTS.

- access: SUBJECTS $\times$ OPS $\times$ OBJECTS $\times$ PURPOSES $\times$ RECIPIENTS $\rightarrow$ DECISION $\times$ OBLIGATIONS $\times$ RETENTIONS, the core part in determining whether a access is granted or denied with any obligations and retention policies according to the subject that invoke the access, operation of the access, the objects that the subject requesting, the purposes for this request, and the recipients of the result generated by the set of collected objects. Formally: access(s, op, $\{o_1, o_2, ..., o_i\}$, $\{pp_1, pp_2, ..., pp_j\}$, $\{rp_1, rp_2, ..., rp_k\}$) = (ALLOW, $\{obl_1, obl_2, ..., obl_m\}$, $\{rt_1, rt_2, ..., rt_i\}$) if subject s can access any object in $\{o_1, o_2, ..., o_i\}$ using operation op for any purpose in $\{pp_1, pp_2, ..., pp_j\}$ with any recipient in $\{rp_1, rp_2, ..., rp_k\}$, (DENY, $\varnothing$, $\varnothing$) otherwise. If the access is granted, a set of obligations $\{obl_1, obl_2, ..., obl_m\}$ and also a set of retention policies $\{rt_1, rt_2, ..., rt_i\}$ for corresponding set of objects $\{o_1, o_2, ..., o_i\}$ are returned to subject s

- object_owner: OBJECTS $\rightarrow$ SUBJECTS, the mapping of an object to its owner. Formally: object_owner(o) = $\{s \in$ SUBJECTS $|(s,o) \in$ OWNER$\}$.

- owner_object: SUBJECTS$\rightarrow 2^{OBJECTS}$, the mapping of a subject to all the objects it owns. Formally: owner_object(s) $\subseteq \{ \forall_{i=1,2,...,n} o_i \subseteq$ OBJECTS $|(s,o_i) \in$ OWNER$\}$.

- To restrict the one-to-many mapping between subjects and objects, we add the following rules:

$\forall s_i s_j \in$ SUBJECTS, $s_i \neq s_j$, obj$\in$ OBJECTS,

If object_owner(obj) = s_i
owner_object(s$_j$) $\subseteq$ OBS \ {obj}.

Figure 2 presents an access control framework of core RBAC with privacy-based extension. When a request arrives at the access control, the core RBAC is enhanced with the privacy-based extension (e.g., purpose, recipient, obligation and retention). Once the decision is made to either grant or deny the permission to the subject according to the request, a set of obligations and a set of retention policies are returned.

With the privacy extension in RBAC model, we revise the general privacy policy

Figure 2. An access control framework of core RBAC with privacy-based extension

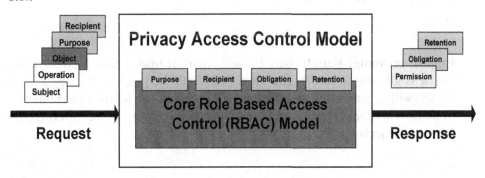

rule based on HIPAA basic principle (HIPPA, 2005) as follows:

```
ALLOW [Subject]
to perform [Operation] on [Object]
only for legitimate [Purposes] to [Recipients]
Carry out [Obligations] and [Retentions].
DENY otherwise.
```

The privacy rule can be described as follows:

A subject only has access to an object if the access is authorized by the core RBAC. In addition, the subject needs to specify the purpose(s) of the access and recipient(s) of the result of access operation. The purpose(s) and recipient(s) must be legitimate in accordance to the access of the object defined by the owner or an authority such as the government. Thus, obligations and retention policy will be returned as a response message if the access is allowed. The subject must also comply with the obligations and retention policy. The access request will be denied otherwise.

HIPAA's six privacy rules can be represented by the above extended RBAC model. Due to the page limit, we only present the first three rules as below:

1.   The right to view and make a copy of a patients own medical records.

$\forall \ s_i \in$ SUBJECTS, subject_user(s_i) $\not\subset \varnothing$,
r = "patient" $\in$ subject_role(s_i) $\subseteq$ ROLES,
subject_user(s_i)$\in$ assigned_user(r) ,
op_1="read" $\in$ OPS,
$\{o_1, o_2, ..., o_k\} \subseteq$ owner_object(s_i)
$\{pp_1, pp_2, ..., pp_j\} \subseteq$ PURPOSES,
$s_i \in$ RECIPIENTS,
$\Rightarrow$
access(s_i, op_1, $\{o_1, o_2, ..., o_k\}$, $\{pp_1, pp_2, ..., pp_j\}$,$\{s_i\}$) = (ALLOW, $\{obl_1, obl_2, ..., obl_m\}$, $\{rt_1, rt_2, ..., rt_k\}$),
$\{obl_1, obl_2, ..., obl_m\} \subseteq$ OBLIGATIONS,

$\{rt_1, rt_2, ..., rt_k\} \subseteq$ RETENTIONS

English meaning: For all users in the system, if his/her has the role "patient," he/she is allowed to read his/her own PHIs with the purpose $\{pp_1, pp_2, ..., pp_j\}$. He/she will be the only person for the PHIs recipient and he/she has to follow a set of obligations $\{obl_1, obl_2, ..., obl_m\}$ and retentions $\{rt_1, rt_2, ..., rt_k\}$ for corresponding set of objects $\{o_1, o_2, ..., o_k\}$.

Note: $\{pp_1, pp_2, ..., pp_j\} \subseteq$ PURPOSES, $\{obl_1, obl_2, ..., obl_m\} \subseteq$ OBLIGATIONS and $\{rt_1, rt_2, ..., rt_k\} \subseteq$ RETENTIONS would need to be defined by the healthcare services provider.

2.   The right to request the correction of inaccurate health information.

$\forall s_i \in$ SUBJECTS, subject_user(s_i) $\not\subset \varnothing$,
r = "patient" $\in$ subject_role(s_i) $\subseteq$ ROLES,
subject_user(s_i)$\in$ assigned_user(r) ,
op$_1$="read" $\in$ OPS, op$_2$="write" $\in$ OPS,
$\{o_1, o_2, ..., o_k\} \subseteq$ owner_object(s_i)
pp$_1$= "Correction of inaccurate information" $\in$ PURPOSES
$s_i \in$ RECIPIENTS,
$\Rightarrow$
access(s_i, op$_1$, $\{o_1, o_2, ..., o_k\}$, $\{pp_1\}$,$\{s_i\}$) = (ALLOW, $\{obl_1, obl_2, ..., obl_m\}$, $\{rt_1, rt_2, ..., rt_k\}$),
access(s_i, op$_2$, $\{o_1, o_2, ..., o_k\}$, $\{pp_1\}$,$\{s_i\}$) = (ALLOW, $\{obl_1, obl_2, ..., obl_m\}$, $\{rt_1, rt_2, ..., rt_k\}$),
$\{obl_1, obl_2, ..., obl_m\} \subseteq$ OBLIGATIONS,

$\{rt_1, rt_2, ..., rt_k\} \subseteq$ RETENTIONS

English meaning: For all users in the system, if his/her has the role "patient," he/she is allowed to create, update and delete his/her own PHIs if they are incorrect or inaccurate. He/she will be the only person for the PHIs recipient and he/she has to follow a set of obligations $\{obl_1, obl_2, ..., obl_m\}$ and retentions $\{rt_1, rt_2, ..., rtk\}$ for corresponding set of objects $\{o_1, o_2, ..., o_k\}$.
Note: $\{obl_1, obl_2, ..., obl_m\} \subseteq$ OBLIGATIONS and $\{rt_1, rt_2, ..., rt_k\} \subseteq$ RETENTIONS would need to be defined by the healthcare services provider.

3.   The right to find out where PHI has been shared for purposes other than care, payment, or healthcare operations.

$\forall s_i \in$ SUBJECTS, subject_user(s_i:SUBJECTS) $\not\subset \varnothing$,
r = "patient" $\in$ subject_role(s_i) $\subseteq$ ROLES,
subject_user(s_i)$\in$ assigned_user(r) ,
op$_1$="read" $\in$ OPS
$\{o_1, o_2, ..., o_k\} \subseteq$ {"Access logs of a subject's own PHIs"}$\subseteq$ owner_object(s_i)
$\{pp_1, pp_2, ..., pp_j\} \subseteq$ PURPOSES,
$s_i \in$ RECIPIENTS,
$\Rightarrow$

access(s_i, op$_1$, {o_1, o_2, ..., o_k},{pp$_1$, pp$_2$, ..., pp$_j$},{s_j}) = (ALLOW, {obl$_1$, obl$_2$, ..., obl$_m$}, {rt$_1$, rt$_2$, ..., rt$_k$}),

{obl$_1$, obl$_2$, ..., obl$_m$} $\subseteq$ OBLIGATIONS,

{rt$_1$, rt$_2$, ..., rt$_k$} $\subseteq$ RETENTIONS

English meaning: For all users in the system, if his/her has the role "patient," he/she is allowed to read the access log of his/her own PHIs with the purpose {pp$_1$, pp$_2$, ..., pp$_j$}. He/she will be the only person for the PHIs recipient and he/she has to follow a set of obligations {obl$_1$, obl$_2$, ..., obl$_m$} and retentions {rt$_1$, rt$_2$, ..., rt$_k$} for corresponding set of objects {o_1, o_2, ..., o_k}.

Note: {pp$_1$, pp$_2$, ..., pp$_j$} $\subseteq$ PURPOSES, {obl$_1$, obl$_2$, ..., obl$_m$} $\subseteq$ OBLIGATIONS and {rt$_1$, rt$_2$, ..., rt$_j$} $\subseteq$ RETENTIONS would need to be defined by the healthcare services provider.

"Access logs of a subject's own PHIs" refers to objects' access decision history.

Implementation in Web Services

In this chapter, we discuss Web services technologies as a platform to realize the privacy access control model for healthcare. A Web service is a software system designed to support interoperable application-to-application interaction over the Internet. Web services are based on a set of XML standards, such as universal description, discovery and integration (UDDI), Web services description language (WSDL), and simple object access protocol (SOAP).

Referring to Figure 3, a multi-layer framework describing the conceptual model, logical model and implementation model is proposed by Hung, Ferrari, and Carminati (2004). It shows the mapping of each layer between the conceptual and logical models with the support of corresponding XML language model for the implementation of Web services. We are particularly interested in the privacy and security layer in the conceptual model. These two layers are referred to access control in the logical model and supported by enterprise privacy authorization language (EPAL) (IBM, 2003)/ Platform for Privacy Preferences Project (P3P) (W3C, 2002)/extensible access control markup language (XACML) (OASIS, 2005) and WS-security (IBM & Microsoft, 2002) in the implementation model. It is believed that XACML is suitable for expressing the privacy policy and access control language because the XACML can implement the RBAC with privacy-based extension and also incorporate with the policy constraint assertion model: WS-PolicyConstraints.

Figure 3. The relation of conceptual model, logical model and implementation model of developing Web services applications

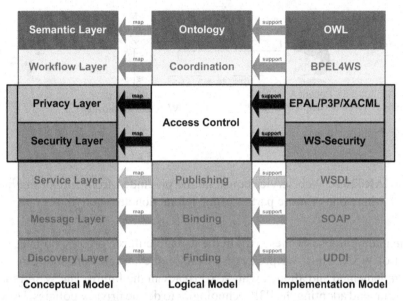

Preliminary Requirements

In this section, we discuss some requirements of Web services architecture (WSA) (IBM & Microsoft, 2002) as the preliminary requirements to develop a Web services privacy framework.

To enable privacy protection for Web service requesters across multiple domains and services, the World Wide Web Consortium (W3C) published a document called "*Web Services Architecture (WSA) Requirements*" (W3C, 2002) to define some specific privacy requirements for Web services, as follows:

- **AR020.1:** The WSA must enable privacy policy statements to be expressed about Web services.

- **AR020.2:** Advertised Web service privacy policies must be expressed in P3P.

- **AR020.3:** The WSA must enable a service requester to access a Web service's advertised privacy policy statement.

- **AR020.5:** The WSA must enable delegation and propagation of privacy policy.

Figure 4. An example scenario for healthcare service request and return messages

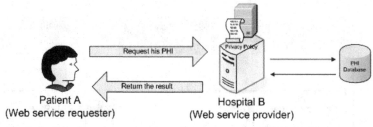

Patient A
(Web service requester)

Hospital B
(Web service provider)

•   **AR020.6:** Web services must not be precluded from supporting interactions where one or more parties of the interaction are anonymous.

The main purpose of these requirements is to enforce privacy policies in the context of WSA. Thus, we present a privacy policy framework that can possibly be complemented and aligned with WS-Privacy in the future. The WSA requirements recommend adopting the P3P technologies to define privacy policies. However, one can imagine that vocabularies vary in different applications like the healthcare sector. It is essential to have an independent privacy vocabulary specification for WSA.

Figure 4 illustrated an example for a patient making a request to view his PHI through Web services provided by the hospital. In this example, patient A is the Web services requestor while the hospital B is the service provider. After receiving the request from patient A, hospital B would check if the request complies with the pre-defined privacy policy and get access to the PHI database. If it is a legitimate request, hospital B returns PHI of patient A from the PHI database.

Referring to the example scenario in Figure 4, we specify the privacy policy that "The Web service is the only recipient collected the data (*Hospital*, *Treatment* and *Pharmacy*) for healthcare purposes" and present the privacy policy XACML in Figure 5.

Figure 6 describes a vocabulary-based Web services privacy framework for supporting healthcare applications. The privacy framework was first proposed by Hung, Ferrari, and Carminati (2004) and further enhanced by Cheng and Hung (2005) to fit into the e-healthcare application domain. In the e-healthcare Web services scenario, Web services providers can be hospitals, insurance companies or any health/financial data repositories. The Web services requestors could be the patients, doctors, physicians, insurance companies' staff, or any legitimate users. After the Web services applica-

Figure 5. An illustrative XACML rule

```
<rule>
 <target>
  <subject>samlp:AuthorizationDecisionQuery/Subject/NameIdentifier/Name</subject>
  <resource>
   <patternMatch>
    <attributeRef>#healthcare_systems</attributeRef>
    <attibuteValue>#hospital.*</attibuteValue>
     <attibuteValue>#treatment.*</attibuteValue>
     <attibuteValue>#pharmacy.*</attibuteValue>
   </patternMatch>
  </resource>
  <actions><saml:Actions><saml:Action>read</saml:Action></saml:Actions></actions>
 </target>
 <condition><equal>
   <attributeRef>healthcare</attributeRef>
   <attributeRef>urn:oasis:names:tc:xacml:2.0:action:purpose</attributeRef>
 </equal></condition>
 <effect>Permit</effect>
</rule>
```

Figure 6. A Vocabulary-based Web services privacy framework for healthcare applications

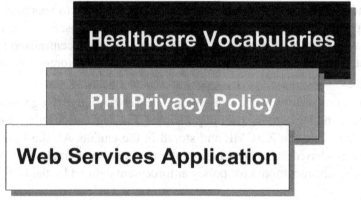

tion receives a request (e.g., viewing a medical record) from a user, the application needs to follow the internal data privacy policy principle.

In the following section, a healthcare Web service architecture will be presented for tackling the privacy principles discussed in an earlier section.

E-Healthcare Privacy Legislation Compliance Architecture

Based on the principles discussed in a previous section, we proposed a technical architecture (Figure 11) by which the privacy legislations and can be tackled properly. The architecture is divided into three major components which are referring to the three concepts (vocabulary, privacy policy and Web service application), as illustrated in Figure 6.

Communication Security Layer

To address the communication-level security protection principle (Principle 2), the bottom layer of the technical architecture is designed to be supported by a security infrastructure. The three core cryptographic components (confidentiality, integrity and authentication) in this infrastructure are required to achieve. The implementation of this layer can be done by using the existing encryption tools such as secure socket layer (SSL), public key infrastructure (PKI) and IP security (IP Sec), which are used to support secure data in transmission and exchange.

E-Healthcare Privacy Policy Layer

This layer is used for describing and specifying the privacy policy. Privacy policy description language is the core component for implementing this layer. According to the XACML 2.0 specification, XACML is intended to be suitable for a variety of application environment. XACML is therefore chosen to specify the privacy policy and it was designed to support centralized or decentralized policy management. XACML can be used for policy presentation, enforcement, negotiation and management.

Application security and privacy enforcement engine is used for governing application specific and legislation specific principles. The legislation rules (e.g., HIPAA) are translated into the XACML and stored in the engine. All the PHI access control decision is based on the rules and an authorization management component. XACML share an abstract model for policy enforcement defined by the IETF (2000):

- **Policy decision point (PDP):** The point where policy decisions are made
- **Policy enforcement point (PEP):** The point where the policy decisions are actually enforced
- **Resource:** Something of value in a network infrastructure to which rules or policy criteria are first applied before access is granted. Examples of resources include the buffers in a router and bandwidth on an interface.

Figure 7. XACML policy enforcement model

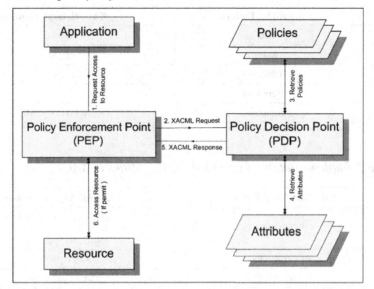

- **Policy:** The combination of rules and services where rules define the criteria for resource access and usage

Figure 7 shows the components of this model. All requests for resources access from application is handled by the PEP. After gathering the necessary information, the PEP formulates a XACML request and sends to PDP. The PDP fetches the necessary policies and attributes for decision making. The PDP then returns the response in XACML back to the PEP. The PEP then enforces the decision by allowing or denying the resources access.

The Authorization Management component is built based on the role-based access control (RBAC) model with privacy enhancement. Within OASIS, the XACML technical committee is developing an RBAC profile for expression of authorization policies in XML, making it easier to build RBAC into Web applications. The RBAC service is defined by the RBAC profile in XACML and the implementations of core RBAC entities are presented in Table 1.

The core RBAC entity *USERS* can be presented in the XACML implementation as the Subjects. The *ROLES* is mapped to the Subject Attributes, either specified in the access message or to be determined by the system. *OBJECTS* is referred to as a Resources in XACML, and the corresponding *OPS* is referred to as Actions. The permission *PRMS* and corresponding access control policies are specified in PolicySet and Policy.

Table 1. Implementation of RBAC entities in XACML

Core RBAC Entities	XACML Implementation
User	`Subjects`
Roles	`Subject Attributes`
Objects	`Resources`
Operations	`Actions`
Permissions	`PolicySet`

Table 2. Implementation of extended RBAC entities in XACML

Extended RBAC Entities	XACML Implementation
PURPOSES	`<resource:purpose>` `<action:purpose>`
RECIPIENTS	`<Subjects>`
OBLIGATIONS	`<Obligations>`
RETENTIONS	`<Retentions>`

Table 2 shows how the privacy access control model can be implemented in XACML.

The extended RBAC entity *PURPOSES* can be presented in the XACML implementation as the `purpose` for accessing a resource, or the purpose of an action. The *RECIPIENTS* can be referred to as `Subjects`. *OBLIGATIONS* are presented in the XACML implementation as `Obligations`. Finally, for the *RETENTIONS*, we extended the response message with a `Retentions` which will make use of the vocabulary `Retentions` we introduced in the privacy access control model, and the current date/time, and duration in the XACML implementation, represented by `environment: current-dateTime` and `duration`, respectively.

Here we illustrate an example of a request from Julius Hibbert; the privacy rules in the privacy access control model may state the following:

Julius Hibbert is allowed to read John Smith's medical record for medical treatment purpose with himself as the only recipient, no disclosure, and no retention.

Based on the XACML implementation of policy, request, and response message with the extended privacy access control model are illustrated in Figures 8, 9, and 10, respectively.

Figure 8. An extended XACML policy for the privacy access control model

```
<Policy RuleCombiningAlgId="urn:oasis:names:tc:xacml:1.0:
                        rule-combining-algorithm:deny-overrides">
    <Description>An extended policy modified from the Draft
                    XACML Conformance Test IIA001 </Description>
    <Rule Effect="Permit">
            <Description>
                Julius Hibbert can read John Smith's medical
                record for medical treatment purpose
                if she follows the obligation "No disclosure"
                and "No retention"
            </Description>
              <Subjects>
                 <Subject>Julius Hibbert</Subject>
              </Subjects>
              <Resources>
                 <Resource>
                     http://medico.com/record/patient/JohnSmith
                 </Resource>
              </Resources>
            <Actions>
                <Action action:purpose = "Medical Treatment">
                    </AttributeValue>read</AttributeValue>
                    <recipients>Individual</recipients>
                </Action>
            </Actions>
            <Obligations>No-disclosure</Obligations>
            <Retentions>No-retention</Retentions>
    </Rule>
</Policy>
```

Figure 9. An extended XACML request message for the privacy access control model

```
<Request>
    <Subject>
        <Attribute>Julius Hibbert</Attribute>
    </Subject>
    <Resource>
        http://medico.com/record/patient/JohnSmith
    </Resource>
    <Action action:purpose = "Medical Treatment">
        <AttributeValue>read</AttributeValue>
        <recipients>Individual</recipients>
    </Action>
</Request>
```

Figure10. An extended XACML response for the privacy access control model

```
<Response>
  <Result>
    <Decision>Permit</Decision>
    <Obligations>No-disclosure</Obligations>
    <Retentions>No-retention</Retentions>
    <Status>
      <StatusCode
        Value="urn:oasis:names:tc:xacml:1.0:status:ok"/>
    </Status>
  </Result>
</Response>
```

Privacy Policy Negotiation Engine is used for privacy policy negotiation. We adopt the idea of using user privacy profile (Cheng & Hung, 2005) to facilitate the negotiation. A user privacy profile is a profile for storing the user's preference of how much information can be disclosed to others. Registered users have the right to create, view, update or delete their own user privacy profiles. It is a dynamic profile that is defined by the user or a group of individuals. Users can create, view, update or delete their privacy profiles. For example, a patient can set his/her privacy profile such that the billing information is visible to all the staff in his/her insurance company or be only visible to his/her corresponding insurance broker. Usually, a Web services provider may have different privacy profiles for different requestors. For example, an insurance company may wish to get all the details of their clients, but one of them may only wish to provide the minimum amount of PHI that is sufficient for the claim. To resolve the conflicts of privacy profiles, this negotiation engine can provide controlled access points in the form of a programmatic interface.

Healthcare Specific Vocabularies Layer

The data-level security protection principle (Principle 1) and the consent require-ment principle (Principle 3) can be embedded inside the consent management engine. Users must first consent to data collection, use, and storage proposals for any PHI. The consent management engine would be responsible for managing all the Hippocratic data and the corresponding data privacy profiles. The Hippocratic data has to be stored securely to follow the data-level security protection principle (Principle 1.1). To achieve data privacy, a data privacy profile is used for each data object and specifies the access views that are exposed to the different Web services. Each PHI would therefore have its own privacy profile to limit the access control for different systems with different purposes. For example, the billing information in the PHI can be transferred to the patients' insurance companies but not a system

Figure 11. Privacy legislation compliance conceptual architecture for e-healthcare Web service application

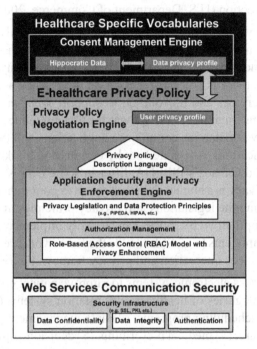

administrator in the hospital. The highest level for viewing PHI is the Hippocratic Data Layer. PHI is presented in a HL7 standardized XML format.

Discussion and Conclusion

Access control is one of the most important aspects of information management because of the disaster of releasing unauthorized content and also the legal issues such as the privacy acts. With the increase in digitalizing health information, one can imagine that the demand for privacy-enhancing technologies, especially based on Web services, is ever increasing. As for legal compliance, effective privacy policy and system architecture is required in countries all over the world. However, because different countries have different requirements, mechanism for facilitating the customization of such policies is essential. Apart from the HIPAA, there are also other legislations such as the European Union Directive on Data Protection (European Union, 1995), Personal Information Protection and Electronic Documents Act (PIPEDA) of Canada and Privacy Act of Australia. According to the U.S.

Department of Commerce, this directive would prohibit the transfer of personal data to non-European Union nations that do not meet the European "adequacy" standard for privacy protection (U.S. Department of Commerce, 2005).

Privacy generally includes the full spectrum of organizational controls of information under security but also covers specific privacy issues such as consent management, unlinkability, unobservability, pseudonymity, and anonymity of data. To the best of our knowledge, there is no prior research on the privacy access control technologies for Web services and no solution to support Web services-based healthcare applications. This framework perhaps was the first guideline setup for implementing national privacy legislations compliance applications and the Web services-based healthcare applications. As pointed out by Perkins and Markel (2004), although the EU directive and Canada's PIPEDA differ in some details, both are based on the premise that privacy is a human right that deserves comprehensive legal protection. After categorizing the legislations into privacy principles, it is believed that multi-legislations compliant Web services can be easily implemented. In fact, most of the technology components (e.g., SSL) inside the framework are not new. However, the idea of Web services integration and privacy framework are new.

To utilize paperless electronic systems to improve patient care and safety, there are generally six categories of healthcare information systems (HISs) in a healthcare institution: (1) scheduling programs, (2) data management programs, (3) medical reference software, (4) medical prescribing, (5) decision-support programs, and (6) billing and charge-capture programs. Further requirements from privacy legislation may cause many healthcare institutions to find it difficult to build HISs that can fully address security and privacy requirements, especially in light of recent changes in health privacy legislative environment. One reason is the lack of clear linkages from security and privacy considerations at a management-level conceptualization to the technology implementations of security and privacy mechanisms and solutions into various HISs. Although the legislations are not discussed in full context, we tried our best to cover the important technical issues required in the legislations. The rest (such as those exceptions) can be implemented by adding rules in the privacy enforcement engine or adding rules in access control decision.

An interesting research issue about e-healthcare application is the owner of PHI. Although a patient should be the primary owner of the PHI, he/she only needs the right to view his/her PHI (unless it is incomplete or incorrect). On the other hand, his/her doctor, physicians, or his/her healthcare providers are responsible for updating the PHI. Only consent is required from the primary owner when updating the PHI. In the real practice, to get the consent from a patient, the doctor needs the patient to sign a consent form. This is a paper-based solution but soon can be moved into an electronic-based solution with the world trend. If we introduce the concept of secondary owner and allow the delegations by using digital signature (or proxy signature) from the primary owner, this can also be a solution to the consent requirement principle.

Consent has always been emphasized in the privacy legislations and it is necessary to handle properly in the future Web service application development. The idea of consent and authorization may perhaps be implemented in the same standard such as WS-authorization. However, according to the WSA, the WS-Authorization has not yet been developed (IBM & Microsoft, 2002). We believe it is possible that RBAC can be one of the WS-authorization components in the future. With WS-authorization being standardized, we believe that the WS-Privacy can be developed and mutually supportive of each other.

In order to implement healthcare Web services applications, it is necessary to be compliant with international legislations. It is believed that emerging Web services would be able to facilitate the integration and collaboration of PHI with privacy compliance. The contributions in this chapter are the categorization of the core part of these legislations into privacy principles and the proposed multi-legislation-compliant Web services for healthcare solution. The privacy principles setup guidelines for developing legislations-compliant Web services for healthcare applications, while the enhanced vocabulary-based framework illustrates the implementation of healthcare Web Services application. We presented that XACML are suitable in the context of expressing privacy policy and access control rules. XACML is the best fit in describing the healthcare domain vocabularies, as well as in the negotiations of different privacy policies.

Web services for healthcare can only succeed if the users are confident that their privacy is protected. We believe that the presented principles and architecture will provide sufficient guidelines for developing HIPAA-compliant privacy access control model for healthcare applications.

References

Anderson, R. (1996). A security policy model for clinical information systems. *Proceedings of the 1996 IEEE Symposium on Security and Privacy.*SP, (p. 30). Washington, D.C.: IEEE Computer Society.

Agrawal, R., Kini, A., LeFevre, K., Wang, A., Xu, Y., & Zhou, D. (2004). Managing healthcare data hippocratically. *Proceedings of the 2004 ACM SIGMOD international Conference on Management of Data,* (pp. 947-948). Paris, France. New York: ACM Press.

Bell Canada. (2005). *Privacy, trust and striking the correct balance.* Retrieved from enterprise.bell.ca/en/resources/uploads/pdf/BSSI_privacy_trust_en.pdf

Canadian Standards Association (CSA). (1996). *Model code for the protection of personal information.* Retrieved from canada.justice.gc.ca/en/news/nr/1998/attback2.html

Cheng, V., & Hung, P. (2005). Health Insurance Portability and Account-ability Act (HIPAA) compliant access control model for Web services. *The International Journal of Health Information Systems and Informatics (IJHIS)*, *1*(1).

Cheng, V., & Hung, P. (2005). Towards an integrated privacy framework for HIPAA-compliant Web services. *Proceedings of the 2005 IEEE International Conference on E-Commerce Technology*, (pp. 480-483).

Dubauskas, N. (2005). Business compliance to changing privacy protections. *Proceedings of the 38t^h Annual Hawaii international Conference on System Sciences (Hicss'05)*. Washington, D.C.: IEEE Computer Society.

European Union. (1995). Directive 95/46/EC of the European Parliament. Retrieved from europa.eu.int/comm/justice_home/fsj/privacy/

Federal Privacy Act (2000). *The office of the Privacy Commissioner.* Retrieved May 3, 2004 from http://www.privacy.gov.au/act/privacyact/index.html.

Ferraiolo, D., Kuhn, D., & Chandramouli, R. (2003). *Role-based access control.* Computer Security Series. Artech House Publishers.

Fischer-Hubner, S. (2001). *IT-security and privacy*. Lecture Notes on Computer Science 1958.

Hachman, M. (2007). *Microsoft launches 'HealthVault' records-storage site.* Retrieved October 4, 2007 from http://www.pcmag.com/article2/0,1759,2191920,00.asp

HealthVault. (2007). Retrieved October 4, 2007 from http://search.healthvault.com

HIPAA. (2005). *Medical privacy—national standards to protect the privacy of personal health information.* U.S. Department of Health & Human Services (HSS). Retrieved April 18, 2005 from www.hhs.gov/ocr/hipaa/

HL7. (2004). *HIPAA claims and attachments preparing for regulation.* Retrieved May 2004 from www.hl7.org/memonly/downloads/Attachment_Specifications/HIPAA_and_Claims_Attachments_White_Paper_20040518.pdf

Hung, P., Ferrari, E., & Carminati, B. (2004). Towards standardized Web services privacy technologies. *Proceedings of the IEEE international Conference on Web Services (Icws'04)*, (pp.174-181). Washington, D.C.:IEEE Computer Society.

IBM. (2003). *Enterprise Privacy Authorization Language (EPAL).* IBM Research Report. Retrieved June 12, 2003 from www.zurich.ibm.com/security/enterprise-privacy/epal

IBM & Microsoft. (2002) *Security in a Web services world: A proposed architecture and roadmap.* White Paper, *Version 1.0.* Retrieved April 7, 2002 from www-106.ibm.com/developerworks/library/ws-secmap/

IMIA. (2001). *A code of ethics for professionals (HIPs)*. International Medical Informatics Association (IMIA). Retrieved March 2001 from www.imia. org/pubdocs/Code_of_ethics.pdf

Jepsen, T. (2003). IT in healthcare: Progress report. *IT Professional, 5*(1), 8-14.

Jones, V., Ching, N., & Winslett, M. (1995). Credentials for privacy and interoperation. *Proceedings of the New Security Paradigms Workshop*, (pp. 92-100).

May, T. (1998). Medical information security: The evolving challenge. *Proceedings of the 32nd Annual 1998 International Carnahan Conference on Security Technology*, (pp. 85-92).

National Privacy Principles (Extracted from the Privacy Amendment (Private Sector) Act 2000). (2000). *The office of the privacy commissioner.* Retrieved from www.privacy.gov.au/publications/npps01.html

NIST. (2005). *Role-based access control standards roadmap*. National Institute of Standard and Technology (NIST). Retrieved May 18, 2005 from csrc.nist. gov/rbac/rbac-stds-roadmap.html

OASIS. (2005). *eXtensible Access Control Markup Language v2.0 Core (XACML)*. Retrieved February 1, 2005 from docs.oasis-open.org/xacml/2.0/access_control-xacml-2.0-core-spec-os.pdf

Osborn, S., Sandhu, R., & Munawer, Q. (2000). Configuring role-based access control to enforce mandatory and discretionary access control policies. *ACM Transactions on Information and Systems Security (TISSEC), 3*(2), 85-106.

Perkins, E., & Markel, M. (2004). Multinational data-privacy laws: An introduction for IT managers. *IEEE Transactions on Professional Communication, 47*(2), 85-94.

PIPEDA. (2000). *Personal Information Protection and Electronic Documents Act. Department of Justice of Canada.* Retrieved August 31, 2004 from laws.justice. gc.ca/en/P-8.6/text.html

Powers, C., Ashley, P., & Schunter, M. (2002). Privacy promises, access control, and privacy management—enforcing privacy throughout an enterprise by extending access control. *Proceedings of the 3rd International Symposium on Electronic Commerce*, (pp.13-21).

Privacy Rights Clearinghouse (PRC). (1998). *Ten privacy principals for healthcare.* Retrieved November 1998 from www.privacyrights.org/ar/privprin.htm

Tan, J., & Hung, P. (2005). E-security: Framework for privacy and security in e-health data integration and aggregation. In *E-healthcare information systems: An introduction for students and professionals* (pp. 450-478). Jossey-Bass.

University of Miami Ethics Programs. (2005). Privacy standard/rule (HIPAA). Retrieved May 12, 2005 from privacy.med.miami.edu/glossary/xd_privacy_stds. htm

U.S. Department of Health & Human Services. (2004). Fact Sheet—protecting the privacy of patients' health information. Retrieved April 14, 2004 from www.hhs.gov/news/facts/privacy.html

U.S. Department of Commerce. (2005). *Safe Harbor Overview.* Retrieved February 3, 2005 from www.export.gov/safeharbor

W3C. (2002). *The platform for privacy preferences 1.0 (P3P1.0) specification.* World Wide Web Consortium (W3C) Recommendation. Retrieved April 16, 2002 from www.w3.org/TR/P3P/

W3C. (2002). *Web services architecture requirements.* Working draft. World Wide Web Consortium (W3C). http://www.w3.org/TR/2002/WD-wsa-reqs-20021114

Yee, G., & Korba, L. (2004). Privacy policy compliance for Web services. *Proceedings of IEEE International Conference on Web Services,* (pp.158-165).

Section II

HISI Methodological Approaches

Chapter IV

The Internet and Managing Boomers and Seniors' Health

Christopher G. Reddick, The University of Texas at San Antonio, USA

Abstract

This chapter examines the use of the Internet for gathering health information by boomers and seniors. This study attempts to determine whether online health seekers (individuals that have Internet access and have searched for health information online) have changed their behavior from the information they found online. Essentially, has online health information helped them manage their health more effectively? This research analyzes the Kaiser Family Foundation e-Health and the Elderly public opinion dataset of access by boomers and seniors to online health information. The major results indicate that boomers marginally use online health information more than seniors for the management of their health. The most significant results indicated that boomers and seniors who are more aware and have positive feelings towards online health information would use it more to manage their health.

Introduction and Background

For baby boomers, the Internet has become the most important source of health information other than consultation with their family doctor (Kaiser Family Foundation, 2005). The focus of this chapter is on both baby boomers, those in the age range of 50 to 64, and seniors or those 65 and older.[1] This study examines the use of online health information by baby boomers and seniors and how they use the information for managing their health. The Internet can empower citizens in their health management (Alpay et al., 2007). The primary objectives of this article are to examine the differences in behavior between boomers and seniors and to test for the presence of a variety of associations between their characteristics and a number of management of health variables.

This study explores five specific questions. First, are there any differences between boomers and seniors and their access to health information for managing health? Second, will healthier boomers and seniors rely less on online health information to manage their health because they would have less need? Third, will the presence of boomers and seniors that have more experience and familiarity with the Internet lead to greater use of online health information to manage health? Fourth, would individuals who are in a lower sociodemographic status rely less on online health information because of lack of resources to access this information? Finally, would avid Internet users use online health information more often to manage their health because they would have greater access to and familiarity with the Internet?

Eighty percent of American Internet users have searched for information on at least 1 of 17 health topics (Fox, 2006). This places health searches at about the same level of popularity on a typical day as paying bills online, reading blogs, or using the Internet to look up a phone number or address. Certain groups of Internet users in 2006 were the most likely to have sought health information online: women, Internet users younger than 65, college graduates, those with more online experience, and those with broadband Internet access at home.

Online health information is especially important given the millions of uninsured Americans trying to get information on their health situation. Individuals can use this online health information to make informed choices on their healthcare needs. They can potentially use information on the Internet to better manage their health. Essentially, has online health information influenced the behaviors of boomers and seniors with respect to their healthcare needs? This influence could be as extensive as visiting a doctor or simply talking to family or friends about health information that a boomer or senior found online.

Access to timely and reliable information on health and healthcare has long been a goal for seniors, who face a greater number of health conditions and use prescription drugs and healthcare services at a higher rate than younger adults (Kaiser Family Foundation, 2005). However, the online behavior of seniors has not been studied as closely as that of health information searches of adolescents (Gray et al., 2005), women (Pandey et al., 2003), cancer patients (Eysenbach, 2003; Ziebland, 2004), those affected by the digital divide (Skinner et al., 2003), and comparing online and off-line behavior (Cotton & Gupta, 2004). There is little empirical research that examines whether online health searches affect the management of health (Nicholas et al., 2001; Lueg et al., 2003), one of the two objectives of this study. This study measures whether Internet health information changed the self-reporting behavior of boomers and seniors and does not specifically address change in health outcomes.

There are two reasons why this study does a comparison of both boomers and seniors. First, baby boomers represent future seniors and by examining this age group, this study can provide some indication about what the future holds for the Internet and health information. Second, both boomers and seniors are in the greatest need of health information since they are more prone to having health problems than other age groups.

This study is different from existing work of Nicholas et al. (2001), Lueg et al. (2003), and Huntington et al. (2004) in that this focuses on the use of online health information in the management of health. This study focuses especially on comparing two groups, boomers and seniors, while the existing empirical work examines the entire Internet population. This study is different from studies that conduct a meta-analysis, which combine published results from different sources (Eysenbach, 2003). This research performs a statistical analysis leading to conclusions that are different from the original dataset (Kaiser Family Foundation, 2005). The aim of this study is not just to learn about the differences between boomers and seniors and access to online health information, it is to discern the magnitude of differences between these groups and the impact of factors such as awareness and feelings on health management.

In order to accomplish the goal of examining online health information and the management of boomers' and seniors' health, this chapter is divided into several sections. First, this research examines the literature on the use of the Internet as a health information source. Second, this chapter outlines how the literature can be summarized into hypotheses that model the most probable impacts on management of boomers' and seniors' health. Third, this research provides details of the Kaiser Family Foundation *e-Health and the Elderly* dataset that is used to model public opinion data of online health information (Kaiser Family Foundation, 2005). The fourth and fifth sections discuss the models and results of tests on the use of online health information for healthcare management. The sixth section provides a discussion, which outlines how the test results confirm or deny the specified hypotheses and shows the broader significance of this work. The last section provides avenues for future research and limitations of this study are presented.

Literature Review

The following section outlines the common themes found in the literature on the Internet and health information and the management of health. They can be divided into the factors of differences between age groups, the health of the individual, online proficiency, sociodemographic characteristics, and awareness and feelings about online health information. Existing research shows that little is known about how Internet usage, health status, and sociodemographic characteristics affect health information seeking (Cotton & Gupta, 2005).

Eysenbach (2003) provides a conceptual framework of the possible link between Internet use and cancer. Some of the important factors according to that author's meta-analysis indicate that Internet use is related to communication, community, and content leading to an impact on cancer outcomes. In a similar line of inquiry, a study by Lueg et al. (2003) provided a conceptual framework of Internet searches for online health information. These authors examine the situation that individuals find themselves confronted with in terms of health needs and frequency of use predicting access to health information. Eysenbach's (2003) conceptual framework is different from Lueg et al. (2003) in that the former examines the social aspect of Internet use and health information, while the latter study focuses on the situation involvement and the frequency of Internet use. The conceptual framework of this study is similar to Eysenbach (2003) and Lueg et al. (2003), but differs in that it examines boomers and seniors and factors such as frequency and satisfaction having an influence on the management of health (Figure 1).

Online Health Information and Managing Boomers' and Seniors' Health

If the Internet can be used to change the behavior of individuals, this is one assessment of the long-term utility of this information resource. If individuals just look at information online and do not use it in any substantial way, it does not make much

Figure 1. Conceptual framework of access to online health information by boomers and seniors

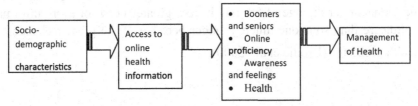

sense to invest in Internet health resources. The Internet suggests a remarkable change from the traditional "doctor knows best" approach (Eysenbach & Jadad, 2001). The Internet can be seen as challenging hierarchical models of information sharing in which the provider of the information decides how the information should be delivered (Ziebland, 2004).

For example, existing research in a 2001 survey showed that 44% of online health information seekers said that the information they found online affected a decision about how to treat an illness or cope with a medical condition (Fox & Rainie, 2002). A majority of respondents to a survey of adolescents and use of Internet health information reported that it helped them to start a conversation with a lay or professional medical person (Gray et al., 2005). Online health information seekers are mostly going online to look for specific answers to targeted questions (Fox & Rainie, 2000). In addition, 4 in 10 young people say they have changed their personal behavior because of health information they obtained online (Rideout, 2002). In an Internet survey, over one-third of respondents said that their condition had improved after having visited a Web site and more than 1 in 4 said that the Web information had resulted in a deferred visit or had actually replaced a visit to the doctor (Nicholas et al., 2001). Therefore, the existing research has examined adolescents' and all age groups' behavioral changes, but has not focused on seniors and their use of the Internet for managing health. There are five factors outlined in the literature, which are differences between boomers and seniors: the health of boomers and seniors, their online proficiency, their sociodemographic characteristics, and awareness and feelings towards online health information that are predicted to have an impact on whether online health information is used.

Boomers' and Seniors' Differences

Existing empirical evidence shows that health seekers are proportionately more middle aged than very young or old, with the highest proportion of usage witnessed in those between the ages 30 and 64 (Fox & Rainie, 2000; Fox, 2006). A more recent survey indicates that 70% of baby boomers have gone online in 2004, while only 31% of seniors have gone online (Kaiser Family Foundation, 2005). Boomers will retire shortly and the amount of online health information they will search for should increase dramatically compared to what seniors are currently consuming. In order to explore both the present and what the future will hold for online health information and seniors, it is important to compare both age groups. In addition, individuals over the age of 50 may have a greater need for more information on healthcare than someone much younger because of the greater chance of facing health problems (Brodie et al., 2000).

Health of Boomers and Seniors

The literature also mentions that individuals who are in worse health will want to search more for online health information. The Internet becomes an additional tool for them to search for health information. Empirical evidence shows that there is a link between an individual's health and his or her need for online health information. Less healthy individuals are more likely to explore different aspects of a Web site and use more health-related interactive features and in doing so improve their well-being (Lueg et al., 2003). Individuals who were suffering with an illness were 2 ½ times as likely, compared to respondents without a standing illness, to say that they had used information from the Internet as an alternative to seeing their general practitioner (Nicholas et al., 2001). In many cases, information seekers were acting on behalf of others such as family and friends. However, access to online health information should also be related to the consumer's ability to use the Internet, not just on whether they are healthy.

Online Proficiency

The ability to use the Internet should also have an impact on whether boomers and seniors use online health information to manage their health (Nicholas et al. 2007). Individuals who use Internet information more to manage their health have broadband Internet access, are frequently online, spend many hours online, and search for information on many different topics. Research shows that individuals using a Web site regularly were more likely to have said that the information was helpful (Nicholas et al., 2001). A survey of adolescents shows that there are issues of the disparity of Internet access and quality of Internet access such as dial-up versus broadband connection (Skinner et al., 2003).

Sociodemographic Characteristics of Online Health Seekers

Another factor explored in the literature that should have an impact on access to online health information is the sociodemographic characteristics of the individual. There is research on the digital divide, between the haves and have-nots of Internet access. This research predicts that those who have greater access to the Internet would have more resources in society. For instance, those groups of individuals who are more disadvantaged economically in the United States would have less access to the Internet and online health resources. Hispanics, the largest minority group in the United States, have traditionally had less Internet access (Fox & Rainie, 2000). Those with medium to high family income should be able to access the Internet more for health information because of greater resources.

Existing research shows that individuals who are older, have lower incomes, minorities, less educated, and males will be less likely to use the Internet for health information seeking (Anderson, 2004; Cotton & Gupta, 2004). In contrast, women increasingly rely on the Internet to supplement health information received from traditional sources (Pandey et al., 2003) and are more likely than men to seek online health information (Fox & Rainie, 2000; Nicholas et al., 2001). Awareness and feelings towards online health information also should have an impact on using this information to manage consumers' health.

Awareness and Feelings Towards Online Health Resources

A final factor that should explain access to Internet health information is the awareness and feelings of the individual towards online health information. If boomers and seniors have more positive feelings about the Internet as a health information resource, they will utilize it more often than someone who harbors more negative feelings towards the Internet. In addition, individuals who go online for health information frequently should use it more to manage their health. If a boomer's or senior's doctor or medical professional recommends or uses the Internet as a communication device, the patient is more likely to use it to manage his or her health. In summary, the prediction is that boomers and seniors who are more aware of online health resources should use these resources more to manage their health. In addition, boomers and seniors who have positive feelings about the benefits of online health information will use this resource more to manage their health.

Empirical evidence shows that there is a relationship between using the Internet more often and accessing access health information (Lueg et al., 2003). Those using the Web once a day were twice as likely to report that it helped a lot in terms of being better informed from health information found on the Web (Nicholas et al., 2001). E-mail is still a new medium for obtaining access to consumer health information and is also explored in the research as a way to manage a consumer's health (Huntington et al., 2004). The literature just outlined can be formally specified with the following hypotheses that demonstrate the relationship between boomers and seniors, the Internet, and the management of health.

Hypotheses

In order to examine whether online health information has affected the choices that individuals make in managing their health and the differences between boomers and seniors, several hypotheses are tested in this chapter. These hypotheses are derived from the literature mentioned in the previous section and they are divided into five areas:

- Boomers' and seniors' differences

    Hypothesis 1: *Online health seekers who are baby boomers are more likely to believe that online health information has helped them manage their health better compared with seniors.*

- Health of boomers and seniors

    Hypothesis 2: *Online health seekers who are healthy or who have family and friends that are healthy will rely less on online health information because of lack of need.*

- Online proficiency

    Hypothesis 3: *Online health seekers who have broadband Internet access will go online more for health information to manage their health*

    Hypothesis 4: *Online health seekers who go online more often and conduct many online activities will use Internet health information more to manage their health.*

- Sociodemographic status

    Hypothesis 5: *Boomers and seniors who are females will rely more on online health information.*

    Hypothesis 6: *Boomers and seniors who are college educated will rely more on online health information.*

    Hypothesis 7: *Boomers and seniors who are Hispanics will go online less for health information.*

    Hypothesis 8: *Boomers and seniors who have family income above $75,000 will go online more for health information.*

- Awareness and feelings towards online health resources

    Hypothesis 9: *Online health seekers who most of the time and always look to see who provides medical information on the Internet would use online health information more to manage their health.*

    Hypothesis 10: *Online health seekers who access health information online once or twice a month would have a greater likelihood of using online health information to manage their health.*

Hypothesis 11: *If a doctor has recommended a Web site to an online health seeker, he or she is more likely to use health information to manage their health.*

Hypothesis 12: *If an online health seeker has communicated with his or her doctor via e-mail, he or she is more likely to use online health information to manage their health.*

Hypothesis 13: *Online health seekers that have more positive feelings about looking for health information on the Internet are more likely to use this information to manage their health.*

These hypotheses are examined with a dataset that surveyed public opinion of both baby boomers and seniors on their use and acceptance of online health information.

Dataset and Methods

The e-Health and the Elderly dataset is a nationally representative random digit dial telephone survey of 1,450 adults age 50 and older.[2] Included in this sample were 583 respondents age 65 and older. The survey was designed by Kaiser Family Foundation (KFF) in consultation with Princeton Survey Research Associates (PSRA) and the survey was administered in the field by PSRA. The survey interviews were conducted between March 5 and April 8, 2004. The entire dataset of 1,450 respondents was first examined to determine the characteristics of boomers and seniors and access to online health information.

Out of the 1,450 responses to the survey, this study also has taken a sub sample of 628 respondents, of which there were 464 boomers and 164 seniors surveyed. Therefore, the original dataset was split and the sample sizes differ for both age groups. The 628 boomers and seniors represent those individuals who are called online health seekers. They have both Internet access and have looked for online health information. This group is of interest since in this study there is a comparison of the characteristics of those that actually look up online health information.

In this study, we use a consumer survey to explore the differences between boomers and seniors and their use of online health information to manage health. This research uses both descriptive statistics and logistic regression to explore differences in access to online health information between boomers and seniors.[3]

Table 1. Boomers and seniors who go online for health information

Go online for health information (Yes or No)	Age group	Frequency	Percent
No	50-64	335	42.5
	65+	454	57.5
	Total	789	100
Yes	50-64	464	78.2
	65+	129	21.8
	Total	593	100

Descriptive Statistics of Boomers and Seniors and Online Health Information

In order to model the relationship between seniors and boomers, online health information, and its impact on managing healthcare needs, this study has specified the following variables that will comprise the models tested.

Table 1 provides information on boomers and seniors who go online for health information. Boomers that go online for health information represent 78.2%, while seniors that go online for health information represent just over 21% of those surveyed in this category. This table generally supports the notion that boomers tend to go online more for health information than seniors. Boomers that do not go online for health information represent 43% and seniors that do not go online represent 58% of those surveyed in this category.

Table 2 outlines demographic information of boomers and seniors that go online and do not go online for health information. The digital divide is very evident with the data presented in this table. For instance, 43% of college educated individuals go online for health information compared with only 15% who are college educated that do not go online for health information. Among females and Hispanics there is not much of a difference in the percentage who go online and do not go online for health information. However, boomers and seniors that have a family income for 2003 above $75,000 were more likely to go online for health information. Finally, age seems to have an impact on accessing online health information. The mean age was 61 years for individuals that go online and 69 years for consumers who do not go online for health information. Higher income implies greater use of online health information and having a college education means a greater likelihood of going online for health information. This finding also indicates that boomers are more likely to go online for health information since the average age range was just over 61 years old.

Table 2. Demographic information of boomers and seniors gong online for health information

Go online for health information (Yes or No)		N	Mean	Standard Deviations
No	College educated	822	0.15	0.36
	Gender is female	822	0.65	0.48
	Race is Hispanic	822	0.03	0.18
	Family income 2003 above $75,000	822	0.07	0.25
	Age	822	68.79	12.41
Yes	College educated	628	0.43	0.50
	Gender is female	628	0.61	0.49
	Race is Hispanic	628	0.03	0.17
	Family income 2003 above $75,000	628	0.27	0.45
	Age	628	60.88	11.81

Table 3. Logistic regression results of sociodemographic variables predicting going-online for health information

Dependent Variable	Go Online for Health Information		
Predictor Variables	Odds Ratio	Wald Statistic	Prob. Sig.
Age	0.95	(301.47)***	0.00
College educated	4.05	(300.72)***	0.00
Gender is female	1.25	(11.49)***	0.00
Race is Hispanic	1.06	0.26	0.61
Family income 2003 above $75,000	2.25	(63.38)***	0.00
Constant	11.34	(139.67)***	0.00
Nagelkerke R-Square	0.25		
*Note: *** significant at the 0.01 level.*			

Logistic regression is used to test whether sociodemographic variables predict whether boomers or seniors go online for health information. Logistic regression was used, since this study models dependent variables that are binary, represented by either a "1" or "0" (Nicholas et al., 2001; Lueg et al., 2003). The odds ratio can be used to interpret the relative impact of the observance of a "1" in the dependent variable. Table 3 shows that almost all of the sociodemographic variables help to explain whether someone goes online for health information, with the only exception being Hispanic. For instance, having a college education means that a boomer or senior is four times more likely to go online for health information. Having a higher income indicates that boomers and seniors are two times more likely to go online for health information. However, as the age of the respondent increases this marginally decreases the likelihood of someone going online for health information.

Dependent Variables

Table 4 provides a list of the dependent and predictor variables and also demonstrates whether there were differences between boomers and seniors in these variables. Perhaps the most important dependent variable is whether "somewhat" or "a lot" of information on the Internet has helped take care of a senior's or boomer's health. The mean score indicates that 59% of boomers and 46% of seniors believed that the Internet has helped them take care of their health, demonstrating some impact on the management of their health.

The second dependent variable measures whether online health seekers had a conversation with family or friend about health information they found online (Table 4). Family and friends who go online for health information may guide someone else as to whether they should see a doctor because of this information (Eysenbach, 2003). The results indicate that 66% of boomers said that they had a conversation with family members or friends and only 48% of seniors said they had this conversation about the information they saw online. There were statistically significant differences between seniors and boomers for this question with the reported F-statistic being significant at the 0.01 level, meaning that boomers were more likely to have a conversation with family and friends about health information they found online.

The third dependent variable measures whether online health information changed the behavior of boomers and seniors (Table 4). Thirty-six percent of boomers' behavior changed as a result of online health information compared with 25% of seniors. This result was also shown to have a statistically significant difference between boomers and seniors at the 0.01 level. Around one-third of boomers changed their behavior, which is a good indication that the information they are finding is affecting their health.

A fourth management of health issue was whether boomers or seniors made a decision on treatment of an illness as a result of the information they found online (Table 4). The results showed that 34% of boomers believed that they made a decision about how to treat an illness because of information they found online, while only 26% of seniors made a decision on treatment. This result also showed a statistically significant difference between the two age groupings at the 0.01 level.

Another dependent variable was visiting a doctor as a result of the health information found online (Table 4). Only 16% of boomers visited a doctor as a result of health information they found online, while 13% of seniors visited a doctor. Visiting a doctor was the least utilized change in behavior as a result of online health information.

Table 4. Difference of means tests of dependent and predictor variables that online health seekers boomers are significantly different from seniors

Variable Name	Mean of Boomers	Standard Deviations Boomers	Mean of Seniors	Standard Deviations Seniors	Probability Significantly Different Boomers and Seniors
Dependent Variables					
Somewhat and a lot of information on Internet helped take care health	0.59	0.49	0.46	0.50	0.07
Had a conversation family or friend about online health information	0.66	0.47	0.48	0.50	0.00
Online health information changed behavior	0.36	0.48	0.25	0.43	0.00
Made a decision about how to treat an illness because of online health information	0.34	0.48	0.26	0.44	0.00
Visited a doctor because of information found online	0.16	0.37	0.13	0.34	0.07
Predictor Variables: Health					
Excellent or very good health	0.58	0.49	0.52	0.50	0.07
Health problems index	3.95	2.45	3.80	2.41	0.48
Predictor Variables: Online Proficiency					
Broadband Internet access	0.43	0.50	0.29	0.45	0.00
Online more than 10 hrs week	0.28	0.45	0.23	0.42	0.00
Online every day	0.57	0.50	0.51	0.50	0.08
Online activities index	2.86	0.97	2.45	1.14	0.00
Predictor Variables: Online Health Information					
Most of the time and always look to see who provides medical information on Internet	0.40	0.49	0.24	0.43	0.00
Access health information online once or twice a month or greater	0.38	0.49	0.34	0.48	0.04
Doctor recommended a health or medical Website	0.06	0.23	0.04	0.20	0.13
Communicated with doctor or other health care provider through email	0.12	0.32	0.11	0.31	0.55
Positive feelings about looking for health information on the Internet Index	2.59	0.73	2.23	0.94	0.00
Negative feelings about looking for health information on the Internet	0.68	0.78	0.71	0.81	0.25

Notes: The number of observations are 464 for boomers and 164 for seniors.

Referring back to Hypothesis 1 on whether online health information has been used to manage a boomer or senior's health, this study has found that overall there were differences between both groups of online health seekers (Table 4). The mean values for all five dependent variables were higher for boomers compared with seniors. In addition, 3 out of the 5 dependent variables showed statistically significant differences between boomers and seniors at the 0.01 level. With these dependent variables outlined, this research should also describe the predictor variables and their characteristics.

Predictor Variables

The predictor variables used to explain how the Internet has managed the healthcare of boomers and seniors are also presented in Table 4. Many of the predictor variables are represented in terms of binary numbers to capture the specific impacts on the dependent variables. As previously noted, this study has divided the hypotheses into the differences between boomers and seniors, the relative health of the individual, his or her online proficiency, and how active he or she is at seeking online health information. This study discerns the impact that these factors have on the management of the healthcare of boomers and seniors.

To see all of the predictor variables refer to Table 4. We will only mention a few of them in this section. For instance, an index was created of the health problems that boomers and seniors have faced in the past year or someone they know has faced. An individual who has more health problems or is concerned with someone else's health problems would score higher on the index. The health problems index indicates less than four issues, that they faced and/or someone they know faced, were indicated by online health seekers (out of nine possible health problems). The nine possible health problems listed were cancer, heart disease, obesity and weight loss, arthritis, diabetes, Alzheimer's, high cholesterol, osteoporosis, and mental health issues.

The online activities index measures the amount of activities that boomers and seniors conduct online, and the average is around two activities (Table 4). The prediction is that health seekers who conduct more online activities have a greater likelihood of using health information to manage their health because of their familiarity and comfort with the Internet. The four online activities that comprised the index were instant messaging, reading news, buying a product, and checking the weather.

The online health information predictor variables also show the capacity of the individual to look up health information on the Internet (Table 4). Seniors are more trusting of the health information that they read online, with only 24% of seniors "most of the time" and "always" looking to see who provides medical information on the Internet. On the other hand, 40% of boomers are looking to see who provides the online health information. This difference was also statistically significant at the 0.01 level. In addition, boomers are more frequent consumers of online health information using it at least once or twice a month as represented by 38% of the sample. Seniors consume online health information marginally less frequently with 34% doing so.

With regards to overall positive feelings towards the Internet there was an average score of 2, on an index scaled from 0 to 3, indicating that boomers and seniors have overall positive feelings towards the Internet as a source of health information. The index was calculated by adding up the specific responses whether the online health seeker agreed that online health information gave them information quickly, it helped them feel more informed when they go to the doctor, and allows them to get information from a lot of different sources.

On an index of 0 being the lowest and 2 being the highest, less than 1 was found indicating very few online health seekers harbor negative feelings towards the Internet as a source of health information. Having positive feelings about online health information also showed a statistically significant difference between boomers and seniors at the 0.01 significance level. Similarly, this negative feelings index was calculated by adding the individual responses if they agreed that online health information was frustrating because it is hard to find what they were searching for and it is confusing because there is too much information. The following section tests the relationship between accessing online health information and managing a boomers and seniors health.

Results of Logistic Regression Models of Online Health Information Managing Health

This study uses logistic regression with five separate management of health dependent variables. A "1" was recorded for each of the five dependent variables if: (1) the online health seeker said "somewhat" or "a lot" of information on the Internet helped them take care of their health; (2) they had a conversation with family or friend about online health information; (3) online health information changed their behavior; (4) they made a decision about how to treat an illness because of online health information; and (5) they visited a doctor because of information found online. A "0" was recorded for each of the five dependent variables if this was not the case.

The results in Table 5 indicate that for four of the five dependent variables, boomers were slightly more likely to use the Internet to manage their health. For instance, an odds ratio of 1.31 for the dependent variable of "somewhat" or "a lot" of information on the Internet has helped to take care of the online health seekers' problem

Table 5. Logistic regression of factors predicting whether online health informatino has managed a boomer's or senior's health

Dependent Variables	Somewhat and a lot of information on Internet helped take care health		Had a conversation family or friend about online health information		Online health information changed behavior		Made a decision about how to treat an illness because of online health information		Visited a doctor because of information found online	
Independent Variables	Odds Ratio	Wald Statistic	Odds Ratio	Wald Statistic	Odds Ratio	Wald Statistic	Odds Ratio	Wald Statistic	Odds Ratio	Wald Statistic
Boomers = 1 (age between 50 to 64)	1.31	(4.49)**	1.49	(10.67)***	1.71	(14.99)***	1.66	(12.63)***	0.90	(0.36)
Health										
Excellent or very good health	1.11	(0.88)	1.64	(21.39)***	1.21	(3.06)	1.36	(7.09)***	1.10	(0.41)
Health problems index	0.99	(0.36)	1.14	(34.51)***	1.04	(3.40)	1.00	(0.00)	1.04	(1.35)
Online Proficiency										
Broadband Internet access	0.82	(2.79)	0.63	(15.51)***	0.90	(0.80)	0.68	(9.37)***	0.89	(0.51)
Online every day	1.55	(13.13)***	1.31	(5.01)**	1.82	(22.22)***	1.43	(7.15)***	1.41	(3.99)**
Online more than 10 hrs week	0.65	(9.62)***	0.89	(0.71)	0.97	(0.05)	1.46	(7.26)***	0.81	(1.39)
Online activities index	1.01	(0.01)	0.93	(1.50)	0.95	(0.55)	0.92	(1.83)	0.80	(7.75)***
Online Health Information										
Access health information online once or twice a month or greater	3.51	(115.95)***	1.59	(17.35)***	2.29	(54.99)***	3.11	(95.83)***	1.82	(16.15)***
Communicated with doctor or other healthcare provider through e-mail	0.91	(0.28)	1.95	(12.45)***	1.58	(7.28)***	2.83	(35.37)***	1.86	(9.94)***
Doctor recommended a health or medical Web site	0.76	(0.97)	0.91	(0.10)	1.17	(0.31)	2.13	(7.10)***	3.68	(22.13)***
Positive feelings about looking for health information on the Internet Index	2.46	(119.44)***	1.63	(46.32)***	1.85	(42.97)***	1.70	(31.68)***	1.84	(19.73)***
Most of the time and always look to see who provides medical information on Internet	1.31	(4.86)**	2.80	(63.13)***	1.61	(15.80)***	1.57	(13.23)***	1.69	(11.21)***
Negative feelings about looking for health information on the Internet	0.75	(16.82)***	0.81	(10.16)***	0.71	(21.06)***	0.70	(20.83)***	0.77	(6.21)***
Constant	0.08	(89.93)***	0.13	(65.14)***	0.03	(122.43)***	0.04	(103.03)***	0.03	(66.25)***
Nagelkerke R-Square	0.27		0.22		0.22		0.26		0.13	

*Notes: ** significcant at the 0.05 level and *** significcant at the 0.01 level.*

implies that consumers are around 1⅓ times more likely to say this is the case if they are a boomer rather than a senior.

Changing behavior for boomers because of information found online registered an odds ratio of 1.71, having a conversation with family or friend about online health information had an odds ratio of 1.49, and making a decision about how to treat an illness had an odds ratio of 1.66 (Table 5). Overall, the results showed that boomers are around 1 1/2 more likely than seniors to change their behavior and use online health information to manage their health, which is not that high given the attention placed on the differences between these age groups (Kaiser Family Foundation, 2005).

In terms of online proficiency, those who had broadband Internet access were less likely to have a conversation with a family member or friend about what they saw online and less likely to make a decision about how to treat an illness. However, for those online health seekers who are online every day this had a consistent impact, across all five dependent variables, if they used online health information to manage their health. For instance, there was a 1.82 times greater chance that daily online users changed their behavior because of online health information. In addition, individuals who go online everyday are 1.41 times more likely to visit a doctor because of information that they found online. In terms of being online more than 10 hours a week, this had a negative likelihood for the dependent variables "somewhat" or "a lot" of information on the Internet helped to take care of their health, but had a positive impact with an odds ratio of 1.46 for making a decision on how to treat an illness. Overall, there was no overwhelming support that being more proficient with the Internet had a substantial impact on using health information to manage an online health seeker's health. The only consistently significant variable that had an impact on managing health was being online everyday.

Boomers and seniors who had excellent or very good health were 1.64 times more likely to have a conversation with a family member or friend about online health information. In addition, the boomer or senior who had more health problems or knows someone who was experiencing health problems was 1.14 times more likely to have a conversation with family or friend about online health information. Individuals who are in excellent and very good health were 1.36 times more likely to use online health information to make a decision about how to treat an illness because of online health information. Generally, the health of the individual was not a strong predictor of using health information to manage a boomers or seniors health.

The strongest predictors of using health information to management health were for the online health information awareness and feelings variables. Frequent consumers of online health information were 3.51 times more likely to use the Internet to take care of their health. It has become a valuable tool for their healthcare management needs. There was also a 3.11 greater likelihood of someone making a decision about treating an illness to use the Internet more than once a month for health information.

In fact, frequently accessing health information registered an impact for all of the dependent variables.

Individuals who had positive feelings about online health information were more likely to use online health information to manage their health. Boomers and seniors who had more negative feelings towards online health information were less likely to use it for health management. This finding was consistently found across all five of the dependent variables. Online health seekers who usually looked to see who provided the health information were more likely to use this to manage their health. For instance, individuals who looked to see who provided the health information were 2.80 times more likely to have a conversation with family or friends about the information that they saw online. If a doctor recommended a health or medical Web site, online health seekers were 2.13 times more likely to make a decision about how to treat an illness because of online health information, and they were 3.68 times more likely to visit a doctor because of information they found online. In addition, individuals who communicated with a doctor or healthcare provider via e-mail were 1.95 times more likely to have a conversation about health information they found online with a family member or friend. Overall, the logistic regression results indicate the most consistent and highest support for increased awareness and positive feelings towards online health information as a driver for helping to manage boomers and seniors' health.

Discussion of Results and Hypotheses

This section will discuss how the empirical results of this study confirm or deny the hypotheses (see Table 6). First, the evidence shows, through the difference of means tests, that boomers and seniors are different in terms of their use of online health information in the management of their health. The mean values scored higher for boomers in using online health information to take care of their health, having a conversation with a family or friend about the health information found online, changing their behavior because of online health information, and making a decision about treating an illness because of online health information. There is some evidence that boomers will use more online health information to manage their health, supporting Hypothesis 1. However, there is no overwhelming support for differences between boomers and seniors and using health information to manage their health, with boomers only utilizing this information one and a half times more than seniors.

The health of the individual or Hypotheses 2 only predicted the use of online health information to manage a boomers' and seniors' health when they had a conversation with a family member or friend about online health information and making

Table 6. Support for hypothesis of boomers and seniors and online health informa-tion

Hypotheses	Supported? (Yes, No, or Partially)	Major Test(s) Performed
Hypothesis 1: Online health seekers who are baby boomers are more likely to believe that online health information has helped them manage their health better compared with seniors.	Yes	Descriptive statistics, difference of means tests, and logistic regression
Hypothesis 2: Online health seekers who are healthy or who have family and friends that are healthy will rely less on online health information because of lack of need.	Partially	Logistic regression
Hypothesis 3: Online health seekers who have broadband Internet access will go online more for health information to manage their health	No	Logistic regression - Evidence found in the opposite direction
Hypothesis 4: Online health seekers who go online more often and conduct many online activities will use Internet health information more to manage their health.	Yes	Logistic regression
Hypothesis 5: Boomers and seniors who are females will rely more on online health information.	Yes	Logistic regression
Hypothesis 6: Boomers and seniors who are college educated will rely more on online health information.	Yes	Logistic regression
Hypothesis 7: Boomers and seniors who are Hispanics will go online less for health information.	No	Logistic regression -No support found in logistic regression
Hypothesis 8: Boomers and seniors who have family income above $75,000 will go online more for health information.	Yes	Logistic regression
Hypothesis 9: Online health seekers who most of the time and always look to see who provides medical information on the Internet would use online health information more to manage their health.	Yes	Logistic regression
Hypothesis 10: Online health seekers who access health information online once or twice a month would have a greater likelihood of using online health information to manage their health.	Yes	Logistic regression
Hypothesis 11: If a doctor has recommended a Web site to an online health seeker, he or she is more likely to use health information to manage their health.	Partially	Logistic regression
Hypothesis 12: If an online health seeker has communicated with his or her doctor via e-mail, he or she is more likely to use online health information to manage their health.	Yes	Logistic regression
Hypothesis 13: Online health seekers that have more positive feelings about looking for health information on the Internet are more likely to use this information to manage their health.	Yes	Logistic regression

a decision about how to treat an illness. In addition, the health variable predicted boomer's and senior's behavior when he or she talked to his or her doctor about information they found online. Overall, there was no overwhelming support that the health of the boomer or senior had an impact on use of online health information to manage their health.

Hypotheses 3 and 4 examine whether being more proficient online means that the online health seeker would use the Internet more to manage his or her health. The results consistently showed that those who go online everyday were more likely to use the Internet to manage their health. There was not much support that being more proficient with the Internet meant that boomers and seniors would use it more often for health information, since many of the other independent variables in this category were not statistically significant. This is most likely explained by what these online health seekers are doing on the Internet; they are looking for information, which does not require, for instance, broadband Internet access since a standard dial-up connection will suffice. Therefore, this research cannot confirm that being more proficient with the Internet means that online health seekers would use this communication media to manage their health more than those that are not as proficient. However, this could change with greater availability of streaming video health information, which is much more suited to a broadband Internet connection.

Boomers and seniors of higher sociodemographic status use the Internet for health information much more than lower sociodemographic status individuals (Hypotheses 5-8). Therefore, this research confirms that there is a digital divide in access to online health information and public policy should attempt to address this issue. It should be noted that one-third of the United States adult population have not gone online and, therefore, would not be able to benefit from online health information (Pew Internet & American Life, 2005).

Hypothesis 10 was confirmed in the logistic regression results that those who are frequent patrons of online health information would actually use it more often to manage their health. The results showed that health seekers who are accessing health information online once or twice a month or greater would be more likely to actually use this information to manage their health. Therefore, these individuals are not just searching for information; they are actually using some of what they find online. Individuals who have positive feelings about online health information would also use it more often to manage their health, and individuals that harbor more negative feelings would use it less often (Hypothesis 13). Online health seekers who are very aware of who provides the medical information on the Internet are more likely to use this information to manage their health (Hypothesis 9). Finally, where there is communication with their doctor via e-mail or at the doctor's office about online health information, boomers and seniors are more likely to use online health information to manage their health (Hypothesis 12). Awareness and feelings towards online health information were generally well-supported predictor variables

(Hypotheses 9-13), having an impact on a boomer's or senior's use of this information to manage their healthcare needs.

Recommendations, Limitations, and Future Research

This chapter examined the use of the Internet for accessing health information by boomers (age 50 to 64) and seniors (age 65 and over). Boomers generally use Internet health information to manage their health more than seniors. However, there were no overwhelming differences between boomers and seniors, which is the main difference in findings from another study (Kaiser Family Foundation, 2005). For instance, boomers are much more likely to talk to a doctor about health information they saw online. Boomers are around 1 ½ more likely than seniors to use online health information to manage their health. This study found that awareness and feelings towards online health information provided the best explanation of health information for management of boomers' and seniors' health.

Since boomers were marginally found to use online health information more than seniors, what are the implications of this observation? Will seniors of tomorrow be similar to seniors of today? Perhaps boomers will continue to seek online health information as they get older. The implication that boomers and seniors may be in greatest need of health information may not be true in the future with the growing obesity epidemic in the United States which affects all age groups.

Some policy recommendations should be noted to bring more seniors online and to enhance the quality of Internet health resources. Healthcare professionals should recommend Web sites, promote more effective search and evaluation techniques, and be more involved in developing and promoting uniform standards for health Web sites (Morahan-Martin, 2004). Since only a minority of seniors have ever gone online, this represents a significant digital divide. These findings confirm that for the foreseeable future, the Internet is less likely to be a primary source of information for most seniors suggesting a need to invest more heavily in education and outreach strategies. This is especially the case for seniors with low or modest income, who are least likely to go online for this information. These recommendations could make seniors more aware and create a positive experience when going online for health information.

In the near future, the Internet will become a decision-making tool for seniors who will need to make choices about the Medicare prescription drug benefits. They will need to decide which plan has the most attractive premium and determine whether it will cover the medications they take and work with the pharmacy they use. Seniors will also need to manage the Internet to make these important decisions. Web site design is part of the solution since seniors have problems scrolling on Web sites and remembering Web pages (Voelker, 2005).

There are some limitations of this research. With any type of public opinion data, especially when asking subjective questions about sensitive topics of consumers' health, respondents may not be as forthcoming with information. Another limitation is that of the general applicability of the results given the proportion of the sample is different for seniors and boomers. In addition, there was no question that specifically addressed whether there was an improvement in the health outcome, just that people felt better informed. Future research could do a longitudinal follow-up of this dataset which, might reveal shifts in the use of Internet health information for managing health with boomers and seniors looking at other measures to see if there is an impact on change in the person's health.

References

Alpay, L., Overberg, R., & Zwetsloot-Schonk, B. (2007). Empowering citizens in assessing health-related Web sites: A driving factor for healthcare governance. *International Journal of Healthcare Technology and Management, 8*(1-2), 141-160.

Anderson, J. (2004). Consumers of e-Health: Patterns of use and barriers. *Social Science Computer Review, 22*(2), 242-248.

Brodie, M., Flournoy, R., Altman, D., Blendon, R., Benson, J., & Rosenbaum, M. (2000). Health information, the Internet, and the digital divide. *Health Affairs, 19*(6), 255-265.

Cotton, S., & Gupta, S. (2004). Characteristics of online and off-line health information seekers and factors that discriminate between them. *Social Science & Medicine, 59*(9), 1795-1806.

Eysenbach, G. (2003). The impact of the Internet on cancer outcomes. *CA A Cancer Journal for Clinicians, 53*(6), 356-371.

Eysenbach, G., & Jadad, A. (2001). Evidence-based patient choice and consumer health informatics in the Internet age. *Journal of Medical Internet Research, 3*(2), e35.

Fox, S. (2006*). Online health search 2006*. Washington, D.C.: Pew Internet & American Life.

Fox, S., & Rainie, L. (2000). *The online healthcare revolution: How the Web helps Americans take better care of themselves*. Washington, D.C.: Pew Internet & American Life.

Fox, S., & Rainie, L. (2002). *Vital decisions: How Internet users decide what information to trust when they or their loved ones are sick.* Washington, D.C.: Pew Internet & American Life.

Gray, N., Klein, J., Noyce, P., Sesselberg, T., & Cantrill, J. (2005). Health information-seeking behavior in adolescence: The place of the Internet. *Social Science & Medicine, 60*(7), 1467-1478.

Huntington, P., Nicholas, D., Homewood, J., Polydoratou, P., Gunter, B., Russell, C., et al. (2004). The general public's use of (and attitudes towards) interactive, personal digital health information and advisory services. *Journal of Documentation, 60*(3), 245-265.

Kaiser Family Foundation. (2005). *E-health and the elderly: How seniors use the Internet for health information.* Washington, D.C.: Kaiser Family Foundation.

Lueg, J., Moore, R., & Warkentin, M. (2003). Patient health information search: An explanatory model of Web-based search behavior. *Journal of End User Computing, 15*(4), 49-61.

Morahah-Martin, J. (2004). How Internet users find, evaluate, and use online health information: A cross-cultural review. *CyberPsychology & Behavior, 7*(5), 497-510.

Nicholas, D., Huntington, P., Williams, P., & Blackburn, P. (2001). Digital health information provision and health outcomes. *Journal of Information Science, 27*(4), 265-276.

Nicholas, D., Huntington, P., Jamali, H., & Dobrowolski, T. (2006). Characterising and evaluating information seeking behaviour in a digital environment: Spotlight on the 'bouncer'. *Information Processing and Management, 43*(4), 1085-1102.

Pandey, S., Hart, J., & Tiwary, S. (2003). Women's health and the Internet: Understanding emerging trends and implications. *Social Science & Medicine, 56*(1), 179-191.

Pew Internet & American Life. (2005). *January 2005 Internet Tracking Survey.* Retrieved May, 10, 2005 from www.pewInternet.org.

Rideout, V. (2002). Generation Rx.com: What are young people really doing online?. *Marketing Health Services, 22*(1), 27-30.

Skinner, H., Biscope, S., & Poland, B. (2003). Quality of Internet access: Barrier behind Internet use statistics. *Social Science & Medicine, 57*(5), 875-880.

Voelker, R. (2005). Seniors seeking health information need help crossing the "digital divide". *JAMA, 293*(11), 1310-1312.

Ziebland, S. (2004). The importance of being expert: The quest for cancer information on the Internet. *Social Science & Medicine, 59*(9), 1783-1793.

Endnotes

[1]   In this study, for simplicity baby boomers are classified as those individuals between the ages of 50 to 64 and seniors are classified as 65 and older.

[2]   This author would like to thank Victoria Rideout, M.A., vice president and director, Program for the Study of Entertainment Media and Health, Kaiser Family Foundation (KFF) for the dataset and documentation used in the statistical analysis of this study.

[3]   For the data analysis the software package used was SPSS version 13.0.

Chapter V

Data Mining Medical Information:
Should Artificial Neural Networks be Used to Analyze Trauma Audit Data

Thomas Chesney, Nottingham
University Business School, UK

David Chesney, Freeman Hospital,
UK

Kay Penny, Napier University, UK

Nicola Maffulli, Keele University of
Medicine, UK

Peter Oakley, The University
Hospital of North Staffordshire, UK

John Templeton, Keele University
of Medicine, UK

Simon Davies, University of
Birmingham Research Park, UK

Abstract

Trauma audit is intended to develop effective care for injured patients through process and outcome analysis, and dissemination of results. The system records injury details such as the patient's sex and age, the mechanism of the injury, various

*measures of the severity of the injury, initial management and subsequent manage-
ment interventions, and the outcome of the treatment including whether the patient
lived or died. Ten years' worth of trauma audit data from one hospital are modelled
as an Artificial Neural Network (ANN) in order to compare the results with a more
traditional logistic regression analysis. The output was set to be the probability that
a patient will die. The ANN models and the logistic regression model achieve roughly
the same predictive accuracy, although the ANNs are more difficult to interpret
than the logistic regression model, and neither logistic regression nor the ANNs
are particularly good at predicting death. For these reasons, ANNs are not seen as
an appropriate tool to analyse trauma audit data. Results do suggest, however, the
usefulness of using both traditional and non-traditional analysis techniques together
and of including as many factors in the analysis as possible.*

Introduction

An artificial neural network (ANN) attempts to model human intelligence using
the neurons in a human brain as an analogy. ANNs have been described numerous
times (Lee & Park, 2001; Bose & Mahapatra, 2001; Setiono, Thong, & Yap, 1998;
Lee, Hung Cheng, & Balakrishnan, 1998), but a brief description is that the network
accepts a series of factors as input, which it processes to output a probability that the
input belongs to a certain class. For example, in the case of the trauma data analysed
in this study, the characteristics of the trauma are the input to the ANN, which then
outputs the probability that the patient will die. The processing is done by layers of
neurons (called hidden layers) which apply a weight to each input factor according to
how important that factor is in calculating the classification probability. The weight
is learned by the network during its training. In training, a series of input factors to
which the correct classification is known is fed into the ANN. The ANN then adjusts
its weights to minimise the error between its predicted classification and the known
correct class. A pictorial representation of an ANN is shown in Figure 1.

An ANN has the potential to discriminate accurately between patients who will live
and those who will die, and can capture complex relationships between factors that
traditional analysis methods may miss. However, there are two potential problems
with using ANNs to analyse trauma data. First, they are affected by imbalances
in the data (Fu, Wang, Chua, & Chu, 2002). A common characteristic of medical
data is its imbalance (Cios & Moore, 2002). What this means is that the attribute
of interest to data miners is likely to be present only in a minority of records in the
dataset. In the case of the trauma data discussed here, a much higher percentage of
patients lived than died. The second disadvantage with neural networks is that it is

Figure 1. Example neural network topology and output equations

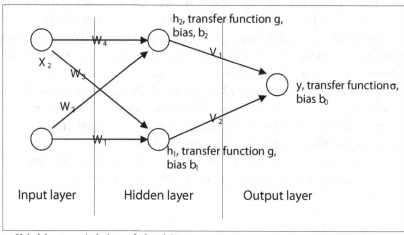

Output of h1, h1out = g(w1x1 + w3x2 + b1)

Output of h2, h2out = g(w2x1 + w4x2 + b2)

Output of node y, the output layer which uses the sigmoid function and is the probability of a certain class, for instance DEATH = 1, given the input vector ,

p(DEATH = 1 |) = s(v1(h1out) + v2(h2out) + b0)

very difficult to explain and to justify the model. In other words, after training, it is difficult to explain why one neuron is weighted in a particular way. The ANN often does not have an underlying probabilistic model (Giudici, 2003), and evaluation of the model usually is done by examining its output — its predictive accuracy. In mining medical data, consideration is also usually given to the model's sensitivity and specificity and less frequently to the model's positive and negative predictive value.

Despite this, ANNs frequently have been used in healthcare. For example, Lee and Park (2001) applied neural networks in order to classify and predict the symptomatic status of HIV/AIDS patients; Baxt, Shofer, Sites, and Hollander (2002) used an ANN to aid in the diagnosis of acute myocardial infarction; Lapuerta, Azen, and LaBree (1995) used neural networks to predict the risk of coronary artery disease. DiRusso, Sullivan, Holly, Nealon Cuff, and Savino (2000) used ANNs to predict survival in trauma patients that was similar to the application in the current study. ANNs are just one of a number of techniques that are known collectively as machine learning. Others long have been used in medical applications to improve decision making (Konomenko & Kular, 1995). Lavrac (1999) lists some applications: diagnosis and prognosis in oncology (Bratko & Konomenko, 1987), liver pathology (Lesmo, Saitta, & Torasso, 1982), neuropsychology (Muggleton, 1990) and gynecology

(Nunez, 1990). Breault, Goodall, & Foss (2002) used a decision tree to examine a diabetic data warehouse. Imberman, Damask, and Thompson (2002) identified association rules in a head trauma dataset. The aim of this chapter is to examine how analysing trauma data with an ANN compares with a more traditional logistic regression analysis.

Trauma Audit and Research Network

In 1991, in response to a report from the Royal College of Surgeons of England, the government supported a pilot system for treating trauma patients at the North Staffordshire Hospital (NSH) in Stoke-on-Trent in the UK (Oakley, MacKenzie, Temppleton, Cook, & Kirby, 2004). At the same time, a system for collecting trauma data from a set of core hospitals in England and Wales was established at the University of Manchester. This project, the Major Trauma Outcome Study (UK), grew in size with more hospitals becoming involved. By the late 1990s, one-half of all trauma-receiving hospitals in England and Wales returned data to the now renamed Trauma Audit & Research Network (TARN). NSH served as a core hospital and has contributed trauma audit data to TARN since that time.

Trauma is the most common cause of death in those under 40, and many of these are preventable (TARN, 2004). Trauma audit is intended to develop effective care for injured patients through process and outcome analysis and through dissemination of results. The system records injury details, such as the patient's sex and age, the mechanism of the injury, various measures of the severity of the injury, initial management and subsequent management interventions, and the outcome of the treatment, including whether the patient lived or died. Several analyses that used traditional statistical techniques have been performed on the data and published (Oakley et al., 2004; Templeton et al., 2000). Oakley et al. (2004) analysed six years of NSH trauma audit data from April 1992 through March 1998 in order to identify factors related to mortality and to examine whether there was a longitudinal trend in mortality. Multiple logistic regression analysis evidenced eight factors as determinants of mortality. In order of importance, these were age, head abbreviated injury score (AIS), chest AIS, abdominal AIS, calendar year of admission, external injury AIS, mechanism of injury, and primary receiving hospital. However, the data from NSH never have been modelled as an ANN.

This chapter continues as follows. The next section describes the method of preparing and analysing the data by ANN and logistic regression. The results are then presented, compared, and discussed.

Method

The study concerned trauma audit data from patients treated at the North Staffordshire Hospital from 1993 to 1999 and from 2001 to 2004 (the gap was due to a lack of resources during this period, which affected data collection). The data were limited to those most severely injured patients, since there should be most to learn from such patients. Patients with an injury severity score (ISS) greater than 15 were included. All the injury scores (Abbreviated Injury Scores, ISS, and Glasgow Coma Scores) were assigned, checked, and entered into the database by trauma audit staff under the guidance of three clinicians (three of the authors) as soon as possible after the injury. All were well-trained in the use of the scoring systems. (For an explanation of all of these scoring techniques, see Baker [1974] and Teasdale and Jennett [1974]) Very little data were missing, as the summary in Table 1 shows.

The criteria for inclusion just described left 1,658 records in the data set with which to train and test different ANN models. The factors shown in Table 1 were included as input, with the output being whether the patient lived or died. If the data are well-balanced with approximately equal numbers of patients who lived and died, learning algorithms will have a better chance of finding patterns that distinguish the two groups. As has been explained already, the trauma audit data are very imbalanced — 79% of patients lived, 21% died. Machine learning techniques usually are biased toward the majority class, as these dominate during training (Fu et al., 2002). For example, a classifier could achieve 79% accuracy with this data by always predicting "live." A number of techniques has been examined to deal with this (Guo & Viktor, 2004): undersampling the majority class (Kubat & Matwin, 1997), oversampling the minority class (Ling & Lee, 1998), doing both together (Chawla, Bowyer, Hall, & Kegelmeyer, 2002), and boosting the learning algorithm (Schapire, 2001). The data were balanced by adjusting the proportion of the patients who died by a factor of 3.685. However, it has been suggested that record balancing has no impact on neural network models (Fu et al., 2002).

The data mining package SPSS Clementine 7.0 was used to create the ANNs. This software allows the user to specify any ANN model (the model consists of the number of hidden layers of neurons and the number of neurons in each hidden layer), and the learning rates (alpha and eta, which specify how the weights change during training). All the neurons are fully connected and each is a feed-forward, multi-layer perceptron that uses the sigmoid transfer function (Watkins, 1997). The learning technique used is back propagation. This means that, starting with the given topology, the network is trained, then a sensitivity analysis is performed on the hidden units, and the weakest are removed (Watkins, 1997). This training/removing is repeated for a set length of time. A k-fold cross-validation technique was used to test the ANN models, with k set to five. This is good practice when building neural networks with medical data (Cunningham, Carney, & Jacob, 2000). Using

Table 1. NSH trauma audit data (note that high AIS relates to an increase in severity, whereas high GCS relates to a decrease in severity)

Input factors	Percentage complete	Count (Percentage)
Sex	Male	100	1244 (75)
	Female		414 (25)
Type of injury	Blunt	99.94	1608 (97)
	Penetrating		50 (3)
Referred from another hospital (yes or no)		100	464 (28) referred
Mechanism group		100	Motor vehicle crash	829 (50)
			Fall greater than 2m	249 (15)
			Fall less than 2m	282 (17)
			Assault	50 (3)
			Other	249 (15)
Age group		99.94	0-15 years	149 (9)
			16-25 years	381 (23)
			26-35 years	265 (16)
			36-50 years	315 (19)
			51-70 years	332 (20)
			71 years and over	216 (13)
Year of admission		100	1992	83 (5)
			1993	166 (10)
			1994	83 (5)
			1995	166 (10)
			1996	216 (13)
			1997	166 (10)
			1998	66 (4)
			2001	166 (10)
			2002	182 (11)
			2003	232 (14)
			2004	116 (7)
			2005	17 (1)

continued on following page

Table 1. continued

Month of admission	100							
		Jan	149 (9)					
		Feb	116 (7)					
		Mar	133 (8)					
		Apr	133 (8)					
		May	166 (10)					
		Jun	133 (8)					
		Jul	149 (9)					
		Aug	133 (8)					
		Sept	116 (7)					
		Oct	149 (9)					
		Nov	133 (8)					
		Dec	149 (9)					
Day of admission	100	Sun	249 (15)					
		Mon	216 (13)					
		Tues	232 (14)					
		Wed	199 (12)					
		Thurs	264 (16)					
		Fri	249 (15)					
		Sat	249 (15)					
Time of admission group	100	0:00-3:00	431 (26)					
		4:00-7:00	50 (3)					
		8:00-11:00	116 (7)					
		12:00-15:00	481 (29)					
		16:00-19:00	265 (16)					
		20:00-23:00	348 (21)					

AIS Score		0	1	2	3	4	5	6
AIS Head	100	348 (21)	50 (3)	99 (6)	199 (12)	415 (25)	564 (34)	0 (0)
AIS Face	100	1111 (67)	265 (16)	232 (14)	66 (4)	0 (0)	0 (0)	0 (0)
AIS Neck	100	1625 (98)	17 (1)	0 (0)	0 (0)	0 (0)	0 (0)	0 (0)
AIS Chest	100	1011 (61)	50 (3)	50 (3)	249 (15)	216 (13)	83 (5)	0 (0)
AIS Abdomen	100	1376 (83)	50 (3)	83 (5)	83 (5)	50 (3)	17 (1)	0 (0)
AIS Spine	100	1310 (79)	0 (0)	166 (10)	116 (7)	33 (2)	17 (1)	0 (0)
AIS Upper limbs	100	1127 (68)	83 (5)	282 (17)	166 (10)	0 (0)	0 (0)	0 (0)

continued on following page

Table 1. continued

	%	V1	V2	V3	V4	V5	V6	V7
AIS Lower limbs	100	1111 (67)	66 (4)	116 (7)	282 (17)	66 (4)	0 (0)	0 (0)
AIS External	100	1227 (74)	381 (23)	17 (1)	0 (0)	17 (1)	17 (1)	0 (0)
AIS CSpine	100	1509 (91)	0 (0)	66 (4)	50 (3)	17 (1)	0 (0)	0 (0)
AIS TSpine	100	1509 (91)	0 (0)	83 (5)	33 (2)	17 (1)	17 (1)	0 (0)
AIS LSpine	100	1525 (92)	83 (5)	33 (2)	17 (1)	0 (0)	0 (0)	0 (0)
Glasgow Coma Score		1	2	3	4	5	6	
GCS Eye	88.24	483 (33)	102 (7)	132 (9)	746 (51)	N/A		
GCS Verbal	88.24	395 (27)	205 (14)	59 (4)	205 (14)	600 (41)	N/A	N/A
GCS Motor	88.24	219 (15)	73 (5)	73 (5)	102 (7)	263 (18)	732 (50)	
Outcomes								
Alive or dead	98.97	344 (21) dead, 1296(79) alive						

this technique, the data were split into five groups. When splitting the dataset, those patients who lived were selected randomly and independently of those patients who died in order to keep the same proportion of live/die outcomes in each set. Four of the sets were used to train each ANN model; the fifth was used to test it. This then was repeated another four times so that each group was used to test the model once. The overall performance of the model was then the average performance of the five tests. Four different ANN models were tested in this way. To decide which ANN models to test, a range of models was trained with a random sample of two-thirds of the data and tested on the remaining one-third. Again, the split was made to keep the same proportion of live/die outcomes in each set. These models differed on the number of hidden layers, neurons, and learning rates. The four best performing models were selected. Specific guidelines on how to choose these parameters were unavailable, as this was dependent upon the underlying data generating process (Berardi, Patuwo, & Hu, 2004), which is unknown, so experimentation like this is a reasonable approach.

The multiple logistic regression model was created using SPSS 11.0, and the factors shown in Table 1 were considered for inclusion. Such a model normally would not be tested using k-fold cross validation. In this case, the logistic regression model was created using the same random two-thirds of the data from before and tested on the remaining one-third.

In many data mining applications, the evaluation criterion is the percentage of correct classifications made by an algorithm. However, in medical data mining, consideration also must be given to the percentages of false positive and false negative classifications. The evaluation criteria for comparing the algorithms here are sensitivity, specificity, positive predictive value (PPV), and negative predictive value (NPV). The sensitivity is the proportion of actual deaths that were correctly predicted to die, whereas the specificity is the proportion of actual survivors who were correctly predicted to survive. The positive predictive value (PPV) is the probability that a subject for whom the model predicts as dying actually will be a true death, and the negative predictive value (NPV) is the probability that a subject predicted as surviving actually will survive.

Results

The number of hidden layers, the number of neurons in each layer, and the learning rates of the four ANN models are shown in Table 2. The results of the k-fold cross validations are shown in Table 3. Also shown in Table 3 are the results of the logistic regression analysis. The logistic regression model itself is shown in Table 4. This model shows that the mechanism group, age group, GCS-motor, Head AIS, Abdomen AIS, and External AIS all are associated independently with survival during a hospital stay. Those patients who have suffered a fall or assault have decreased odds of death compared to those involved in a motor vehicle crash. Those suffering a fall greater than two meters in height compared to those involved in a motor vehicle

Table 2. Model characteristics

	ANN1	ANN2	ANN3	ANN4
Number of hidden layers	2	1	3	3
Number of neurons in layer 1	30	30	30	30
Number of neurons in layer 2	20	N/A	20	20
Number of neurons in layer 3	N/A	N/A	10	10
Alpha	0.5	0.5	0.3	0.4
Initial eta	0.5	0.5	0.5	0.5
High eta	0.9	0.9	0.8	0.8
Low eta	0.01	0.01	0.05	0.05
Eta decay	30	30	20	20

Table 3. K-fold cross validation results (note that for the analysis, death was considered the positive outcome)

	ANN1	ANN2	ANN3	ANN4	LR
True positives	44	41	41	44	84
True negatives	219	219	221	219	286
False positives	38	38	37	39	86
False negatives	26	30	29	26	23
Sensitivity	63	57	58	62	79
Specificity	87	85	86	85	77
Predictive accuracy	80	79	80	80	77
Positive predictive value	54	53	53	55	49
Negative predictive value	89	88	88	89	92

crash have much decreased odds of death (odds ratio = 0.27; 95% confidence interval is 0.13 to 0.53). A less severe GCS motor score is associated with decreased odds of death compared to a more severe injury. Those suffering abdominal or external injuries have increased odds of death during a hospital stay. Correcting for the other factors included in the model, those with a head AIS of five or six have an odds ratio of 1.68 of death compared to those with a score of 0; however, those with head AIS scores of 1-4 appear to have decreased odds of death compared to those with a score of 0. Increasing age is associated with increased odds of death, especially for those over 70 years old. A cut-point of 0.2 was used in the logistic regression in order to increase the sensitivity (and thereby decrease the specificity).

All of the ANNs achieved roughly 80% overall predictive accuracy and slightly outperformed the logistic regression model in this respect, although this finding is examined more closely in the next section. There is no one agreed procedure for presenting ANN architectures with their weights, and in this case, it is not possible to show the four neural networks, since each was trained five times, and for each

Table 4. Logistic regression model (note that high AIS relates to a increase in sever-
ity, whereas high GCS relates to a decrease in severity, and odd ratios refer to odds
of death as opposed to survival)

Factor	No. of Patients	Odds Ratio (95% CI)	p-value
Mechanism			
Motor Vehicle Crash	497	1.00	0.004
Fall < 2m	145	0.68 (0.36 – 1.29)	0.234
Fall > 2m	159	0.27 (0.13 - 0.53)	0.000
Assault	33	0.34 (0.09 - 1.30)	0.115
Other	130	0.60 (0.31 - 1.15)	0.124
Age group			
0 - 15 years	89	1.00	<0.001
16 - 25 years	221	4.25 (1.45 – 12.50)	0.009
26 - 35 years	153	6.46 (2.09 - 20.00)	0.001
36 - 50 years	177	5.83 (1.90 – 17.86)	0.002
51 - 70 years	193	18.42 (6.06 - 56.02)	<0.001
71 years or over	131	87.27 (26.86 – 283.55)	<0.001
Arrival GCS - Motor			
1	151	1.00	<0.001
2	46	0.47 (0.21 – 1.02)	0.055
3	51	0.14 (0.06 – 0.32)	<0.001
4	70	0.07 (0.03 – 0.16)	<0.001
5	170	0.08 (0.04 – 0.15)	<0.001
6	476	0.03 (0.02 – 0.07)	<0.001
AIS – Head			
0	199	1.00	<0.001
1 – 2	84	0.31 (0.10 – 0.99)	0.048
3	116	0.28 (0.12 – 0.66)	0.004
4	247	0.38 (0.18 – 0.77)	0.008
5 – 6	318	1.68 (0.90 – 3.12)	0.101
AIS - Abdomen			
0	797	1.00	
1 – 5	167	2.31 (1.35 – 3.96)	0.002
AIS - External			
0	721	1.00	
1 – 6	243	1.85 (1.17 – 2.94)	0.009

Table 5. Factors important in each model

Order of importance	ANN1	ANN2	ANN3	ANN4
1	Abdomen AIS	Head AIS	Abdomen AIS	Abdomen AIS
2	Age group	Neck AIS	Chest AIS	Chest AIS
3	Chest AIS	Face AIS	Age group	External AIS
4	Arms AIS	Chest AIS	External AIS	Cervical spine AIS
5	External AIS	Abdomen AIS	Cervical spine AIS	Age group
6	Cervical spine AIS	Spine AIS	Arms AIS	Arms AIS
7	Mechanism group	Year of admission	Mechanism group	Motor GSC
8	Motor GSC	Month of admission	Referred from another hospital	Verbal GCS
9	Verbal GCS	Time of admission	Face AIS	Mechanism group
10	Referred from another hospital	Day of admission	Penetrating injury	Face AIS

training session, the final weights were different. However, in an attempt to illustrate the ANNs, Table 5 shows the 10 most important factors in each when trained with two-thirds of the data used to create the logistic regression model. Apart from ANN2, these appear very similar.

Discussion and Conclusion

Implications for Practice

Interpreting Table 5 is difficult. While three of the four ANN models show Abdomen AIS to be the most important factor in determining whether a patient lives or dies, it should be remembered that it is a network of factors that calculates the output, and Abdomen AIS can be used only to make a prediction in conjunction with all the other factors. As the following demonstrates, the ANN is not designed to analyse individual factors in the way that logistic regression can. Apart from ANN2, the models show reasonable agreement in the most important factors. ANN2, however, suggests that time, day, and month of admission are important determinants of death. This appears counter-intuitive, although when these factors are removed as inputs and then the ANNs are retrained, the predictive accuracy of each drops to around 73%. Clearly, therefore, these factors do have an impact on building the classifier. It is possible to suggest ideas about why this might be (staff will be affected by tiredness at difference times of the day, staff and patients may be affected by the seasons, and staff turnover may have an impact from year to year). It seems far-fetched to suggest that these have a real impact on mortality, and in fact, when chi-squared tests were performed to examine the relationship between these factors and death, no significant association was found. So, it is known that these factors have some influence, but it is not clear what that influence is. Perhaps there are complex cross-correlations between these factors and others that can be modelled by the ANN but not explained. Discussions on how to deal with peculiarities like this are scarce in the ANN literature. One way of trying to examine these cross-correlations is to list the meaningful factors with which day, month, and year could be correlated. In this instance, there do not appear to be any. This goes back to one of the two big disadvantages of using ANNs: it is not possible to show why a neuron is weighted in a certain way after training. Without this, the usefulness of ANNs is severely impaired, and, in the case of trauma audit data, illustrates the limitations of an ANN as an analysis tool.

While ANNs may not be suitable alone for analysing trauma audit data, they may have a place alongside more traditional techniques. The results demonstrate the value of recording as much data about the trauma as possible and including it in an exploratory analysis. An analysis by ANN may be valuable for identifying factors that previously have not or normally would not be identified as having an impact on outcomes, such as time of day, which was identified in this study by an ANN but not by logistic regression. These factors then can be investigated by traditional techniques in order to examine their impact.

The implication of this is that the goal of using ANNs in analysing trauma data can only ever be one of prediction. The ANN cannot be used to analyse the individual factors that are important in making this prediction. If the goal is to analyse these factors, then logistic regression is more suitable. If an ANN is used for survival prediction, this will have implications for treatment (e.g., if carers believe a patient will die, their care changes from one of treatment to one of making the patient's last moments as comfortable as possible). Such systems already exist and are currently in use. For instance APACHE is used to predict an intensive care patient's risk of dying, although its advocates claim that it is used only to help carers consider the issue of whether their treatment is making a difference (http://www.openclinical. org/aisp_apache.html, retrieved October 17, 2005) rather than deciding on what treatment to give.

Comparison with Logistic Regression

The ANN models appear to support the findings of Oakley et al. (2004) and the current logistic regression model about which factors have an impact on mortality, but they also demonstrate that outcomes are dependent on a complex interplay among a large number of factors and cannot be predicted easily or very accurately. While the ANN overall predictive accuracy is better than that of the logistic regression model, the logistic regression model is better at predicting death than all four ANN models; the sensitivity is 79% for the logistic model and ranges between 57% and 63% for the ANN models. Although the logistic regression model outperforms all the ANNs in sensitivity, it has a lower specificity (this is probably due to the cut-point being moved from the default of 0.5 to 0.2). The positive predictive value of the logistic regression model is slightly lower than the ANNs, showing that fewer than half of those predicted to die actually did die during their hospital stay. The results of analysing the trauma audit data show that the ANN is a relatively poor predictor of death and is of limited use in examining the determinants of death.

Concluding Remarks

The management of multiple-injured patients remains difficult with input from a number of surgical and medical specialities. Trauma scoring systems are a useful research tool, permitting comparison of multiple-injured patients in different centres around the world. Mortality remains a favoured outcome to study in trauma data mining, but others may be considered. Length of stay in hospital is one, although this really measures the process of care rather than anything specific about the injury. Disability as a result of the injury is another worthwhile outcome to study, but it is difficult to measure, especially when comparing different injury patterns. Future research should be directed at producing a scoring method to measure disability, similar to the AIS. Research to follow up patients after discharge from a hospital also would be useful in order to measure their outcome in terms of both continuing morbidity and quality of life. Trauma audit systems such as TARN take time to evolve; the data grow at a slower rate than some other medical databases, which means that improvements in patient care cannot be expected immediately. The University Hospital of North Staffordshire is starting to see a reduction in deaths; hopefully, studies such as the present one will help to continue this trend.

References

Baker, S. P. et al. (1974). The injury severity score: A method for describing patients with multiple injuries and evaluating emergency care. *J Trauma, 14*, 187-196. Retrieved January 18, 2005, from http://www.trauma.org/scores/iss.html

Baxt, W. G., Shofer, F. S., Sites, F. D., & Hollander, J. E. (2002). A neural computational aid to the diagnosis of acute myocardial infarction. *Annals of Emergency Medicine, 39*(4), 366-373.

Berardi, V. L., Patuwo, B. E., & Hu, M. Y. (2004). A principled approach for building and evaluating neural network classification models. *Decision Support Systems, 38*(2), 233-246.

Bose, I., & Mahapatra, R. K. (2001). Business data mining — A machine learning perspective. *Information & Management, 39*(3), 211-225.

Bratko, I., & Konomenko, I. (1987). Learning diagnostic rules from incomplete and noisy data. In B. Phelps (Ed.), *AI methods in statistics* (pp. 67-83). London: Gower Technical Press.

Breault, J. L., Goodall, C. R., & Fos, J. (2002). Data mining a diabetic data warehouse. *Artificial Intelligence in Medicine, 26*(1, 2), 37-54.

Chawla, N., Bowyer, K., Hall, L., & Kegelmeyer, W. (2002). SMOTE: Synthetic minority over-sampling technique. *Journal of Artificial Intelligence Research, 16*, 321-357.

Cios, K. J., & Moore, G. W. (2002). Uniqueness of medical data mining. *Artificial Intelligence in Medicine, 26*(1, 2), 1-24.

Cunningham, P., Carney, J., & Jacob, S. (2000). Stability problems with artificial neural networks and the ensemble solution. *Artificial Intelligence in Medicine, 20*(3), 217-225.

DiRusso, S., Sullivan, T., Holly, C., Nealon Cuff, S., & Savino, J. (2000). An artificial neural network as a model for prediction of survival in trauma patients: Validation for a regional trauma area. *The Journal of Trauma Injury, Infection and Care, 49*(2), 212-223.

Fu, X., Wang, L., Chua, K. S., & Chu, F. (2002). Training RBF neural networks on unbalanced data. In *Proceedings of the 9th International Conference on Neural Information Processing, Volume 2*. Retrieved from http://sci2s.ugr.es/keel/monografia/unbalanced/01198214.pdf

Giudici, P. (2003). *Applied data mining.* Chichester: Wiley.

Guo, H., & Viktor, H. L. (2004). Learning from imbalanced data sets with boosting and data generation: The DataBoost-IM approach. *ACM SIGKDD Explorations Newsletter Archive, 6*(1), 30-39.

Imberman, S. P., Damask, B., & Thompson, H. W. (2002). Using dependency/association rules to find indications for computed tomography in a trauma dataset. *Artificial Intelligence in Medicine, 26*(1, 2), 55-68.

Konomenko, I., & Kular, M. (1995). Machine learning for medical diagnosis. In *Proceedings of the CADAM-95* (pp. 9-30), Bled.

Kubat, M., & Matwin, S. (1997). Addressing the curse of imbalanced training sets: One sided selection. In *Proceedings of the 14th International Conference on Machine Learning*, San Francisco, CA (pp. 179-186).

Lapuerta, P., Azen, S. P., & LaBree, L. (1995). Use of neural networks in predicting the risk of coronary artery disease. *Computers and Biomedical Research, 28*(1), 38-52.

Lavrac, N. (1999). Selected techniques for data mining in medicine. *Artificial Intelligence in Medicine, 16*(1), 3-23.

Lee, A., Hung Cheng, C., & Balakrishnan, J. (1998). Software development cost estimation: Integrating neural network with cluster analysis. *Information & Management, 34*(1), 1-9.

Lee, C. W., & Park, J. (2001). Assessment of HIV/AIDS-related health performance using an artificial neural network. *Information & Management, 38*(4), 231-238.

Lesmo, L., Saitta, L., & Torasso, P. (1982). Learning of fuzzy production rules for medical diagnosis. In M. Gupta, & E. Sanchez (Eds.), *Approximate reasoning in decision analysis* (pp. 249-260). Amsterdam: Elsevier

Ling, C., & Li, C. (1998). Data mining for direct marketing: Problems and solutions. In *Proceedings of the ACM SIGKDD International Conference on Knowledge Discovery and Data Mining (KDD-98)* (pp. 73-79).

Muggleton, S. (1990). *Inductive acquisition of expert knowledge*. Wokingham: Addison-Wesley.

Nunez, M. (1990). Decision tree induction using domain knowledge. In B. Wielinga, J. Boose, B. Gaines, G. Schreiber, & M. van Someren (Eds.), *Current trends in knowledge acquisition* (pp. 276-288). Amsterdam: IOS Press.

Oakley, P. A., MacKenzie, G., Templeton, J., Cook, A. L., & Kirby, R. M. (2004). Longitudinal trends in trauma mortality and survival in Stoke-on-Trent 1992-1998. *Injury, 35*(4), 379-385.

Schapire, R. E. (2001, March 19-29). The boosting approach to machine learning: An overview. In *Proceedings of the MSRI Workshop on Nonlinear Estimation and Classification*, Berkeley, CA. Retrieved from http://citeseer.ist.psu.edu/schapire02boosting.html

Setiono, R., Thong, J. Y. L., & Yap, C. (1998). Symbolic rule extraction from neural networks: An application to identifying organizations adopting IT. *Information & Management, 34*(2), 91-101.

TARN. (2004). *The first decade*. Retrieved from http://www.tarn.ac.uk/introduction/FirstDecade.pdf

Teasdale, G., & Jennett, B. (1974). *LANCET*, (ii), 81-83. Retrieved from http://www.trauma.org/scores/gcs.html

Templeton, J., Oakley, P. A., MacKenzie, G., Cook, A. L., Brand, D., Mullins, R. J., et al. (2000). A comparison of patient characteristics and survival in two trauma centres located in different countries. *Injury, 31*(7), 493-501.

Watkins, D. (1997). *Clementine's neural networks technical overview*. Retrieved from http://www.cs.bris.ac.uk/~cgc/METAL/Consortium/secure/neural_overview.doc(Note that high AIS relates to an increase in severity, whereas high GCS relates to a decrease in severity.)

This work was previously published in International Journal of Healthcare Information Systems and Informatics, Vol. 1, Issue 2, edited by J. Tan, pp. 51-64, copyright 2006 by IGI Publishing, formerly known as Idea Group Publishing (an imprint of IGI Global).

Chapter VI

Diagnostic Cost Reduction Using Artificial Neural Networks:
The Case of Pulmonary Embolism

Steven Walczak, University of Colorado at Denver, USA

Bradley B. Brimhall, Tricore Reference Laboratory, USA;
University of New Mexico, USA

Jerry B. Lefkowitz, Weill Cornell College of Medicine, USA

Abstract

Patients face a multitude of diseases, trauma, and related medical problems that are difficult and costly to diagnose with respect to direct costs, including pulmonary embolism (PE). Advanced decision-making tools such as artificial neural networks (ANNs) improve diagnostic capabilities for these problematic medical conditions. The research in this chapter develops a backpropagation trained ANN diagnostic model to predict the occurrence of PE. Laboratory database values for 292 patients who were determined to be at risk for a PE, with 15% suffering a confirmed PE, are collected and used to evaluate various ANN models' performance. Results indicate that using ANN diagnostic models enables the leveraging of knowledge gained from standard clinical laboratory tests, significantly improving both overall positive predictive and negative predictive performance.

Introduction

Medical and surgical patients today face a variety of conditions that are both difficult and costly to diagnose and treat. With ever skyrocketing medical costs (Benko, 2004), the use of information technology is seen as a much-needed means to help control and potentially reduce medical direct costs (Intille, 2004). Deep vein thrombosis (DVT) and pulmonary embolism (PE) are medical conditions that are particularly difficult to diagnose in the acute setting (Mountain, 2003). Frequent usage of costly clinical laboratory tests to screen patients for further treatment is commonplace. All too commonly hospitals provide treatment to patients without PE as a preventative measure (Mountain, 2003). Furthermore, patient mortality, morbidity, and both direct and indirect costs for delayed diagnosis of these conditions may also be substantial. Recent studies show that 40 to 80 percent of patients that die from a PE are undiagnosed as having a potential PE (Mesquita et al., 1999; Morpurgo et al., 1998).

DVT may occur as the result of patient genetic and environmental factors or as a side effect of lower extremity immobility (e.g., following surgery). When a blood clot in the veins of a lower extremity breaks away, it may travel to the lungs and lodge in the pulmonary arterial circulation causing PE. If the clot is large enough it may wedge itself into the large pulmonary arteries leading to an acute medical emergency with a significant mortality rate. Approximately 2 million people annually experience DVT, with approximately 600,000 developing a PE and approximately 10% of these PE episodes result in mortality (Mesquita et al. 1999; Labarere et al., 2004). Documented occurrence of DVT in postoperative surgical populations ranges from 10% (Hardwick & Colwell, 2004) to 28% (Blattler et al., 2004).

Direct costs associated with DVT and PE come from the expensive diagnostic and even more expensive treatment protocols. It may be possible to lower these direct costs, especially when additional testing or treatment may be ruled out due to available knowledge. Artificial neural network (ANN) systems enable the economic examination (Walczak, 2001) and nonlinear combination of various readily available clinical laboratory tests. Laboratory tests typically performed on surgical patients, for example, blood chemistry, form the foundation for analysis and diagnostic model development..

One such test is the D-dimer assay that measures patient plasma for the concentration of one molecular product released from blood clots. When blood vessels are injured or when the movement of blood is too slow through veins of lower extremities, blood may begin to clot by initiating a series of steps in which fibrin molecules are crossed linked by thrombin to form a structure that entraps platelets and other coagulation molecules—a blood clot. As healing begins to occur, plasmin begins to break down the clot and releases, among other things, D-dimer molecules. Ddimers are actually small fragments of cross-linked fibrin and provide the basis for assessing blood clotting activity. Patients with DVT and PE frequently have elevated levels of D-dimer in their plasma. Consequently, many hospitals now employ the D-dimer assay as a first test in the diagnostic pathway for these conditions. Usage of the results of a D-dimer assay effectively reduces the direct costs of DVT by reducing the requirement for downstream testing and treatment, specifically Doppler ultrasound tests (Wells, 2003). The use of nonparametric models enables the analysis of laboratory tests without regard to the population distribution, which may be a problematic factor when combining more than one laboratory test for the diagnostic prediction. Additionally, ANNs provide nonlinear modeling capabilities that may be beneficial in combining pathology tests.

The research reported in this chapter will examine the efficacy of using ANN models to predict the likelihood of a PE in surgical patient populations. A corollary research question is whether less invasive and less costly diagnostic methods are both available and reliable in predicting PE. The benefit of the reported research is twofold. First, the reported research examines new combinations of laboratory tests to determine if a combined model may be more reliable than currently used single variable medical models. Second, the research evaluates the viability of utilizing an ANN model to predict PE (and potentially DVT). The ANN provides improved positive predictive performance of the combined laboratory test model over the more traditional step-wise logistic regression models that are currently employed in medical modeling (León, 1994; Tran et al., 1994; Walczak & Scharf, 2000). The cost effectiveness of utilizing the described neural network pathology tool is determined by examining the direct costs to patients, where direct costs represent the costs of diagnostic work ups and the costs of any goods, services, and other resources utilized in any subsequent intervention (Wildner, 2003; Patwardhan et al., 2005). Implementing the described ANN-based PE predictive model is capable of reducing patient evaluation direct costs by well over $1,200 per patient suspected of having a potentially life-threatening PE, as well as reducing medical risks associated with some of the more advanced diagnostic methods.

The organization of the remainder of this chapter follows. The next section gives background on some of the issues associated with diagnosing and treating PE and DVT as well as examining the utilization of ANN systems in medicine and issues surrounding the design of ANN systems. The methodology section describes the patient population and development of the neural network models for predicting PE occurrence. The next section performs an analysis of the ANN system's performance and consequent savings in direct costs. The last section concludes with a summary of the research findings and directions for future research.

Background

Diagnostic Difficulties of PE

Various tests exist for attempting to detect the presence of a DVT or PE and are commonly administered to patients viewed as being at risk based on medical history as well as patient signs and symptoms. For example, leg pain or swelling may indicate a patient with DVT; however, such symptoms are far from specific. Venography (x-ray with injected intravenous radioactive contrast dye) of the legs, Doppler ultrasound scans, plethysmography (measuring differential blood pressure between arms and legs), and the D-dimer assay blood test are some of the tests that may be employed in the evaluation of DVT (see http://www.nlm.nih.gov/medlineplus/ency/article/000156.htm). Venography is the "gold standard" for diagnosing DVT, which is commonly treated with anticoagulant therapy such as intravenous heparin, requiring hospitalization, or injected low molecular weight heparin combined with oral warfarin medication, which may be continued for six months.

Patients with a sudden onset of chest pain or tachycardia or rapid shallow breathing may have a PE, but these are also general signs of a wide variety of medical conditions (Mesquita et al., 1999; Mobley et al., 2005). PE's are often first evaluated using ventilation perfusion scanning (costing $300-$500 and involving the injection of radioactive-tagged material) and chest x-rays that may be followed by pulmonary angiography (see http://www.nlm.nih.gov/medlineplus/ency/ article/000132.htm). If the diagnosis of PE is made, the patient requires emergency treatment, typically thrombolytic therapy to dissolve the clot, and hospitalization.

While the pulmonary angiogram is considered the "gold standard" for determining PE presence (Evanders et al., 2003; Mountain, 2003), it has a direct cost between $800 and $1,200 and involves injecting contrast through a catheter that has been threaded into major coronary blood vessels, with associated morbidity and mortality risks. If use of the D-dimer assay can better determine the likelihood or absence of a PE, then a significant reduction in risks to the patient and costs ensues. The D-dimer assay has a direct cost of less than $7. Another factor that encourages the use of the D-dimer and other blood tests is the timeliness of the test, which average approximately 30 minutes total time including acquisition of the sample, transportation, analysis, and delivery of results. Improved detection of PE and early management will decrease the mortality and morbidity associated with PE (Stein et al., 2004b).

Currently, the D-dimer assay has strong negative predictive reliability that is excluding DVT or PE patients who are exceedingly unlikely to benefit from further invasive testing (e.g., angiography) or very few false negatives. Unfortunately, the test does not appear to have reliable positive predictability (Stein et al., 2004a), leaving the diagnostic role of the D-dimer uncertain. Maximizing both the positive and negative predictive values of laboratory tests should be a goal of diagnostic tests (Kara & Güven, 2007).

A potential cause of the lack of positive predictability is that due to the potential life-threatening outcome of PE, the screening threshold for the D-dimer result is set very low (e.g., 400 or 450) to avoid false negative tests. As a result, many patients who do not have a PE must undergo a pulmonary angiogram or other expensive testing procedure to determine if a PE exists. Additionally, no standard for the D-dimer result threshold has been established allowing for a wide-range of cutoff values between hospitals (Stein et al., 2004a) and subsequent variation, though usually high, of patient population percentages undergoing unnecessary treatment.

Neural Networks in Medicine

The issues related to the use of D-dimer assay results: lack of standardized cutoff value, lack of positive predictive capability, and other influencing factors, pose a modeling problem. ANNs provide strong modeling capabilities when population dynamics of the independent variables are unknown or nonlinear (Smith, 1993; Walczak & Cerpa, 2002), as would happen when using multiple laboratory test results to perform a diagnosis.

Before examining the factors that affect ANN development (in the next section), a brief review of ANN applications in medical domains is provided in this section. Neural networks or artificial neural networks applied to solve or provide decision support for a variety of medical domain problems started two decades ago (Leese, 1986).

Many physicians are reluctant to utilize artificial intelligence technologies including ANN, especially neural networks that attempt to perform diagnosis or treatment in other than a decision support role (Kleinmuntz, 1992; Hassoun et al., 1994; Baxt, 1995; Baxt & Skora, 1996; Hu et al., 1999; Walczak, 2003). The reluctance of physicians to adopt neural networks has led to the usage of neural networks as primarily image processing and laboratory test analysis tools. Table 1 provides a brief overview of historic and more recent neural network applications in medicine. A full review of all neural network applications in medicine is beyond the scope of this chapter[1], and as such Table 1 only provides a representative sample of research over the past decade.

Although representative and not comprehensive, Table 1 indicates that ANN applications in medical domains tend to be used in either imaging or laboratory settings (Walczak & Scharf, 2000), with diagnostic neural networks occurring rarely. Of interest from Table 1 for the research presented in this chapter are the three PE-related ANN applications. Each of these ANN research applications (Fisher et al., 1996; Evander et al., 2003; Serpen et al., 2003) examines the improvement in

Table 1. Types of artificial neural network applications in medicine

Classification	ANN applications research
Imaging (detect indicators in images)	Breast disease (Khuwaja & Abu-Rezq, 2004; Papadopoulos et al., 2005), Coronary artery disease (Baxt, 1991; Dorffner & Porenta, 1994; Lapuerta et al., 1995; Baxt & Skora, 1996; Scott et al., 2004), Electromyography (Hassoun, 1994), Lung disease (Suzuki et al., 2004; Lin et al., 2005), Pulmonary embolism (Fisher et al., 1996; Evander et al., 2003; Serpen et al., 2003), Tomography (Tourassi & Floyd, 1995; Bruyndonckx et al., 2004; Durairaj et al., 2007; Dokur, 2008)
Laboratory (produce test results)	Breast disease (Mattfeldt et al., 2004), EEG (Walczak & Nowack, 2001; Nowack et al., 2002; Güler et al., 2005b), General blood test pathology (Liparini et al., 2005), Head injury (Erol et al., 2005), Heart disease (Haraldsson et al., 2004; Andrisevic et al., 2005; Mobley et al., 2005), Hematology (Zini, 2005), Lung disease (Folland et al., 2004; Güler et al., 2005a)
Resource Planning	Blood transfusions (Ruggeri et al., 2000; Walczak & Scharf, 2000; Covin et al., 2003; Pereira, 2004; Walczak, 2005), Pharmacology (Polak et al., 2004; Gaweda et al., 2005)
Diagnostic	Acute Appendicitis (Sakai et al., 2007), Breast cancer (Übeyli, 2005), Eye disease (Kara & Güven, 2007)
Other	Medical cost estimation (Goss & Vozikis, 2002; Polak et al., 2004; Crawford et al., 2005), Medical data mining (Petrovsky & Brusic, 2004), Patient Outcomes Assessment (Buchman et al., 1994; Frye et al., 1996; Izenberg et al., 1997; Orunesu et al., 2004; Yeong et al., 2005)

identification or validation of PE from chest x-ray images or pulmonary angiogram data. Thus, each of these existing methods still requires the usage of and incurrence of the direct costs associated with these more costly diagnostic methods.

While ANNs previously performed image analysis to confirm a diagnosis of PE, the use of ANNs to predict a PE from standard low direct cost blood tests is a novel application of this nonparametric modeling paradigm. The next section examines factors impacting the development of ANN models, with an emphasis on the medical domain application of predicting PE.

Neural Network Design Issues

Patient treatment information must necessarily be of high quality (Silverman, 1998), since the consequences of prediction error can lead to increased morbidity and even mortality. ANNs have been shown to outperform various statistical modeling methods in medical domains with respect to the accuracy of results (White, 1992; Buchman et al., 1994; León, 1994; Dybowski & Gant, 1995; Lapuerta et al., 1995; Stair & Howell, 1995; Baxt & Skora, 1996; Walczak & Scharf, 2000; Walczak, 2005)ANN design can be problematic and should account for the following influencing design factors (Walczak & Cerpa, 1999; Walczak & Cerpa, 2002): training algorithm selection, input variable selection, and hidden layer architecture.

Various ANN training algorithms exist, however Alpsan et al. (1995) have claimed that the backpropagation training algorithm produces classification and prediction models that generalize (on out of sample data) as well as or better than most other ANN training algorithms, at least for their specific medical domain problem. Backpropagation trained ANN in particular have been proven to be robust models of arbitrary complex equations (Hornik et al., 1989; White, 1990; Hornik, 1991). Backpropagation trained ANNs are commonly used to provide solutions to business and engineering problems and also are the most common ANN type for medical domain applications which facilitates cross research comparison of methodologies (Cherkassky & Lari-Najafi, 1992; Dorffner & Porenta, 1994; Montague & Morris, 1994; Alpsan et al., 1995; Baxt, 1995; Dybowski & Gant, 1995; Rodvold et al., 2001).

A reason for selecting another training algorithm besides backpropagation, such as the radial basis function, is to overcome problems with very noisy input data in the training sets (Barnard & Wessels, 1992; Carpenter et al., 1995). Since the proposed ANN prediction model utilizes the results of laboratory tests, many already controlled by computers and robotics, the resultant error rate in the input data is minimal and should not require a training algorithm that may not generalize well in order to alleviate error-prone data problems. Generally considered the best and most robust training method for ANN classification and prediction models, backpropagation works well when low-noise input data exists (Walczak & Cerpa, 2002). The backpropagation algorithm has been widely discussed in literature and readers should see Hertz et al. (1991), Fu (1994), Jain et al. (1996), and Rodvold et al. (2001) for further details on the function of the backpropagation ANN training methodology.

A critical step in the design of any ANN model and especially in medical applications is the selection of high quality predictive input (independent) variables that are not highly correlated with each other (Smith, 1993; Pakath & Zaveri, 1995; Tahai et al., 1998; Walczak & Cerpa, 1999). Domain expert physicians identify all available data that is related to the PE diagnosis problem.

The final influencing factor from above in developing ANN models is the determination of the hidden node architecture (Smith, 1993; Walczak & Cerpa, 1999). The quantity of hidden nodes has a direct effect on generalization performance (Hung et al., 1996), with both too few and too many hidden nodes decreasing performance. The number of hidden layers also affects the smoothness and closeness of fit of the solution surface (Barnard & Wessles, 1992). A common heuristic method to determine the optimal number of hidden nodes is to start with a small quantity of hidden nodes (commonly ¼ to ½ the quantity of input nodes) and increment the hidden node quantity by one until generalization performance begins to deteriorate. This method will safeguard against under-fitting and over-fitting the model (Walczak & Cerpa, 1999).

The research reported below will evaluate the efficacy of utilizing an ANN methodology for developing a diagnostic model of PE that utilizes tests with a lower direct cost.

Methodology: An ANN Model for Diagnosing PE

As stated above, the evaluation mechanisms for determining if a patient has a PE and requires treatment currently have high direct costs (e.g., ventilation perfusion scan costing from $300 to $500 and pulmonary angiogram costing from $800 to $1,200). In addition to other demographic and medical risk factors, the purpose of this research is to determine if less costly evaluation mechanisms for PE are available, especially using the D-dimer assay results which has a direct cost of under $7 and is commonly used to negatively screen out patients for PE (Stein et al., 2004a).

Research Population Description

The patient population in this research is 292 surgical patients admitted to a large Midwest teaching hospital during a 9½ month period. All patients during the period of the study diagnosed by physicians as being 'at risk' for either DVT or PE are included in the study with no exclusions. Database records maintained by the hospital clinical laboratory as well as clinical information provided from radiology and chart records provide the data used in the ANN input vector (independent variables). Patient records used in this study only come from patients clinically identified as being 'at risk' for a DVT or possible PE by attending physicians based on signs (e.g., swelling in legs or irregular breathing) and symptoms (e.g., report of pain in legs for DVT or chest for PE). Just over 15% of this patient population, 44 out of 292, suffered a confirmed PE, which is consistent with other findings on the rate of DVT occurrence in surgical populations and consequent occurrence of PE (Blattler et al., 2004; Hardwick & Colwell, 2004). A pulmonary angiogram confirmed or negated the presence of PE.

The 'at risk' population of surgical patients for DVT and a possible PE has some basic statistical measures that are displayed in Table 2. From Table 2, it can be seen that the D-dimer results alone are not significantly different between patients with

Table 2: Typical D-dimer surgical population values

	D-dimer minimum	D-dimer maximum	D-dimer μ (average)	D-Dimer σ (std dev)	Age μ Age σ	Gender
Patients w/ confirmed PE	145	35450	4218.7	5862.75	48.45 22.38	47.5 % male
Patients w/o PE	124	22375	1782.63	1264.16	53 16.64	38.34 % male

PE and patients without PE, although the PE patients have a much larger average D-dimer result and also a wider distribution. High D-dimer values may result from a variety of causes in addition to DVT or PE, which further confuses the application of the D-dimer for diagnosing PE.

ANN Design of a PE Diagnosis Model

The focus of this study is on the use of the D-dimer assay results in possible combination with other values to improve the overall positive predictive performance to reduce false positives, which lead to unnecessary PE evaluation direct costs. As discussed in a previous section, the small error associated with laboratory tests and because of the reported robustness of the backpropagation training algorithm implied selection of backpropagation as the training algorithm for implementing the ANN-based PE diagnosis model. Radial basis function (RBF) neural networks and step-wise logistic regression (LR) models were also implemented simultaneously to produce multiple models for comparison and to evaluate if a backpropagation trained neural network would produce the optimal model. Using the model selection perspective (Swanson & White, 1995), comparison of each of the independent model types yielded the backpropagation ANN model as the optimal model. The backpropagation models outperformed, with regard to overall accuracy (the sum of true positives and true negatives divided by all cases) both of the other model types ($p < .01$ against the RBF-trained ANN and $p < 0.10$ for the LR models).

Domain-expert physicians identified blood test results with minimal direct costs that would be available for suspected DVT and PE patients prior to the performance of an angiogram. Since the research question of trying to determine if one or more of these test results could improve the PE diagnosis accuracy, a correlation matrix of all blood chemistry and other blood test results is performed to determine those variables that appear to be correlated with a positive diagnosis of PE. The variables include: D-dimer, reactive glucose (Glu-R), blood urea nitrogen, serum creatinine, serum sodium, serum potassium, serum chloride, serum carbon dioxide level, serum calcium, white blood cell count, red blood cell count, hemoglobin, hematocrit, mean corpuscular volume, mean corpuscular hemoglobin, mean corpuscular hemoglobin concentration, red cell distribution width, and platelet count. Other values including: mean platelet volume, absolute neutrophil count (and %), absolute lymphocyte count (and %), absolute monocyte count (and %), absolute eosinophil count (and %), and absolute basophile count (and %) were considered for use but eliminated due to missing data for many of the patients (i.e., the tests had not been ordered by their attending physician). The predictive correlation of different blood test results measured by a Pearson's correlation matrix indicated that the D-dimer had the highest correlation with a validated PE for those test results included in the matrix and that randomized glucose (Glu-R) and CO2 also both had significant ($p < 0.05$) predictive correlations with the PE dependent variable. The age and sex of the patient are also included as independent variables to determine if these may be predictive when combined with blood test results[2]. Different backpropagation trained ANN models use various combinations of these five variables: age, sex, D-dimer, Glu-R, and CO2 as the input vector of independent variables, producing 23 different sets of input variables and corresponding diagnosis models.

ANN models for each of the 23 different input vectors each start with a single hidden processing node. Both one and two hidden layer architectures are evaluated since the complexity of the diagnosis solution surface is unknown (Fu, 1994). When a second hidden layer is implemented it is also started with a single hidden processing node. The quantity of processing nodes in each layer is incremented independently of the other layer and by a quantity of one. Re-initialization of each new, larger, model produces random interconnection weights before training occurs. Hidden node expansion stops once the generalization performance begins to deteriorate and the model with the best generalization performance is kept.

Training of each ANN model uses one sample of data and then validation uses a separate hold out sample. Due to the relatively small size of the population data, we use an 8-fold cross validation technique to increase the quantity of hold out samples analyzed in the results to the full population of 292. The majority of the ANNs evaluated performed similarly to just using the D-dimer result alone, meaning they had very good specificity (identifying positive PE cases) but very poor sensitivity (identifying negative PE cases). The finding that the sex-independent variable did not influence the performance of the various neural supports the findings of Stein et al. (2003b) who found that sex was not a factor in the diagnosis of PE.

The best performing ANN model utilized both the D-Dimer and GLU-R result for each patient. The name of the ANN PE diagnosis model is PEDimeNet, since it utilizes the D-dimer laboratory test in combination with another test to maximize positive PE predictive performance. The hidden node architecture for this backpropagation trained ANN is 2 input nodes representing the D-dimer and Glu-R results, 4 hidden nodes, and 1 output node, as shown in Figure 1. This ANN is the one discussed in the next section.

Figure 1. PEDimeNet ANN architecture

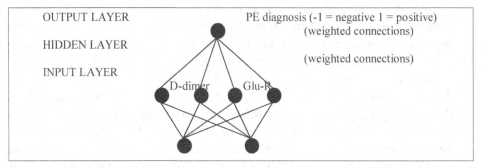

Results and Discussion

Backpropagation trained ANNs provide a real number output between -1 and 1 (though some ANN shell tools allow this range to be extended) and not a true or false result for predicting the occurrence of a PE in a patient. These real number output values require interpretation to determine the optimal cutoff point for partitioning the solution space into the two desired groups: probable PE and unlikely PE. A ROC (Receiver Operating Characteristic) curve analysis is commonly performed by those involved in medical diagnostics to determine the optimal threshold cutoff value for maximizing positive predictive performance on the generalization sample (Kamierczak, 1999; Obuschowski et al, 2004) and this technique is used with the ANN training sample output values to determine the optimal real number threshold value for performing the classifications. A similar and independent ROC curve analysis for the RBF and LR models reported in the previous section determines each model's cutoff value. The area under the ROC curve for the training data was 0.79. Once the ROC threshold value is determined, it is then applied universally to all out-of-sample output values produced by the ANN to determine the ANN's PE diagnosis for the corresponding patient.

Table 3 displays the prediction results of the resulting ANN model. Similar to increasing the D-dimer cutoff value to include more of the patient population in the group that undergoes further evaluation via an angiogram or other PE verification method, a tradeoff exists between the positive predictive accuracy and the negative predictive accuracy using the ANN model. Lowering the PE cutoff point causes the positive predictive accuracy to increase and creates a corresponding decrease in the negative predictive accuracy will be seen. Due to the possible outcome of mortality for PE patients, a positive predictive performance of 90% sensitivity is desired as specified by the domain-expert physicians (where the TP rate in Table 3 is the sensitivity and the TN rate is the specificity). The overall diagnosis accuracy ([TP+TN]/Total) performance of the PEDimeNet ANN model is 62.33%, with almost

Table 3. ANN diagnostic prediction results for PE

	ANN positive PE	ANN negative PE
Actual PE (positive)	TP = 40 (90.91%)	FN = 4 (9.09%)
No PE (negative)	FP = 107 (43.15%)	TN = 141 (56.85%)

(TP = True Positive, FN = False Negative, FP = False Positive, and TN = True Negative)

91% of all PE patients identified and also nearly 57% of patients that do not have a PE and therefore do not require any additional testing for PE with subsequent reduction in direct costs.

Recall that traditional usage of the D-dimer, with a relatively low threshold values, produces a false negative (FN) rate very close to 0%. As a result, a negative PE test result usually means that the patient will truly not have a PE. The false positive rate for the standard D-dimer test is very high, which leads to the increased medical costs through unnecessary costly procedures for follow up evaluation (e.g., pulmonary angiogram).

For the test population used in the research reported in this chapter, a simulation of adjusting the D-dimer cutoff value to produce a false negative rate identical to the proposed ANN model, produced a false positive rate of 91.53% (227 patients that require unnecessary evaluation tests), meaning that only 21 of 248 patients did not have further costly PE evaluation procedures recommended. Whereas the PEDimeNet ANN was able to save additional laboratory testing for 141 patients, as opposed to just 21 when using the traditional D-dimer only diagnosis. Therefore, an ANN model of PE that utilizes both D-dimer and Glu-R test results provides a high-quality positive predictor. The ANN PE prediction model exceeds using a non-ANN D-dimer-based evaluation mechanism with respective to true negatives (patients without PE) by well over 600%, resulting in significant cost savings for the patients. Direct cost savings would be approximately $96,000 to $144,000 for the 9½ month period of the research study, which translates to a $121,000 to $182,000 direct cost annualized savings.

A possible limitation of this study is that although the ANN was evaluated using data from a large urban hospital with a demographically diverse population, regional differences in pathological values for PE patients may exist (Stein et al., 2004b). As such, the methodology described would require each hospital to independently train their own ANN model and to establish their own ROC cutoff threshold value for interpreting the generalization (out-of-sample) diagnosis values of the ANN in order to establish confidence in the ANN's values fro specific regions of the world.

Utilizing the proposed ANN system would require only very minor workflow changes in the emergency department and clinical laboratory of the studied hospital and would integrate similarly at most hospitals that follow similar diagnostic methodologies.

Medical user acceptance of new decision support technology is highly dependent on two factors: first that the decision support technology not be perceived as attempting to make diagnosis (Baxt, 1995; Baxt & Skora, 1996; Walczak & Scharf, 2000) and second that the new information technologies not disrupt normal workflows (Walczak, 2003; Kirkley & Stein, 2004). Physicians receive laboratory results at most hospitals either electronically or on paper after encoding and storing the results in a pathology database. The PEDimeNet ANN-based decision support system would architecturally be positioned in the pathology departments IT framework as displayed in Figure 2. This integration of the PEDimeNet ANN diagnostic tool would then appear seamless to physicians, integrating with their existing workflow by simply adding the analysis to the pathology report already received by the physician.

The PEDimeNet PE diagnosis decision support tool is composed of the PEDimeNET ANN, an interface that allows the entry of D-dimer and Glu-R laboratory test results (which may be handled electronically through an EDI interface or performed manually at a keyboard), a backend program that contains the ROC curve analysis-based decision cutoff value (which may also be read from a database to allow for movement in the cutoff value over time perhaps due to new pathology equipment sensitivity) and produces the go/no go diagnostic recommendation for probable PE in a patient. Future enhancements would include a database or agent-oriented Web browser to recommend additional tests if necessary and treatment protocols.

The following scenario presents an illustration of the functioning of the proposed PEDimeNet system within a hospital setting. A physician would request a diag-

Figure 2. PEDimeNet relative to other pathology IT systems

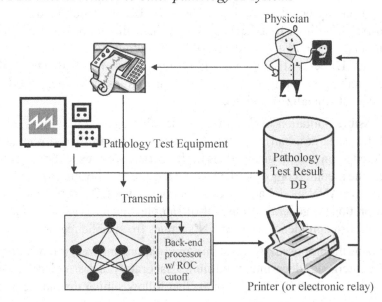

nostic workup including a patient blood draw. The clinical laboratory receives the patient's blood sample. Laboratory tests are completed using the existing laboratory equipment. The results are delivered to the physician either electronically (with EDI requiring a small hardware modification to interface with the existing pathology instrumentation) or on paper (after entering the results into the laboratory database with a simultaneous transmission to the PEDimeNet). A software interface to the database or other peripheral devices (in C# or Java) encodes the received value into the format required by the ANN. The PEDimeNet diagnostic decision support system would then interpret the ANN's results based on a cutoff value established by applying the ROC curve analysis determined threshold. The backend analysis of the ANN output provides a report of the interpreted ANN prediction in either electronic or printed format for the attending physician, who would then determine if any further evaluation was required. Other than the step in the lab necessary to transmit the results to the PEDimeNet decision support system, the automated process is similar to standard decision-making processes for evaluating the need to screen for a PE. From the physician's perspective, there is no change in workflow from the traditional receipt of the original non-interpreted D-dimer assay results.

Conclusion

The research presented in this chapter demonstrates the efficacy of utilizing ANNs for predicting the occurrence of PE in patients presenting to the emergency department and those at risk of PE following surgery. The reported results were able to match the very low false negative rate of a more traditional test that relied on the D-dimer alone. Although the usage of a D-dimer screening test is questioned in cases of PE (Stein et al., 2004a), it has proved reliable for evaluating the presence of DVT (Wells et al., 2003), a leading cause of PE. Furthermore, over a 600% increase in true negative predictions with a corresponding decrease in associated medical risks to patients and decreased medical costs of hundreds of thousands of dollars per hospital per year demonstrates the benefits of using a nonlinear and nonparametric modeling technique such as the backpropagation trained ANN.

Another benefit derived from this research is the identification of the superior positive predictive performance for PE when using the combination of the D-dimer result value in combination with the Glu-R result value. The D-dimer, individually, was unable to reliably distinguish between positive PE cases and negative ones, creating a high corresponding false positive assessment rate so that only a very small number of actual PEs would be misdiagnosed. The utilization of an ANN as the statistical analysis component of the PEDimeNet ANN decision support system enabled the rapid combination of input values in nonlinear ways without regard to population distribution characteristics. A potential drawback of using ANNs as a model determination mechanism to evaluate the contribution of various independent variables is the need to determine the ideal architecture. While the current research utilized a brute force incremental process to analyze both single and two hidden layer networks, new neural network shell tools are able to automate some or all of the ANN node architecture optimization process.

While the research reported in this chapter focused on the prediction of PE, the relationship between PE and DVT and previous research has indicated a strong positive correlation between the D-dimer assay results and accurate DVT diagnosis (Wells et al., 2003), which indicates that a similar ANN model would be able to accurately predict DVT. This would permit the operation of two side-by-side (or possibly one) ANNs in the PEDimeNet decision support system to evaluate both PE and DVT simultaneously and is a topic of future research.

In addition to the specific research benefits just described above, generalizing the research method and results provides implications for both researchers and practitioners. Future research efforts will benefit by realizing that nonparametric modeling techniques in general and neural networks specifically are a viable method for analyzing complex and potentially ill-defined (unknown population and error distributions) problems. Researchers should embrace the most advanced modeling techniques available, especially since neural networks have repeatedly demonstrated increased performance over more traditional parametric statistical methods. The data set for the presented ANN PE diagnosis application is relatively error-free. Researchers should note that designing optimal neural network models has many implementation factors and careful attention in selecting input variables, selecting the training algorithm, and determining the hidden layer and hidden node architecture will help to produce the optimal ANN model (Smith, 1993; Walczak & Cerpa, 1999; 2002).

An implication for practice is to challenge existing protocols and heuristics. The addition of a low direct-cost variable to the PE diagnosis model significantly increases the accuracy and reduces direct costs. Other medical diagnostic and assessment problems may derive benefit from examining new sets of variables. The ANN modeling method provides an inexpensive and reliable way to rapidly asses the impact of adding new variables or removing existing decision variables (Walczak, 2008).

The research reported in this chapter demonstrates the impact of ANN diagnosis models through the reduction of direct costs. Future research is needed to realize the overall benefit gained from ANN diagnosis models by examining the impact on indirect costs, such as reduced patient healing times and overall quality of care received.

References

Alpsan, D., Towsey, M., Ozdamar, O., Ah, C., & Ghista, D. (1995). Efficacy of modified backpropagation and optimization methods on a real-world medical problem. *Neural Networks, 8*(6), 945-962.

Andrisevic, N., Ejaz, K., Rios-Gutierrez, F., Alba-Flores, R., Nordehn, G., & Burns, S. (2005). Detection of heart murmurs using wavelet analysis and artificial neural networks. *Journal of Biomechanical Engineering, 127*(6), 899-904.

Barnard, E., & Wessels, L. (1992). Extrapolation and interpolation in neural network classifiers. *IEEE Control Systems, 12*(5), 50-53.

Baxt, W. (1991). Use of an artificial neural network for the diagnosis of myocardial infarction. *Annals of Internal Medicine, 115*(11), 843-848.

Baxt, W. (1995). Application of artificial neural networks to clinical medicine. *The Lancet, 346,* 1135-1138.

Baxt, W., & Skora, J. (1996). Prospective validation of artificial neural network trained to identify acute myocardial infarction. *The Lancet, 347,* 12-15.

Benko, L. (2004). Going retro. *Modern Healthcare, 34*(33), 14-15.

Blattler, W., Martinez, I., & Blattler, I. (2004). Diagnosis of deep venous thrombosis and alternative diseases in symptomatic outpatients. *European Journal of Internal Medicine, 15*(5), 305-311.

Bruyndonckx, P., Léonard, S., Tavernier, S., Lemaître, C., Devroede, O., Wu, Y., & Krieguer, M. (2004). Neural network-based position estimators for PET detectors using monolithic LSO blocks. *IEEE Transactions on Nuclear Science, 51*(5), 2520-2525.

Buchman, T., Kubos, K., Seidler, A., & Siegforth, M. (1994). A comparison of statistical and connectionist models for the prediction of chronicity in a surgical intensive care unit. *Critical Care Medicine, 22*(5), 750-762.

Carpenter, G., Grossberg, S., & Reynolds, J. (1995). A Fuzzy ARTMAP nonparametric probability estimator for nonstationary pattern recognition problems. *IEEE Transactions on Neural Networks, 6*(6), 1330-1336.

Cherkassky, V., & Lari-Najafi, H. (1992). Data representation for diagnostic neural networks. *IEEE Expert, 7*(5), 43-53.

Covin, R., O'Brien, M., Grunwald, G., Brimhall, B., Sethi, G., Walczak, S., et al. (2003). Factors impacting transfusion of fresh frozen plasma, platelets, and red blood cells during elective coronary artery bypass graft surgery. *Archives of Pathology & Laboratory Medicine, 127*(4), 415-423.

Crawford, A., Fuhr Jr., J., Clarke, J., & Hubbs, B. (2005). Comparative effectiveness of total population versus disease-specific neural network models in predicting medical costs. *Disease Management, 8*(5), 277-287.

Dokur, Z. (2008). A unified framework for image compression and segmentation by using an incremental neural network. *Expert Systems with Applications, 34*(1), 611-619.

Dorffner, G., & Porenta, G. (1994). On using feedforward neural networks for clinical diagnostic tasks. *Artificial Intelligence in Medicine, 6*(5), 417-435.

Durairaj, D., Krishna, M., & Murugesan, R. (2007). A neural network approach for image reconstruction in electron magnetic resonance tomography. *Computers in Biology and Medicine, 37*(10), 1492-1501.

Dybowski, R., & Gant, V. (1995). Artificial neural networks in pathology and medical laboratories. *The Lancet, 346,* 1203-1207.

Erol, F., Uysal, H., Ergün, U., Barişçi, N., Serhathoğlu, & Hardalaç, F. (2005). Prediction of minor head injured patients using logistic regression and MLP neural network. *Journal of Medical Systems, 29*(3), 205-215.

Evander, E., Holst, H., Järund, A., Ohlsson, M., Wollmer, P., Åström, K., & Edenbrandt, L. (2003). Role of ventilation scintigraphy in diagnosis of acute pulmonary embolism: An evaluation using artificial neural networks. *European Journal of Nuclear Medicine and Molecular Imaging, 30*(7), 961-965.

Fisher, R., Scott, J., & Palmer, E. (1996). Neural networks in ventilation-perfusion imaging. *Radiology, 198*(March), 699-706.

Folland, R., Hines, E., Dutta, R., Boilot, P., & Morgan, D. (2004). Comparison of neural network predictors in the classification of tracheal—bronchial breath sounds by respiratory auscultation. *Artificial Intelligence in Medicine, 31*(3), 211-220.

Frye, K., Izenberg, S., Williams, M., & Luterman, A. (1996). Simulated biologic intelligence used to predict length of stay and survival of burns. *Journal of Burn Care and Rehabilitation, 17*(6), 540-546.

Fu, L. (1994). *Neural networks in computer intelligence.* New York, NY: McGraw-Hill.

Gaweda, A., Muezzinoglu, M., Aronoff, G., Jacobs, A., Zurada, J., & Brier, M. (2005). Individualization of pharmacological anemia management using reinforcement learning. *Neural Networks, 18*(5-6), 826-834.

Goss, E., & Vozikis, G. (2002). Improving healthcare organizational management through neural network learning. *Healtcare Management Science, 5*(3), 221-227.

Güler, I., Polat, H., & Ergün, U. (2005a). Combining neural network and genetic algorithm for prediction of lung sounds. *Journal of Medical Systems, 29*(3), 217-231.

Güler, N., Übeyli, E., & Güler, I. (2005b). Recurrent neural networks employing Lyapunov exponents for EEG signals classification. *Expert Systems with Applications, 29*(3), 506-514.

Hardwick, M., & Colwell Jr., C. (2004). Advances in DVT prophylaxis and management in major orthopaedic surgery. *Surgical Technologist, 12,* 265-268.

Hassoun, M., Wang, C., & Spitzer, A. (1994). NNERVE: Neural network extractions of repetitive vectors for electromyography - Part II: Performance analysis. *IEEE Transactions on Biomedical Engineering, 41*(11), 1053-1061.

Hertz, J., Krogh, A., & Palmer, R. (1991). *Introduction to the theory of neural computation.* Reading, MA: Addison Wesley.

Hornik, K. (1991). Approximation capabilities of multilayer feedforward networks. *Neural Networks, 4,* 251-257.

Hornik, K., Stinchcombe, M., & White, H. (1989). Multilayer feedforward networks are universal approximators. *Neural Networks, 2*(5) 359-366.

Hu, P., Chau, P., Sheng, O., & Tam, K. (1999). Examining the technology acceptance model using physician acceptance of telemedicine technology. *Journal of Management Information Systems, 16*(2), 91-112.

Hung, M., Hu, M., Shanker, M., & Patuwo, B. (1996). Estimating posterior probabilities in classification problems with neural networks. *International Journal of Computational Intelligence and Organizations, 1*(1), 49-60.

Intille, S. (2004). A new research challenge: Persuasive technology to motivate healthy aging. *Plant Physiology, 136*(1), 235-237.

Izenberg, S., Williams, M., & Luterman, A. (1997). Prediction of trauma mortality using a neural network. *American Surgeon, 63*(3), 275-281.

Jain, A., Mao, J., & Mohiuddin, K. (1996). Artificial neural networks: A tutorial. *IEEE Computer, 29*(3), 31-44.

Kamierczak, S. (1999). Statistical techniques for evaluating the diagnostic utility of laboratory tests. *Clinical Chemistry and Laboratory Medicine, 37,* 1001-1009.

Kara, S., & Güven, A. (2007). Neural network-based diagnosing for optic nerve disease from visual-evoked potential. *Journal of Medical Systems, 31*(5), 391-396.

Khuwaja, G., & Abu-Rezq, A. (2004). Bi-modal breast cancer classification system. *Pattern Analysis & Applications, 7*(3), 235-242.

Kirkley, D., & Stein, M. (2004). Nurses and clinical technology: Sources of resistance and strategies for acceptance. *Nursing Economics, 22*(4), 195, 216-222.

Kleinmuntz, B. (1992). Computers as clinicians: An update. *Computers in Biology and Medicine, 22*(4), 227-237.

Labarere, J., Bosson, J., Brion, J., Fabre, M., Imbert, B., Carpentier, P., & Pernod, G. (2004). Validation of a clinical guideline on prevention of venous thromboembolism in medical inpatients: A before-and-after study with systematic ultrasound examination. *Journal of Internal Medicine, 256*(4), 338-348.

Lapuerta, P., Azen, S., & LaBree, L. (1995). Use of neural networks in predicting the risk of coronary artery disease. *Computers in Biomedical Research, 28*(1), 38-52.

Leese, S. (1986). Computer advances towards the realization of a cybernated health-science diagnostic system. *American Journal of Psychotherapy, 40*(3), 321-323.

León, M. (1994). Binary response forecasting: Comparison between neural networks and logistic regression analysis. *World Congress on Neural Networks, 2,* 244-247.

Lin, D-W., Yan, C-R., & Chen, W-T. (2005). Autonomous detection of pulmonary nodules on CT images with a neural network-based fuzzy system. *Computerized Medical Imaging & Graphics, 29*(6), 447-458.

Liparini, A., Carvalho, S., & Belchior, J. (2005). Analysis of the applicability of artificial neural networks for studying blood plasma: Determination of magnesium ion concentration as a case study. *Clinical Chemistry & Laboratory Medicine, 43*(9), 939-946.

Mattfeldt, T., Kestler, H., & Sinn, H-P. (2004). Prediction of the axillary lymph node status in mammary cancer on the basis of clinicopathological data and flow cytometry. *Medical & Biological Engineering & Computing, 42*(6), 733-739.

Mesquita, C., Morandi Júnior, J., Perrone, F., Oliveira, C., Barreira, L., Nascimento, S., Pareto Júnior, R., & Mesquita, E. (1999). Fatal pulmonary embolism in hospitalized patients—clinical diagnosis versus pathological confirmation. *Arquivos Brasileiros de Cardiologia, 73*(3), 255-258.

Mobley, B., Schechter, E., Moore, W., McKee, P., & Eichner, June E. (2005). Neural network predictions of significant coronary artery stenosis in men. *Artificial Intelligence in Medicine, 34*(2), 151-161.

Montague, G., & Morris, J. (1994). Neural-network contributions in biotechnology. *Trends in Biotechnology, 12*(8), 312-324.

Morpurgo, M., Schmid, C., & Mandelli, V. (1998). Factors influencing the clinical diagnosis of pulmonary embolism: Analysis of 229 postmortem cases. *International Journal of Cardiology, 65*(Supplement 1), S79-S82.

Mountain, D. (2003). Diagnosing pulmonary embolism: A question of too much choice?. *Emergency Medicine, 15*(3), 250-262.

Nowack, W., Walczak, S., & Janati, A. (2002). Clinical correlate of EEG Rhythmicity. *Journal of Clinical Neurophysiology, 19*(1), 32-36.

Obuschowski, N., Lieber, M., & Wians, F. (2004). ROC curves in clinical chemistry: Uses, misuses, and possible solutions. *Clinical Chemistry, 50,* 1118-1125.

Orunesu, E., Bagnasco, M., Salmaso, C., Altrinetti, V., Bernasconi, D., Del Monte, P., et al. (2004). Use of an artificial neural network to predict Graves' disease outcome within 2 years of drug withdrawal. *European Journal of Clinical Investigation, 34*(3), 210-217.

Pakath, R., & Zaveri, J. (1995). Specifying critical inputs in a genetic algorithm-driven decision support system: An automated facility. *Decision Sciences, 26*(6), 749-779.

Papadopoulos, A., Fotiadis, D., & Likas, A. (2005). Characterization of clustered microcalcifications in digitized mammograms using neural networks and support vector machines. *Artificial Intelligence in Medicine, 34*(2), 141-150.

Patwardhan, M., Matchar, D., Samsa, G., McCrory, D., Williams, R., & Li, T. (2005). Cost of multiple sclerosis by level of disability: A review of literature. *Multiple Sclerosis, 11*(2), 232-239.

Pereira, A. (2004). Performance of time-series methods in forecasting the demand for red blood cell transfusion. *Transfusion, 44*(5), 739-746.

Petrovsky, N., & Brusic, V. (2004). Virtual models of the HLA class I antigen processing pathway. *Methods, 34*(4), 429-435.

Polak, S., Skowron, A., Mendyk, A., & Brandys, J. (2004). Artificial neural network in pharmacoeconomics. *Studies in Health Technology and Information, 105,* 241-249.

Rodvold, D., McLeod, D., Brandt, J., Snow, P., & Murphy, G. (2001). Introduction to artificial neural networks for physicians: Taking the lid off the black box. *The Prostate, 46*(1), 39-44.

Ruggeri, A., Comai, G., Belloni, M., & Zanella, A. (2000). A simulation study for the design of a control system for the blood concentration process in autotransfusion. *Annals of Biomedical Engineering, 28*(4), 470-482.

Sakai, S., Kobayashi, K., Toyabe, S., Mandai, N., & Kanda, T. (2007). Comparison of the levels of accuracy of an artificial neural network model and a logistic regression model for the diagnosis of acute appendicitis. *Journal of Medical Systems, 31*(5), 357-364.

Scott, J., Aziz, K., Yasuda, T., & Gewirtz, H. (2004). Integration of clinical and imaging data to predict the presence of coronary artery disease with the use of neural networks. *Coronary Artery Disease, 15*(7), 427-434.

Serpen, G., Iyer, R., Elsamaloty, H., & Parsai, E. (2003). Automated lung outline reconstruction in ventilation-perfusion scans using principal component analysis techniques. *Computers in Biology and Medicine, 33*(2), 119-142.

Silverman, B. (1998). The role of Web agents in medical knowledge management. *M.D. Computing, 15*(4), 221-231.

Smith, M. (1993). *Neural networks for statistical modeling*. New York, NY: Van Nostrand Reinhold.

Stair, T., & Howell, J. (1995). How long will it take? How much will it cost?: Multiple regression and neural network programs at ED triage. *American Journal of Emergency Medicine, 13*, 118-119.

Stein, P., Hull, R., Patel, K., Olson, R., Ghali, W., Alshab, A., & Meyers, F. (2003a). Venous thromboembolic disease: Comparison of the diagnostic process in blacks and whites. *Archives of Internal Medicine, 163*(15), 1843-1848.

Stein, P., Hull, R., Patel, K., Olson, R., Ghali, W., Alshab, A., & Meyers, F. (2003b). Venous thromboembolic disease: Comparison of the diagnostic process in men and women. *Archives of Internal Medicine, 163*(14), 1689-1694.

Stein, P., Hull, R., Patel, K., Olson, R., Ghali, W., Brant, R., et al. (2004a). D-dimer for the exclusion of acute venous thrombosis and pulmonary embolism. *Annals of Internal Medicine, 140*(8), 589-602.

Stein, P., Kayali, F., & Olson, R. (2004b). Estimated case fatality rate of pulmonary embolism, 1979 to 1998. *American Journal of Cardiology, 93*(9), 1197-1199.

Suzuki, K., Horiba, I., Sugie, N., & Nanki, M. (2004). Extraction of left ventricular contours from left ventriculograms by means of a neural edge detector. *IEEE Transactions on Medical Imaging, 23*(3), 330-339.

Swanson, N., & White, H. (1995). A model-selection approach to assessing the information in the term structure using linear models and artificial neural networks. *Journal of Business and Economic Statistics, 13*(3), 265-275.

Tahai, A., Walczak, S., & Rigsby, J. (1998). Improving artificial neural network performance through input variable selection. In: P. Siegel, K. Omer, A. deKorvin, & A. Zebda, (Eds.), *Applications of fuzzy sets and the theory of evidence to accounting II* (pp. 277-292). Stamford, CT: JAI Press.

Tran, D., VanOnselen, E., Wensink, A., & Cuesta, M. (1994). Factors related to multiple organ system failure and mortality in a surgical intensive care unit. *Nephrology Dialysis Transplantation, 9*(4 Supp), 172-178.

Übeyli, E. (2005). A mixture of experts network structure for breast cancer diagnosis. *Journal of Medical Systems, 29*(5), 569-579.

Walczak, S. (2008). Evaluating medical decision-making heuristics and other business heuristics with neural networks. In: G. Phillips-Wren & L. Jain (Eds.), *Intelligent decision making: An AI-based approach* (chap. 10). New York, NY: Springer.

Walczak, S. (2005). Artificial neural network medical decision support tool: Predicting transfusion requirements of ER patients. *IEEE Transactions on Information Technology in Biomedicine, 9*(3), 468-474.

Walczak, S. (2003). A multi-agent architecture for developing medical information retrieval agents. *Journal of Medical Systems, 27*(5), 479-498.

Walczak, S. (2001). Neural networks as a tool for developing and validating business heuristics. *Expert Systems with Applications, 21*(1), 31-36.

Walczak, S., & Cerpa, N. (1999). Heuristic principles for the design of artificial neural networks. *Information and Software Technology, 41*(2), 109-119.

Walczak, S., & Cerpa, N. (2002). Artificial neural networks. In: R. Meyers (Ed.), *Encyclopedia of physical science and technology,* (3rd ed., vol. 1, pp. 631-645). San Diego, CA: Academic Press.

Walczak, S., & Nowack, W. (2001). An artificial neural network approach to diagnosing epilepsy using lateralized bursts of theta EEGs. *Journal of Medical Systems, 25*(1), 9-20.

Walczak, S., &.Scharf, J. (2000). Reducing surgical patient costs through use of an artificial neural network to predict transfusion requirements. *Decision Support Systems, 30*(2), 125-138.

Wells, P., Anderson, D., Rodger, M., Forgie, M., Kearon, C., Dreyer, J., et al. (2003). Evaluation of D-dimer in the diagnosis of suspected deep-vein thrombosis. *New England Journal of Medicine, 349*(13), 1227-1235.

White, H. (1990). Connectionist nonparametric regression: Multilayer feedforward networks can learn arbitrary mappings. *Neural Networks, 3,* 535-549.

White, H. (1992). Consequences and detection of misspecified nonlinear regression models. In: H. White (Ed.), *Artificial neural networks: Approximations and learning theory* (pp. 224-258), Oxford, UK: Blackwell.

Wildner, M. (2003). Health economic issues of screening programmes. *European Journal of Pediatrics, 162*(Suppl.), S5-S7.

Yeong, E.-K., Hsiao, T-C., Chiang, H., & Lin, C-W. (2005). Prediction of burn healing time using artificial neural networks and reflectance spectrometer. *Burns, 31*(4), 415-420.

Zini, G. (2005). Artificial intelligence in hematology. *Hematology, 10*(5), 393-400.

Endnotes

[1]   A database inquiry on EBSCO using the terms "neural network" AND (medicine OR medical) produced 997 articles. A similar query on PubMed, the NIH article database, produced 6,120 articles.

[2]   The occurrence of PE between blacks and whites has been found to be comparable (Stein et al., 2003a) and as such is not included in the variables considered

for the ANN input vector. Additionally, this variable is subjective being either self-reported by patients or reported as an observation by the admitting nurse in the studied hospital and as such may have a higher than acceptable error rate for use in a backpropagation trained ANN.

Chapter VII

Information Technology in Primary Care Practice in the United States

James G. Anderson, American College of Medical Informatics, USA & Purdue University, USA

E. Andrew Balas, Old Dominion University, USA

Abstract

The objective of this study was to assess the current level of information technology used by primary care physicians in the U.S. Primary care physicians listed by the American Medical Association were contacted by e-mail and asked to complete a Web-based questionnaire. A total of 2,145 physicians responded. Overall between 20% and 25% of primary care physicians reported using electronic medical records, e-prescribing, point-of-care decision support tools and electronic communication with patients. This indicates a slow rate of adoption since 2000-2001. Differences in adoption rates suggest that future surveys need to differentiate primary care and office-based physicians by specialty. An important finding is that one-third of the physicians surveyed expressed no interest in the four IT applications. Overcoming this barrier may require efforts by medical specialty societies to educate their members as to the benefits of IT in practice. The majority of physicians perceived benefits of IT, but they cited costs, vendor inability to deliver acceptable products and concerns about privacy and confidentiality as major barriers to implementation of IT applications. Overcoming the cost barrier may require that payers and the federal government share the costs of implementing these IT applications.

Introduction

The adoption of information technology (IT) to support the delivery of healthcare is increasingly recognized in many countries as an essential tool in improving patient care (Leaning, 1993; Dick & Steen, 1997; President's Information Technology Advisory Committee, 2004). One study of ten countries that belong to the Organization for Economic Cooperation and Development (OECD) found that over 90% of the general practitioners had computers in their offices and, in almost all cases, used them in practice (Protti, 2007). Until recently, IT products available for healthcare providers were mostly designed for large organizations, were business- oriented, complex to implement, and costly. Recent advances in technology have made IT applications more available to primary care physicians in smaller practices. Products are available that are modular; able to be integrated with different systems, and are designed to fit the physicians practice pattern without substantial investments in hardware software and maintenance (McDonald & Metzger, 2002).

As a result, the introduction of computers and IT applications into primary care in countries with favorable government policies and financial incentives has been rapid (Thakurdas, Coster, Guirr & Arroll, 1996; Purves, Sugden, Booth & Sowerby, 1999; Kidd, 2000; Mount, Kelman, Smith & Douglas, 2000). A number of English-speaking countries have experienced widespread implementation of information technology. The Harvard School of Public Health and the Commonwealth Fund's International Symposium survey of primary care physicians found that the proportions of primary care physicians in the following countries who were using electronic medical records were: U.S. (17%), Canada (14%), Australia (25%), New Zealand (52%), and the UK (59%). The survey also found that use of electronic prescribing by primary care physicians was: U.S. (9%), Canada (8%), Australia (44%), New Zealand (52%), and the UK (87%) (Harris Interactive, 2001a).

The U.S. trails European countries in the use of information technology in patient care. A recent study of primary care physicians in seven countries (Australia, Canada, Germany, New Zealand, the Netherlands and the UK) revealed striking differences in the implementation of clinical information systems. U.S. physicians were the least likely to have clinical information systems in their offices (Schoen, Osborn, Huynh, Doty, Peugh & Zapert, 2006). Overall, 29% of general practitioners in the Eurropean Union use electronic medical records compared to only 11% in the U.S. Only three countries from the Organization for Economic Cooperation and Development (OECD), Portugal, France and Spain, lag behind the U.S. (Harris Interactive, 2002b). Despite its potential to improve efficiency and quality of care, use of information technology in healthcare lags behind other sectors of the economy in the U.S. In 2001, most of the $20 million invested in healthcare information technology was used to computerize financial systems (Goldsmith, Blumenthal & Rishel, 2003). Other nations have a significant head start in implementing information technology in healthcare. In comparison to six countries, the U.S. total investment in health information technology per capita in 2005 was $0.43. This compares to $4.93 in Australia and $192.79 in the UK (Anderson, Frogner, Johns & Reinhardt, 2006). Adoption of information technology such as EMRs and computerized physician order entry by U.S. hospitals has also been limited (AHA, 2005).

Given the increasing public attention to the importance of health information technology, the rate of IT adoption among primary care providers is important (Hillestad, Bigelow, Bower, Girosi, Meili, Scoville & Taylor, 2005). Accurate estimates of the adoption rate for information technology form the basis for policy regarding how to stimulate its use by physicians. The overall aim of this study was to determine primary care physicians' use of information technology in patient care. The specific objectives included the following:

1. Estimating the proportion of primary care physicians who have adopted information technology applications in their practices
2. Determining physician perceptions of the benefits of these IT applications
3. Determining physician perceptions of the barriers to the adoption of IT applications in their practices

Primary care in the U.S. is delivered by physicians who comprise several different specialties; namely, family practice (FP), internal medicine (IM), pediatrics (PEDS), and obstetricians and gynecologists (OBGYN). One other group of physicians was included in the survey comprising medical specialties such as geriatrics, and occupational medicine.

Four IT applications were selected for investigation. First, electronic medical records (EMRs) are promoted as more comprehensive and accessible to healthcare providers. Studies have shown that EMRs have the potential to reduce medical errors especially when integrated with other applications such as decision support (Bates et al., 1998). Electronic prescribing involves the use of computers or hand-held devices to submit prescriptions to pharmacies electronically. E-prescribing has the potential to improve efficiency, reduce prescription errors and improve compliance with managed care formularies (Schiff & Rucker, 1998; Miller, Gardner, Johnson & Hripcsak, 2005). Third, point-of-care decision support tools can improve the quality of patient care, for example, an antibiotic decision support system (Evans et al., 1998) and automated decision support alerts for contraindicated medications (Galanter, Didomenico & Polikaitis, 2005). Fourth, patients have consistently expressed a strong desire for online communication with physicians (Harris Interactive, 2005). This may involve e-mail queries as well as online consultations. Electronic communication allows physicians to deliver better care and patients to assume greater responsibility for their own care.

Methods

Survey Method

A Web-based survey was developed to investigate primary care physicians' use of the four IT applications described above. These applications were selected because healthcare providers in the U.S. and the E.U. find them helpful and effective (Harris Interactive, 2003; 2005). Comparative data exist from earlier surveys on the use, perceived benefits and barriers to these applications. At the same time, earlier studies failed to differentiate primary care physicians by specialty.

We describe the design and administration of the survey. A Web-based survey method was chosen because it permitted us to survey a national sample of primary care physicians with a reasonable budget (Lazar & Preece, 1999; Wyatt 2000; Eysenbach, 2005). Also, we wanted to sample an Internet-literate population who are most likely to be early adopters in their practices (Rogers, 1983).

Survey Design

The study was sponsored by the Quality Improvement Working Group of the American Medical Informatics Association and the School of Public Health at St. Louis University. The e-mail that was sent out inviting primary care physicians to participate in the study contained a link to the Web-based survey (See Appendix).

In order to facilitate comparisons to earlier surveys, items were adapted from other widely cited surveys; in particular, the annual Healthcare Information and Management Systems Society (HIMSS) Leadership Survey (HIMSS, 2002) and the Harris Interactive polls that were conducted in the U.S. and the E.U. (Harris Interactive, 2002b; 2003).

The questionnaire was divided into seven sections. The first section included information about the physician's specialty and practice. The second section asked physicians to rate the priority of a number of Internet technologies. The next three sections listed specific financially focused, clinically focused and patient-focused

IT applications. The physician was asked to indicate for each IT application if they (1) had implemented, (2) planned to implement within one year, (3) had no plans to implement but was interested in learning more, or (4) had no interest. Physicians could also respond by indicating that they did not know or that they chose not to answer that question. The sixth section asked physicians to rate the benefits of using IT applications on a Likert scale. Responses ranged from (1) high benefit to (4) not a benefit. The final section asked about barriers to implementing IT applications. Responses ranged from (1) not a barrier to (5) insurmountable barrier. A copy of the survey is included in the Appendix.

Factor analyses were performed on the items that measured perceived benefits of the IT application and on the perceived barriers to implementation. A single factor accounted for 63% of the variance in the benefits items. The reliability based on Chronbach's Alpha was 0.93. For the barriers items, a single factor accounted for 48% of the variance. The reliability was 0.86 based on Chronbach's Alpha.

Sample

We contracted with SK & A Information Services to broadcast an e-mail invitation to primary care physicians to participate in the study. This company maintains a comprehensive list of physicians based on the AMA Physician Masterfile. The list is updated weekly through the use of surveys, publication mailings and the U.S. Postal services Address Correction Services. E-mail invitations to participate in the study were sent out to 31,743 primary care physicians. Of these e-mails, 1,101 were rejected due to invalid e-mail addresses. A total of 2,145 physicians responded representing a 7.3% response rate to the survey. The software prevented respondents from completing the survey more than one time. Questionnaires from physicians who were not currently practicing or who were not currently engaged in primary care were eliminated as were questionnaires with significant missing data. This resulted in a final sample of 1,665 that was used in the analysis.

Table 1 presents demographic data and practice information about the study sample. Sixty percent of the physicians were between 41 and 60 years of age while 29% were younger. Three-fourths of the responding physicians were male. Almost 75% practiced family medicine, internal medicine, or pediatrics, while 15% practiced obstetrics and gynecology and 9% other medical specialties. Over 88% of the respondents were primarily clinicians. The other 12% held primarily administrative positions in their practices and were excluded from the final analysis.

About 14% of the respondents were hospital-based. Almost 18% of the physicians were in group practices of 10 or more; over one-third of the respondents were in small group practices with less than 10 physicians; and 20% of the physicians were in solo practice. The remaining 12% were in integrated health delivery service organizations, managed care organizations, and so forth.

Table 1. Physician characteristics of the study sample

Characteristic	N	%
Age		
30 or less	16	1.1%
31-40	259	17.9%
41-50	537	27.0%
51-60	484	33.4%
61-70	108	7.4%
70 or above	46	3.2%
Gender		
Male	1134	74.5%
Female	388	25.5%
Specialties		
Family Practice	448	29.8%
Internal Medicine	368	24.5%
Pediatrics	324	21.5%
Obstetrics and Gynecology	225	15.0%
Other Medical Specialties	138	9.2%
Role		
Physician	1972	88.4%
Administrative	176	11.6%
Type of Organization		
Hospital	232	13.9%
Group: 10 or more	298	17.9%
Group: Less than 10	607	36.5%
Solo	327	19.6%
Other Settings	201	12.1%

Results

Use of Information Technology

Table 2 shows the extent to which physicians in each specialty have implemented each of the four IT applications. Overall, only 1 out of 4 has implemented electronic medical records and report using point of care decision support tools. About 23% communicate electronically with patients. Only 1 out of 5 primary care physicians utilizes electronic prescribing. A surprisingly high number of physicians indicated no interest in all of the IT applications. Thirty-six percent indicated no interest in decision support tools; while 31.3% and 23.5% evidenced no interest in electronic prescribing and electronic medical records, respectively. Almost 30% stated that they were not interested in electronic communication with patients.

A greater proportion of internists reported having implemented all four of the IT applications in practice ($p<0.05$) than other primary care physicians. Thirty-one

Table 2. Use of information technology by primary care specialty (%)

Application	FP	IM	PEDS	OB/ GYN	Other	Total
Electronic Medical Records						
Implemented	23.2	31.2	23.0	16.4	40.6	25.8
Plan to implement	16.9	13.9	12.5	16.0	12.8	14.4
Interested in	26.7	23.7	33.4	23.7	19.5	26.4
No interest	24.8	21.2	19.7	31.5	21.8	23.5
NA	8.4	10.0	11.5	12.3	5.3	9.5
Electronic Prescribing						
Implemented	17.7	26.4	20.4	13.3	24.0	20.1
Plan to implement	18.2	16.7	13.0	14.3	15.2	16.2
Interested in	21.5	15.5	21.8	17.6	12.0	18.6
No interest	31.1	30.2	30.6	35.2	34.4	31.3
NA	11.6	11.2	14.1	19.5	14.4	13.8
Decision Support Tools						
Implemented	27.6	25.7	24.0	15.6	30.8	25.1
Plan to implement	16.6	11.1	9.4	10.1	8.7	12.0
Interested in	11.2	11.5	9.4	15.6	11.5	12.2
No interest	33.9	35.9	35.6	43.6	35.6	35.9
NA	10.7	15.8	21.5	15.1	13.5	14.8
Electronic Communication						
Implemented	25.5	26.6	20.4	21.2	26.2	23.2
Plan to implement	11.4	7.1	8.2	10.1	1.6	8.7
Interested in	9.3	6.5	12.1	11.1	9.5	9.9
No interest	29.0	28.1	28.9	31.7	29.4	28.9
NA	24.8	31.7	30.4	26.0	33.3	29.4

NA=don't know or choose not to answer

percent have implemented electronic medical records; about 26% have implemented, electronic prescribing, decision support tools and e-mail communication with patients. In general, OBGYNs are the least likely to have implemented any of the IT tools with the exception of electronic communication with patients ($p<0.05$). Less than 1 out of 6 of these physicians have implemented electronic medical records, electronic prescribing or decision support tools and only 1 out of 5 have implemented electronic communication with patients. OBGYNs also expressed the least interest in IT applications ($p<0.05$). Over 30% indicated no interest in electronic medical records, electronic prescribing and e-mail communication with patients. More than 40% indicated no interest in implementing decision support tools. Major reasons for this low use of IT and lack of interest by OBGYNs may be due to several reasons. Most of the IT applications are general and may not meet the specific needs of this specialty. Also there appear to be few published studies involving the use of IT by OBGYNs.

Perceived Benefits and Barriers

Overall, the majority of primary care physicians surveyed perceived benefits from implementing IT applications (see Table 3). Almost 75% indicated that these applications could reduce errors; 70% perceived IT as potentially increasing their productivity; over 60% indicated that IT tools have the potential to reduce costs and help patients assume more responsibility. Physicians are less certain about some of the other potential benefits of IT applications. About half of the physicians surveyed evidenced skepticism that IT applications would shorten consultations and reduce the number of patients who seek unnecessary healthcare. Over 40% felt that IT is unlikely to reduce unnecessary tests and treatments.

More than 80% of primary care physicians report the lack of financial support for IT applications as a major barrier to adoption. This is followed by their perceptions that vendors fail to deliver acceptable products as primary barriers to implementing these tools (79.3%) (see Table 4). In general, physicians perceive these barriers as difficult to overcome. Almost ⅔ of the physicians surveyed also cited the lack of a strategic plan for implementing applications and difficulty in recruiting experienced IT personnel as major barriers; while over ½ cited lack of sufficient knowledge of IT as a barrier to implementation. At the same time, physicians indicated that these last three barriers could be easily overcome.

Predictors of IT Implementation

Table 5 provides the logistic regression models and predictors for implementing each of the IT applications. Demographic factors specifically age and gender, were not significantly associated with the implementation of the four IT applications. In only

Table 3. Perceived benefits of implementing IT applications (%)

Benefit	High	Medium	Low	None
Patients assume responsibility for monitoring symptoms/disease	23.6	38.7	22.1	15.6
Shorter consultations	17.0	29.1	20.9	32.9
Patients not seeking medical care when it was not needed	22.5	28.2	24.4	25.0
Patients coming in sooner for necessary treatment	33.8	29.6	18.4	18.3
Fewer unnecessary tests	29.4	27.9	16.1	26.5
Fewer unnecessary treatments	32.8	24.9	16.9	25.4
Fewer errors	53.4	21.4	10.5	14.7
Increased productivity	39.2	30.3	14.2	16.3
Reduced costs	37.5	25.5	15.4	21.6

Table 4. Perceived barriers to implementing IT applications (%)

Barriers	No Barrier	Easily Overcome	Overcome some effort	Overcome great effort	Insurmountable
Lack of financial support	7.6	5.0	35.3	41.3	10.7
Vendors inability to deliver acceptable products	12.4	8.3	34.8	36.3	8.2
Acceptance by staff	17.8	23.9	41.6	15.3	1.3
Difficulty proving quantifiable benefits	14.8	18.0	38.7	24.6	3.9
Lack of strategic plan for implementing	19.7	15.2	35.7	25.3	4.1
Recruiting experienced IT personnel	22.0	17.6	31.7	24.0	4.8
Retaining experienced personnel	24.6	17.9	36.6	18.1	2.8
Insufficient knowledge of IT applications	15.0	22.5	41.4	19.3	1.7
Considerable investment in IT applications	6.1	6.9	28.8	47.6	10.6

one instance was there a significant difference between male and female physicians. Males were almost twice as likely to implement e-prescribing as females.

Physicians' specialties did predict whether or not they had implemented certain IT applications. Pediatricians and obstetricians and gynecologists were significantly less likely to have implemented electronic medical records. In contrast, family practitioners were almost three times more likely to have implemented point-of-care

Table 5. Predictors of the implementation of IT applications (odds ratios)

Characteristic	EMR	e-Prescribing	Decision Support	e-Commun-ication
Age				
30 or less	1.000	1.000	1.000	1.000
31-40	0.668	1.474	0.761	1.360
41-50	0.421	0.401	0.760	1.614
51-60	0.568	0.392	0.660	1.157
61-70	0.530	0.503	0.606	1.393
70 or above	0.503	0.706	0.499	1.393
Gender				
Male	1.175	1.942**	1.094	1.066
Female	1.000	1.000	1.000	1.000
Specialties				
FP	1.420	1.433	0.591**	0.924
IM	0.712	1.125	0.957	0.851
Pediatrics	0.513**	0.622	1.206	0.616
OBGY	0.406**	0.957	1.180	0.586
Other	1.000	1.000	1.000	1.000
Benefits				
Fewer Errors	1.541**	1.574**	1.238*	1.086
Increased Productivity	1.023	1.282*	1.157	0.919
Reduced Costs	0.804*	0.724**	0.788*	0.868
Barriers				
Lack of Financial Support	1.591**	1.452**	1.296*	0.960
Vendors Failure to Deliver	1.169	1.211*	1.309**	1.108
Considerable Investment	1.207	1.271*	1.221	1.278

**p<0.01 *p<0.05

decision support tools. Specialty was not a significant predictor of implementation of electronic prescribing and communication with patients.

Perceived benefits and barriers appear to be consistent predictors of whether or not primary care physicians implemented 3 of the 4 IT applications. Physicians who perceived that IT can reduce medical errors were 1 ½ times more likely to have implemented electronic medical record, e-prescribing and decision support tools. In contrast, physicians who cited lack of financial support and the considerable investment required to implement these applications as significant barriers were less likely to have implemented all three of these IT applications. Physicians who perceived vendors as failing to deliver useful and acceptable products were significantly less likely to have implemented decision support tools. The decision to implement electronic communication with patients did not appear to be affected by demographic characteristics, specialty or perceptions of benefits or barriers.

Discussion

Adoption of electronic medical record has been the most widely surveyed IT application. A review of 22 studies of outpatient electronic medical record (EMR) adoption from 1998 to 2002 suggested a utilization rate of 20% to 25% at the time of the surveys (Brailer & Terasawa, 2003). A more recent study of 36 surveys conducted between 1995 and 2005 revealed widely different estimates of use of EMRs. On the basis of studies of high or medium quality, the investigators estimated that by 2005 23% of physicians used electronic health records in the ambulatory setting (Jha, Ferris, Donelan, DesRoches, Shields, Rosenbaum & Blumenthal, 2006). At the same time, data from the U.S. National Ambulatory Medical Care Survey (NAMCS) indicated that by 2005 23.9% of physicians reported using full or partial EMRs in their office-based practice, a 31% increase from 18.2% reported in 2001 (Burt & Hing, 2005; Burt, Hing & Woodwell, 2006).

These studies vary considerably in terms of how respondents were selected and their generalizability to a physician population. Many of the studies are unscientific and utilized surveys of meeting attendees. Only three of the 22 studies reviewed by Brailer and Terasawa (2003) were rated as generalizable. Of the 36 studies reviewed by Jha and others (2006), only ten received a high quality methodology rating. Also, most of these studies do not differentiate among physicians by specialty. Consequently, there is only limited data on adoption of EMRs by specialty. The 2002 Healthcare Information and Management Systems Society survey (HIMSS, 2002) administered to attendees and exhibitors at the annual conference found that 42% of internal medicine practice and 30% of family medicine practices reported using EMRs. These rates show little change from the HIMSS survey in 2001. However, since only meeting attendees were surveyed, it is impossible to extrapolate these results to the U.S. primary care physician population as a whole.

There are fewer studies of the adoption of other IT applications such as electronic prescribing and online communication between physicians and patients. The National Ambulatory Medical Care Survey (NAMCS) indicated that only 8% of office-based physicians in 2001 ordered prescriptions electronically (Burt & Hing, 2005). The Harris Interactive study that compared use of IT by U.S. general practitioners to European physicians found that 17% of physicians in primary care practices reported that they used EMRs and 9% reported using electronic prescribing (Harris Interactive, 2002a). This survey also dates back to 2000-2001. Neither study differentiates physicians by specialty.

   More recent information is needed about the extent to which primary care physicians use information technology for patient care, patterns of use and perceived barriers to use of IT. Many of the surveys discussed earlier were undertaken before the year 2000. The NAMCS statistics on uses of computerized clinical support systems in medical settings are based on office-based physician practices rather than only on primary care physicians (Burt & Hing, 2005; Burt, Hing & Woodwell, 2006). The Harris Interactive study reports aggregate statistics for primary care physicians and specialists. Our survey examined IT applications that appear to offer the greatest potential to primary care physicians in providing high-quality patient care. It also differentiates primary care physicians by specialty.

The study reported in this chapter provides evidence from a large sample of U.S. primary care physicians that there is limited implementation of clinical and patient care IT applications. Overall, only about 25% of primary care physicians have implemented electronic medical records, e-prescribing, point-of-care decision support tools or electronic communication with patients. These results are similar to those from a Harris Interactive survey of 400 U.S. physicians conducted in 2001, the NAMCS surveys and other earlier studies indicating a slow rate of adoption However, the proportion of physicians who have implemented e-prescribing has almost doubled from 11% to 20% since 2001. Protti's (2007) study of IT use in general practice in ten OECD countries found the most common clinical application to be the automation of medication prescriptions. This may in part be due to the fact that this clinical application provides one of the largest benefits to practicing physicians as it addresses legibility problems, can save time especially for refills of prescriptions and can be coupled with decision support systems. The increased utilization of e-prescribing may also be due to improvements in technology such as the use of wireless devices.

Of concern is the finding that almost 1 out of 3 primary care physicians surveyed expressed little or not interest in the four IT applications. This may indicate that while ⅔ of primary care physicians perceive that implementation of IT can reduce costs and errors and help patients assume more responsibility for their medical conditions, a significant number of these physicians do not perceive the advantages of implementing IT technologies to provide patient care. One way of overcoming this barrier may be for medical specialty societies to offer seminars, short courses and/or Web seminars on IT for continuing medical education (CME) credit with a focus on those features that are most useful to physicians in that specialty.

Age and gender on the whole do not appear to predict implementation of these four IT applications. This finding, however, differs from that of the NAMCS survey. Results from the 2005 survey indicated that physicians under 35 years of age were more likely to use full or partial EMR s in their practice (Burt, Hing & Woodwell, 2006). Our study indicated that there are significant differences in implementation among the specialties. A greater proportion of internists report having implemented all four IT applications than other primary care physicians. Pediatricians and obstetricians and gynecologists are less likely to have implemented EMRs; while family practitioners are more likely to have implemented decision support tools. OBGYNs, in particular, have been slow to adopt IT in practice. Only 16% have implemented EMRs and decision support tools. Even less, 13% have implemented electronic prescribing. The slow adoption of IT applications by this specialty group may be due to the fact that these tools fail to address the special needs of this group of physicians. Also, OBGYNs may need to see more studies that demonstrate how these tools can help them improve their practices.

This finding suggests that future surveys that assess adoption of IT applications by physicians need to differentiate by specialty rather than treating primary care physicians or office-based physicians as homogeneous groups. Efforts to encourage IT adoption by physicians need to be tailored to specific specialty groups by emphasizing features of the technology that are particularly useful to that specialty.

Perceptions of benefits and barriers are significant predictors of implementation of 3 of the 4 applications. Physicians who perceive that EMRs, e-prescribing, and decision support tools can help them reduce medical errors are significantly more likely to have implemented these technologies. At the same time, perception of barriers is a significant impediment to implementation (Anderson, 1997; 1999; Harris Interactive, 2001b). Those physicians who perceived lack of financial support and high investment cost required were much less likely to have implemented these three IT applications. Also, physicians cited lack of experience and knowledge of IT as barriers. This may indicate that physicians might feel that learning to use IT applications in practice may require too much time and energy by them and their staff in order to achieve the perceived benefits. Consequently, a key to increased use of patient care IT applications by primary care physicians may be to convince them that the benefits significantly outweigh the barriers, primarily cost. Also, physicians do not perceive vendors as delivering acceptable IT products that meet their needs. Over 70% of physicians who responded to the survey perceived vendors' unresponsiveness as a barrier to implementation of IT. It may be necessary for vendors to more thoroughly examine the needs of primary care physicians and how their IT applications fit into clinical practice in order to convince physicians to adopt them.

Other studies have indicated that lack of funding and costs are the largest barriers to adoption of EMRs. Surveys have found that 50% or more of respondents cited lack of adequate funding as the major barrier to implementation (Management Association, 2001; HIMSS, 2002; Medical Records Institute, 2002; Medical Group Miller & Sims, 2004). This perception is based on the fact that implementation of some IT applications such as EMRs requires large up-front investment and ongoing maintenance costs. A study by the California Healthcare Foundation (2003) estimated the cost of implementing a computerized physician order entry (CPOE) system in an ambulatory care practice ranges from $15,000 to $50,000 per physician with a median cost of $30,000 per physician.

Overcoming the cost barrier will be difficult and may require incentives by payers and the government. An example is New Zealand, Australia and the UK that have introduced government funding programs to stimulate adoption and use of EMRs (Bates, Ebell, Gotlier, Zapp & Mullins, 2003). Professional associations can also facilitate adoption of IT. The American Academy of Family Physicians, through a non-profit foundation, is developing low-cost, open-source EMR software that will be available to physicians with no licensing fee.

Decisions to implement electronic communication with patients appear to be independent of perceptions of benefits and barriers. Barriers to electronic communication with patients may be different than barriers to the other IT applications. Physicians generally express concerns about the legal status of these communications and concern about the security of patient information sent over the Internet.

One of the limitations of this study is the low response rate (7.3 %). Low response rates are one of the major limitations of Web-based surveys in general (Eysenbach, 2005). A systematic review of 17 Internet-based surveys of health professionals found that reported response rates ranged from, 9% to 94% (Braithwaite, Emery, de Lusignan & Sutton, 2003). Most of these studies utilized professional e-directories. Some used commercial organizations' e-mail directories or recruited volunteers via Web sites of electronic discussion groups. Six of the 17 studies reviewed did not report response rates. A meta-analysis of response rates in Web- and Internet-based surveys found that the mean response rate for 68 surveys was 39.6% with a standard deviation of 15.7% (Cook, Heath & Thompson, 2000). Other researchers have reported similarly low response rate of 18% for a study of physicians in Hong Kong (Leung, Johnston, Ho, Wong & Cameo, 2001).

One study of general practitioners' use of decision support for management of familial cancer sent five separate e-mail reminders and achieved a response rate of 52.4% (Braithwaite, Sutton, Smithson & Emery, 2002). In the case of our study, the high cost of sending additional reminders to physicians precluded our doing so.

Since our survey was administered online and did not include an alternative mail survey, there is a risk of over sampling respondents who are more likely to utilize computers in their practices. Our sample was drawn from physicians with e-mail addresses listed by the American Medical Association (AMA). These physicians may be knowledgeable about IT applications and more likely to implement them in patient care. This sample design was adopted since we wanted to sample an Internet and computer-literate population of primary care physicians. These physicians are most likely to be early adopters of IT applications in their practices. Consequently, estimates of implementation reported in this study are likely to be higher than for the entire population of primary care physicians.

At the same time, limitations on the generalizability of the results apply to many of the earlier reported studies of IT adoption by physicians (Brailer & Terasawa, 2003). The HIMSS surveys were voluntary surveys administered to conference attendees (HIMSS, 2002). The MediNetwork 2002 Medical Group Office Management Systems Survey was voluntary and reported a 7.52% response rate. The AHA Most Wired Survey 2002 and the Medical Records Institute Survey of Electronic Health Record Trends and Usage sponsored by SNOMED were online voluntary surveys and do not report response rates. Comparative data for the U.S. and E.U. reported by Harris Interactive do not report response rates. Data on the E.U. countries were based on the EuroBarometer 104 conducted in June/July 2001. U.S data were collected by Harris Interactive. Our study is an improvement over a number of these earlier studies where there are serious questions about the reliability and the generalizability of results due to flawed study design or industry sponsorship (e.g., the HIMSS Leadership Survey). Also earlier studies with few exceptions failed to differentiate primary care physicians or office-based physicians by specialty.

In this study, no attempt was made to specify specific features of each of the four IT applications. Physicians were simply asked if they had implemented or intended to implement each application. However, features of each application vary considerably from practice to practice. For example, an EMR in addition to patient problem lists, medications, allergies, tests and personal information and medical history may be linked to an electronic prescribing system and evidence-based decision support tools.

Conclusion

In general, lack of information technology to support efficient care in the U.S. appears to be one of the reasons why the U.S. healthcare system's performance relative to benchmarks for healthy lives, quality, access and equity averages 66, well below the scores of many other developed countries (Schoen, Davis, How & Schoenbaum, 2006). The present study has documented the extent to which primary care physicians use IT in providing patient care. Variation among different primary care specialty groups is an important finding as is the finding that 1 out of 3 primary care physicians expressed no interest in using any of the four IT applications for patient care. Moreover, the finding that perceived benefits and barriers are the most significant predictors of IT implementation has implications for strategies to promote implementation of IT in clinical practice. Primary care physicians will need to be convinced that the benefits of these tools outweigh their costs. Also, vendors will need to be more responsive to the needs of primary care physicians. Finally, overcoming the costs barrier will require incentives and/or cost-sharing by payers and the federal government.

Acknowledgment

This study was supported by the Center for Education and Research in Information Assurance and Security (CERIAS). Data were collected by the Purdue University Social Research Institute. Marilyn Anderson, Don Malott, and Heather Rodriquez assisted with the data analysis and manuscript preparation.

References

American Hospital Association. (2005). Forward momentum: Hospital use of information technology. Retrieved June 19, 2007 from http://www.aha.org/aha/content/2005/pdf/FINALNonembITSurvey105.pdf.

Anderson, G., Frogner, B., Johns, R., & Reinhardt, W. (2006). Healthcare spending and use of information technology in OECD countries. *Health Affairs, 25*(3), 819-831.

Anderson, J. (1997). Clearing the way for physicians' use of clinical information systems. *Communications of the ACM, 40,* 83-90.

Anderson, J. (1999). Increasing the acceptance of clinical information systems. *MD Computing, 16,* 62-65.

Bates, D., Ebell, M., Gotlier, E., Zapp, J., & Mullins, H. (2003). A proposal for electronic medical records in U.S. primary care. *Journal of the American Medical Informatics Association, 10,* 1-10.

Bates, D., Leape, L., Cullen, D., Laird, N., Petersen, L., Teich, J., et al. (1998). Effect of computerized physician order entry and a team intervention on prevention of serious medication errors. *Journal of the American Medical Association, 280,* 1311-1316.

Brailer, D., & Terasawa, E. (2003). *Use and adoption of computer-based patient records.* Oakland, CA: California Healthcare Foundation.

Braithwaite, D., Sutton, S., Smithson, W., & Emery J. (2002). Internet-based risk assessment and decision support for the management of familial cancer in primary care: Survey of GP's attitudes and intentions. *Family Practice, 20*(5), 545-551.

Braithwaite, D., Emery, J., de Lusignan, S., & Sutton, S. (2003). Using the Internet to conduct surveys of health professionals: A valid alternative? *Family Practice, 19,* 587-590.

Burt, C., & Hing, E. (2005). *Use of computerized clinical support systems in medical settings: United States 2001-03. Advanced data from vital and health statistics, No. 353.* Hyattsville, MD: National Center for Health Statistics.

Burt, C., Hing, E., & Woodwell, D. (2006). Electronic medical record use by office-based physicians: United States, 2005. Retrieved June 18, 2007 from http://www.cdc.gov/nchs/prodcuts/pubs/pubd/hestats/electornic/electronic.htm.

California HealthCare Foundation. (2003). Electronic medical records: Lessons from small physician practices. *ihealthreports,* October 2003.

Cook, C., Heath, F., & Thompson, R. (2000). A meta-analysis of response rates in Web- and Internet-based surveys. *Educational and Psychological Measurement, 60*(6), 821-836.

Dick, R., & Steen, E. (1997). *The computer-based patient record: An essential technology for healthcare.* Washington D.C.: National Academy Press, Institute of Medicine.

Evans, R., Pestotnik, S., Classen, D., Clemmer, T., Weaver, L., Orme, J., et al. (1998). A computer-assisted management program for antibiotics and other anti-infective agents. *New England Journal of Medicine, 338,* 232-238.

Eysenbach, G. (2005). Using the Internet for surveys and research. In: J. Anderson & C. Aydin (Eds.), *Evaluating the organizational impact of healthcare information systems,* (2nd ed., pp. 129-143). New York: Springer.

Galanter, W., Didomenico, R., & Polikaitis, A. (2005). A trial of automated decision support alerts for contraindicated medications using computerized physician order entry. *Journal of the American Medical Informatics Association, 12*(3), 269-274.

Goldsmith, J., Blumenthal, D., & Rishel, W. (2003). Federal health information policy: A case of arrested development. *Health Affairs, 22*(4), 44-55.

Harris Interactive. (2001a). U.S. trails other English-speaking countries in use of electronic medical records and electronic prescribing. *HarrisInteractive Healthcare News, 1*(28).

Harris Interactive. (2001b). The increasing impact of eHealth on physician behavior. *HarrisInteractive Healthcare News, 1*(31).

Harris Interactive. (2002a). The future use of the Internet in 4 countries in relation to prescriptions, physician communication and health information. *HarrisInteractive Healthcare News, 2*(13).

Harris Interactive. (2002b). European physicians especially in Sweden, Netherlands and Denmark lead U.S. in use of electronic medical records. *HarrisInteractive Healthcare News, 2*(16).

Harris Interactive. (2003). eHealth influence continues to grow as usage of the Internet by physicians and patients increases . *HarrisInteractive Healthcare News, 3*(6).

Harris Interactive. (2005). Many nationwide believe in the potential benefits of electronic medical records and are interested in online communication with physicians. *HarrisInteractive Healthcare News, 4*(4).

Hillestad, R., Bigelow, J., Bower, A., Girosi, F., Meili, R, Scoville, R., et al. (2005). Can electronic medical record systems transform healthcare? Potential health benefits, savings, and costs. *Health Affairs, 24*(5), 1103-1117.

HIMSS 13th Annual HIMSS Leadership Survey. (2002). http://www.himss.org/ 2002survey.

Jha, A., Ferris, T., Donelan, K., DesRoches, C., Shields, A., Rosenbaum, S., & Blumenthal, D. (2006). How common are electronic health records in the United States? A summary of the 3 evidence. *Health Affairs, 25*(5), w496-w507.

Kidd, M. (2000). Clinical practice guidelines and the computer on your desk. *Medical Journal of Australia, 173*, 373-375

Lazar, J., & Preece, J. (1999). Designing and implementing Web-based surveys. *Journal of Computer Information Systems, 39*(4), 63-67.

Leaning, M. (1993). The new information management and technology strategy of the NHS. *British Medical Journal, 307*, 217.

Leung, G., Johnston, J., Ho, L., Wong, F., & Cameo, S. (2001). Computerization of clinical practice in Hong Kong. *International Journal of Medical Informatics, 62*, 143-154.

Medical Group Management Association. (2001). Medical Group Management Association Survey 2001.

Medical Records Institute. (2002). 4th Annual Medical Record Institute's Survey of Electronic Health Record Trends and Usage.

McDonald, K., & Metzger, J. (2002). Achieving tangible IT benefits in small physician practices. *California HealthCare Foundation, ihealth Report,* September.

Miller, R., Gardner, R., Johnson, K., & Hripcsak, G. (2005). Clinical decision support and electronic prescribing systems: A time for responsible thought and action. *Journal of the American Medical Association, 12*(4), 403-409.

Miller, R., & Sims, I. (2004). Physicians' Use of electronic medical records: Barriers and solutions. *Health Affairs, 23*(2), 116-126.

Mount, C., Kelman, C., Smith, L., & Douglas, R. (2000). An integrated electronic health record and information system for Australia. *Medical Journal of Australia, 172,* 25-27.

President's Information Technology Advisory Committee. (2004). *Revolutionizing healthcare through information technology.* Arlington, VA: National Coordination Office for Information Technology Research and Development.

Protti, D. Comparison of information technology in general practice in 10 countries. *Healthcare Quarterly, 10*(2), 107-116.

Purves, I., Sugden, B., Booth, N., & Sowerby, M. (1999). The PRODIGY Project—the iterative development of the Release One Model. *Proceedings AMIA Annual Symposium,* (pp. 359-363).

Rogers, E. (1983). *Diffusion of innovation,* (3rd ed.). New York, NY: Free Press.

Schiff, G., & Rucker, D. (1998). Computerized prescribing: Building the electronic infrastructure for better medication usage. *Journal of the American Medical Association, 280,* 516-517.

Schoen, C., Davis, K., How, S., & Schoenbaum, S. (2006). U.S. health system performance: A national scorecard. *Health Affairs, 25*(5), w457-w475.

Schoen, C., Osborn, R., Huynh, P., Doty, M., Peugh, J., & Zapert, K. (2006). On the front lines of care: Primary doctors' office systems, experiences, and views in seven countries. *Health Affairs, 25*(6), w555-w571.

Thakurdas, P., Coster, G., Guirr, E., & Arroll, B. (1996). New Zealand general practice computerisation: Attitudes and reported behavior. *New Zealand Medical Journal, 109,* 419-422.

Wyatt, J. (2000). When to use Web-based surveys. *Journal of the American Medical Informatics Association, 7*(4), 426-430.

Appendix

Dr. <name>

The Quality Improvement Working Group of the American Medical Informatics Association in conjunction with the School of Public Health at St. Louis University is undertaking a survey of physician experience with information technology at the point of care.   The survey is being performed under contract with the Social Research Institute at Purdue University and funded by the Center for Education and Research in Information Assurance and Security.

To participate, simply click on the link below and you will be directed to the Social Research Institute Web site at Purdue University. Please complete the short survey. Your responses will be kept strictly confidential and will be used solely for academic research purposes. We are grateful for your willingness to provide your valuable perspective on the real implementation experience of a physician using information technology at the point of care.

If you have any questions, please contact:

James G. Anderson, PhD
Professor of Medical Sociology
Purdue University
Chair Elect, Quality Improvement Working Group
American Medical Informatics Association
Andersonj@soc.purdue.edu

E. Andrew Balas, MD
Dean and Professor
School of Public Health
St. Louis University
Chair, Quality Improvement Working Group
American Medical Informatics Association
balasea@slu.edu

CLICK HERE <Web site Address>

Which of the following best describes your role within your Organization:

1.   Physician
2.   Director
3.   Scientist
4.   President
5.   Chief of Executive officer
6.   Medical Director
7.   Chief Medical Officer
8.   Vice President of Medical Services
9.   Other
    a.   Don't know
    b.   Choose not to answer

Which of the following best describes the environment where you spend most of your workday:

1.   Hospital
2.   Medium or large group practice or clinic (10 or more physicians)
3.   Small group practice or clinic (less than 10 practicing physicians)
4.   Solo Practice
5.   Integrated Health Delivery Service Organization
6.   Long Term Care
7.   Managed Care Organization (MCO)
8.   Mental and Behavioral Services
9.   Other
    a.   Don't know
    b.   Choose not to answer

Which of the following Internet technologies are priorities during the next year:

Upgrading Security of medical information for HIPAA compliance

1.   High Priority
2.   Medium Priority
3.   Low Priority
4.   Not a Priority
    a.   Don't know
    b.   Choose not to answer

Reducing Medical Errors

1.   High Priority
2.   Medium Priority
3.   Low Priority
4.   Not a Priority
    a.   Don't know
    b.   Choose not to answer

Promoting Patient Safety

1.   High Priority
2.   Medium Priority
3.   Low Priority
4.   Not a Priority
    a.   Don't know
    b.   Choose not to answer

Reducing Costs

1.   High Priority
2.   Medium Priority
3.   Low Priority
4.   Not a Priority
    a.   Don't know
    b.   Choose not to answer

Increasing Productivity

1.   High Priority
2.   Medium Priority
3.   Low Priority
4.   Not a Priority
      a.   Don't know
      b.   Choose not to answer

Internet Tools

Which of the following financial-focused Internet technology tools have/do you plan to implement:

Connectivity to payers

1.   Have implemented
2.   Plan to implement within 1 year
3.   No plans to implement but interested in learning more
4.   No interest
      a.   Don't know
      b.   Choose not to answer

Assistance in coding patient visits

1.   Have implemented
2.   Plan to implement within 1 year
3.   No plans to implement but interested in learning more
4.   No interest
      a.   Don't know
      b.   Choose not to answer

Electronic charge capture

1. Have implemented
2. Plan to implement within 1 year
3. No plans to implement but interested in learning more
4. No interest
   a. Don't know
   b. Choose not to answer

Which of the following clinically-focused Internet tool have or do you plan to implement:

Document scanning/imaging

1. Have implemented
2. Plan to implement within 1 year
3. No plans to implement but interested in learning more
4. No interest
   a. Don't know
   b. Choose not to answer

Transcription/voice recognition

1. Have implemented
2. Plan to implement within 1 year
3. No plans to implement but interested in learning more
4. No interest
   a. Don't know
   b. Choose not to answer

Electronic team messaging between clinic staff

1. Have implemented
2. Plan to implement within 1 year

3. No plans to implement but interested in learning more
4. No interest
    a. Don't know
    b. Choose not to answer

Electronic lab order entry

1. Have implemented
2. Plan to implement within 1 year
3. No plans to implement but interested in learning more
4. No interest
    a. Don't know
    b. Choose not to answer

Electronic routing of test results

1. Have implemented
2. Plan to implement within 1 year
3. No plans to implement but interested in learning more
4. No interest
    a. Don't know
    b. Choose not to answer

Electronic medical record

1. Have implemented
2. Plan to implement within 1 year
3. No plans to implement but interested in learning more
4. No interest
    a. Don't know
    b. Choose not to answer

Electronic Prescribing

1. Have implemented
2. Plan to implement within 1 year
3. No plans to implement but interested in learning more
4. No interest
    a. Don't know
    b. Choose not to answer

Point–of-Care decisions support tools

1. Have implemented
2. Plan to implement within 1 year
3. No plans to implement but interested in learning more
4. No interest
    a. Don't know
    b. Choose not to answer

Which of the following patient-focused Internet tools do you have or plan to implement:

Incoming telephone call management

1. Have implemented
2. Plan to implement within 1 year
3. No plans to implement but interested in learning more
4. No interest
    a. Don't know
    b. Choose not to answer

Automated telephone appointment reminders

1. Have implemented
2. Plan to implement within 1 year

3. No plans to implement but interested in learning more
4. No interest
    a. Don't know
    b. Choose not to answer

Automated patient notification of test results

1. Have implemented
2. Plan to implement within 1 year
3. No plans to implement but interested in learning more
4. No interest
    a. Don't know
    b. Choose not to answer

Automated telephone patient reminders for health prevention

1. Have implemented
2. Plan to implement within 1 year
3. No plans to implement but interested in learning more
4. No interest
    a. Don't know
    b. Choose not to answer

Electronic communication between physicians and patients

1. Have implemented
2. Plan to implement within 1 year
3. No plans to implement but interested in learning more
4. No interest
    a. Don't know
    b. Choose not to answer

Internet site with health information links for patients

1. Have implemented
2. Plan to implement within 1 year
3. No plans to implement but interested in learning more
4. No interest
   a. Don't know
   b. Choose not to answer

In general, what have been the benefits for the health service of your patients using IT applications:

Patients assuming more responsibility for monitoring their symptoms/disease?

1. High Benefit
2. Medium Benefit
3. Low Benefit
4. Not a Benefit
   a. Don't know
   b. Choose not to answer

Shorter consultations

1. High Benefit
2. Medium Benefit
3. Low Benefit
4. Not a Benefit
   a. Don't know
   b. Choose not to answer

Patients not seeking medical help when it was not needed

1. High Benefit
2. Medium Benefit

3. Low Benefit
4. Not a Benefit
    a. Don't know
    b. Choose not to answer

Patients coming in sooner for necessary treatment

1. High Benefit
2. Medium Benefit
3. Low Benefit
4. Not a Benefit
    a. Don't know
    b. Choose not to answer

Fewer unnecessary tests

1. High Benefit
2. Medium Benefit
3. Low Benefit
4. Not a Benefit
    a. Don't know
    b. Choose not to answer

Fewer unnecessary treatments

1. High Benefit
2. Medium Benefit
3. Low Benefit
4. Not a Benefit
    a. Don't know
    b. Choose not to answer

Fewer errors

1. High Benefit
2. Medium Benefit
3. Low Benefit
4. Not a Benefit
    a. Don't know
    b. Choose not to answer

Increased productivity

1. High Benefit
2. Medium Benefit
3. Low Benefit
4. Not a Benefit
    a. Don't know
    b. Choose not to answer

Reduced costs

1. High Benefit
2. Medium Benefit
3. Low Benefit
4. Not a Benefit
    a. Don't know
    b. Choose not to answer

Barriers to Implementation

To what extent are the following barriers to implementing IT applications:

Lack of Financial Support

1. Not a barrier
2. Barrier easily overcome
3. Barrier overcome with some effort
4. Barrier overcome with great effort
5. Insurmountable barrier
   a. Don't know
   b. Choose not to answer

Vendors inability to effectively deliver an acceptable product

1. Not a barrier
2. Barrier easily overcome
3. Barrier overcome with some effort
4. Barrier overcome with great effort
5. Insurmountable barrier
   a. Don't know
   b. Choose not to answer

Acceptance by the staff

1. Not a barrier
2. Barrier easily overcome
3. Barrier overcome with some effort
4. Barrier overcome with great effort
5. Insurmountable barrier
   a. Don't know
   b. Choose not to answer

Difficulty proving quantifiable benefits

1.   Not a barrier
2.   Barrier easily overcome
3.   Barrier overcome with some effort
4.   Barrier overcome with great effort
5.   Insurmountable barrier
     a.   Don't know
     b.   Choose not to answer

Lack of a strategic plan for introducing application

1.   Not a barrier
2.   Barrier easily overcome
3.   Barrier overcome with some effort
4.   Barrier overcome with great effort
5.   Insurmountable barrier
     a.   Don't know
     b.   Choose not to answer

Recruiting experience IT personnel

1.   Not a barrier
2.   Barrier easily overcome
3.   Barrier overcome with some effort
4.   Barrier overcome with great effort
5.   Insurmountable barrier
     a.   Don't know
     b.   Choose not to answer

Retaining experience personnel

1.   Not a barrier
2.   Barrier easily overcome

3. Barrier overcome with some effort
4. Barrier overcome with great effort
5. Insurmountable barrier
    a. Don't know
    b. Choose not to answer

Insufficient knowledge of IT applications

1. Not a barrier
2. Barrier easily overcome
3. Barrier overcome with some effort
4. Barrier overcome with great effort
5. Insurmountable barrier
    a. Don't know
    b. Choose not to answer

Requirement of a considerable investment in IT applications

1. Not a barrier
2. Barrier easily overcome
3. Barrier overcome with some effort
4. Barrier overcome with great effort
5. Insurmountable barrier
    a. Don't know
    b. Choose not to answer

Chapter VIII

A Case Study of Health Information Systems Adoption:
An Adaptive Structuration Theory Approach

Dana Schwieger, Southeast Missouri State University, USA

Arlyn Melcher, Southern Illinois University, USA

Ranganathan Chandreasekaran, University of Illinois at Chicago, USA

H. Joseph Wen, Southeast Missouri State University, USA

Abstract

Adaptive structuration theory (AST) is rapidly becoming an important theoretical paradigm for comprehending the impact of advanced information technologies. In this chapter, a modified AST model was designed to illustrate the changing inter-relationships among the variables affecting the adoption and application of a new technology into a medical organization setting. Using findings from a case study conducted over a 10-month period, the authors apply the case to the model to illustrate the complex interactions between medical billing technology and organizational processes. As the organization attempted to install and implement the new system, it found that in order to maintain daily operations, it would have to modify and adapt several aspects of the organization, technology and operations. As the system was slowly integrated into operations and the organization's needs evolved through the adaptation process, the study, in turn, found that different iterations of the model could emphasize different structures. The case illustrated that the capacity to manage health information systems (HIS) often requires the organization to prioritize its needs and focus its energies on a critical structure while temporarily disregarding others until the primary healthcare processes are under control.

Introduction

Driven by a need to improve utilization of information and productivity, information technology (IT) has become pervasive in the healthcare industry. Some of the areas in clinical medicine in which technology has been successfully employed include billing and scheduling, practice management, laboratory result reporting and diagnostic systems. The use of computer technology and information technology in healthcare and its delivery is called medical informatics, which began with the computerization of hospital administration tasks in the 1960s. These systems are best thought of as cost-reducing and/or quality-improving technologies.

Increased demands for electronic exchange of data have been driven by both internal and external pressures. Hospitals are comprised of a multitude of specialized departments and suppliers requiring that large amounts of clinical as well as financial data be exchanged. External forces consisting of insurance company regulations and guidelines (Hagland, 1998) government mandates and restrictions as well as Medicare deadlines (Straub, 1998) have pushed organizations to adopt technologies to automate their operations. Automating these processes may reduce costs as less paper is generated, as fewer mistakes are made and as information is transferred faster.

Health information system (HIS) can also increase the quality of medical care. This was the goal of many of the pioneers in medical informatics or clinical systems development. The quality improvements from hospital information systems would emerge from the improved record-keeping and decreased mistakes engendered by more administrative systems, as well as from clinical systems designed to aid in the provision of medical care.

Today, the role of HIS in medical care has expanded at an ever-increasing pace. As a result, healthcare professionals' familiarity with medical informatics as well as the adoption of HIS is crucial for the delivery of higher quality care. However, the challenges of applying IT to healthcare are very real. Concerns of privacy and confidentiality of data, lack of national standards for protecting medical data, the need for large-scale investments and the requirement for behavioral adaptations on the part of patients, physicians and organizations are just a few of the impediments to the adoption and use of IT in healthcare.

Rural area medical practices are especially feeling squeezed by the demands being placed upon the use of technology in the medical field. Although their use of HIS is limited, governmental regulations and the demands of insurance clearinghouses are forcing these clinics to adopt automated billing technologies. Some clinics, unable to afford billing technology capable of electronic data exchange, have been forced to merge with other practices or close their doors. Those clinics that could afford the technology experienced the challenges associated with adopting this new billing system into their business operations.

This chapter uses a version of adaptive structuration theory (AST) to examine the challenges faced by a rural medical clinic as it adopts new billing technology. AST provides a conceptual change model that helps capture the longitudinal change process. This chapter proposes a modified AST model which provides a theoretical framework that explains the appropriation process of medical electronic billing systems (MEBS). In recent years, MEBS has become a critical tool for supporting healthcare services. The appropriation of MEBS in a medical center involves a great deal of change, which, if not carefully considered, could result in significant difficulties. Using a case study approach, this research identifies appropriation issues when planning and evaluating MEBS usage in medical centers.

Literature Review

Changes in information technologies cannot be viewed as isolated events; rather, one must be mindful of the interdependent, reciprocally structuring relationships that exist between the information technology and the organization (Lucas & Baroudi, 1994; Orilikowski & Baroudi, 1996; Burkhard & Horan, 2006). One strand of research dealing with this type of incorporative change process is adaptive structuration theory originally posited by DeSanctis and Poole (DeSanctis & Poole, 1994) as an extension of Anthony Giddens' structuration theory (Gidden, 1979). Adaptive structuration theory focuses upon the interrelated dynamics embedded in the application/creation of the technology that is in use by the organization through the combined processes of human interaction, technology and organizational social structures (Lucas & Baroudi, 1994; Griffith, 1999; Furumo & Melcher, 2006). This study attempts to extend the research in adaptive structure theory through the de-

Figure 1. Research model (Adapted from DeSanctis and Poole's 1994 model)

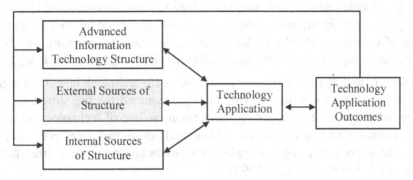

velopment of a modified version of DeSanctis and Poole's 1994 model. The model is depicted in Figure 1.

DeSanctis and Poole found that adaptive structuration theory over time, led to changes in the rules, processes and procedures that were used within group decision support system social interactions. In their study, DeSanctis and Poole defined adaptive structuration theory as "an approach for studying the role of advanced information technologies in organization change" (DeSanctis & Poole, 1994, p. 121). Their research, however, focused upon a "snapshot" of a meeting in which group decision support systems were being used to study interaction at the micro or individual level of the organization rather than at the institutional level. In light of their definition, adaptive structuration theory could best be applied from a longitudinal perspective rather than just an instance in time.

This study extends the scope of research in the area of emergent organizational structure by applying a modified version of DeSanctis and Poole's model to a management information system at the macro level of organization structure. Case study research is applied to describe and analyze the intraorganizational structural changes that develop in a multi-clinic Midwest-based medical organization as a result of the introduction and implementation of medical billing technologies into daily operations.

Structuration theory has been approached from three different schools of thought: institutional, decision-making, and socio-technical. The institutional school of thought viewed technology as an opportunity for change rather than as a causal agent of change (Kling, 1980; Barley & Tolbert, 1997; Rouge & Webb, 2004). Under this perspective, technology did not determine behavior. Instead, people generated social constructions of technology (Orlikowski, 1992; DeSanctis & Poole, 1994; Thatcher, Brower & Mason, 2006).

The literature focusing on the decision-making school of thought emphasized the cognitive processes associated with rational decision-making and adopted a psychological approach to the study of technology and change (DeSanctis & Poole, 1994). The socio-technical school of thought combined the institutional and decision-making perspectives by incorporating the power of existing social practices with the influence of advanced technologies for shaping interaction. This, in turn, was thought to bring about organizational change (DeSanctis & Poole, 1994; Bardhan, 2007).

DeSanctis and Poole continued along the socio-technical line of thought with adaptive structuration theory. This theory accounted for the structural potential of technology while maintaining focus upon the use of technology as a primary determinant of technology impacts. Their study examined the effects that occurred when advanced technologies were brought into social interaction to affect behavioral change (DeSanctis & Poole, 1994).

Few studies have examined the affects of the diffusion process from the perspective of adaptive structuration theory. The diffusion process was considered from beginning to end using the diffusion model posited by Kwon and Zmud (1987) and later modified by Cooper and Zmud (1990). Diffusion literature was applied in parallel to the foundational constructs of the adapted research model to define structure of advanced information technology, external sources of structure, internal sources of structure, technology application, and finally, technology application outcomes.

Figure 2. Research model

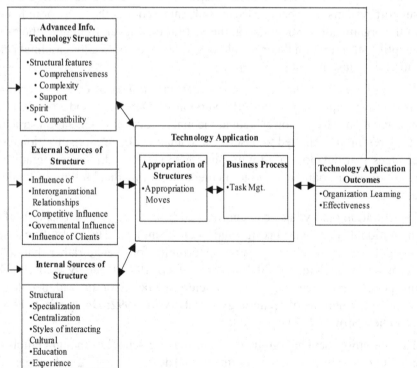

Research Model

By combining adaptive structuration theory (DeSanctis & Poole, 1994) with diffusion theory (Kwon & Zmud, 1987), a model encompassing both areas is proposed. The constructs of the model are defined, for the most part, using Kwon and Zmud's literature review on diffusion theory (Kwon & Zmud, 1987) and a simplification of DeSanctis and Poole's original model. The research model displaying construct definitions is presented in Figure 2. Each construct of the model is defined in the following paragraphs and illustrated in the accompanying tables associated with each variable.

Advanced Information Technology Structure

Advanced information technology structure is defined as the structural features and the spirit of the technology that outline the expected use of technology within an organization. One of the two elements of structural features includes the technology's comprehensiveness in terms of the number and variety of features and capabilities that users are offered. These resources direct how information is gathered, managed and manipulated by users (DeSanctis & Poole, 1994). The second element is the level of complexity defined as the degree of difficulty that users experience in using the new technology (Kwon & Zmud, 1987; Peters, 2006). Complexity can be affected by the ease of use of the application, ease of learning through tutorials, user-friendly screens, help screens, documentation as well as customer service and support.

Spirit of the technology is defined as the "general intent of the technology with regard to values and goals underlying the structural features" (DeSanctis & Poole,

Table 1. Advanced information technology structure construct definition range

Advanced Information Technology Structure			
	Traditional	———————	Customizable
Structural Features	Basic	———————	Full-featured
Comprehensiveness	Basic	———————	All-Inclusive
Complexity	Elementary	———————	Advanced
Support	Poor	———————	Rich
Spirit	Unfavorable	———————	Favorable
Compatibility	Unsuited	———————	Well-suited

1994, p. 126). Spirit defines the behaviors appropriate in using the technology and helping users understand and interpret its meaning to the organization (DeSanctis & Poole, 1994). The spirit of advanced information technology is defined by compatibility. Compatibility is related to the 'fit' of an innovation to an organization in relation to the organization's needs and its underlying goals and values (Kwon & Zmud, 1987; Avolio & Dodge, 2001). The construct ranges defining Advanced Information Technology Structure are illustrated in Table 1.

External Sources of Structure

External sources of structure consist of interorganizational relationships, governmental influence, competitive influence and client influence. Interorganizational relationships examine the influence exerted on an organization through affiliations with other organizations. Governmental influence examines the effect that government has on technology application decisions. Competitive influence explores the effect that competitive organizations have on technology application decisions. Client influence assesses the influence patients have on the organization. Thus, the external environment is related to the variability of the environment in regards to instability and turbulence provided by outside sources and the actions taken in regards to these variations (Kwon & Zmud, 1987). (See Table 2.)

Internal Sources of Structure

Internal sources of structure are divided into two parts: structural and cultural (Table 3). Structural sources of structure consist of specialization and centraliza-

Table 2. External sources of structure construct definition range

External Sources of Structure	Reactive		Proactive
Influence of Interorganizational Relationships	Reactive		Proactive
Influence of Competition	Reactive		Proactive
Influence of Government	Reactive		Proactive
Influence of Clients	Reactive		Proactive

Table 3. Internal sources of structure construct definition range

Internal Sources of Structure	Less Developed	————————	Developed
Structural	Less Developed	————————	Developed
Specialization	Generalized	————————	Functional
Centralization	Low	————————	High
Cultural	Less knowledgeable	————————	Knowledgeable
Education	High School Diploma/GED	————————	Advanced Degree
Experience	Little	————————	Extensive
Styles of interacting	Informal	————————	Formal

tion. Specialization is defined as a diversity of specialists within an organization in which individuals or groups of individuals have special functional skills (Kwon & Zmud, 1987). Centralization relates to the concentration of decision-making activity (Kwon & Zmud, 1987). A centralized focus increases the decision-making activity of upper management while a more decentralized organization can increase the decision-making capabilities of lower level employees.

Cultural sources of structure consist of education, experience and styles of interacting. The organization members' style of interacting can be influenced by a centralized structure, the formality of management operations and the boundaries of hierarchical or functional levels. Members of the organization are influenced by the knowledge, education and experience with technology, both actual and perceived, that others in the organization have.

Technology Application

Technology application is defined as the means by which the technology application outcomes are formulated. This portion of the model consists of two interacting variables: appropriation of structures and business processes (Table 4). The technology application process of the model is influenced by, and likewise influences, advanced information technology structure, external sources of structure, and internal sources of structure and technology application outcomes.

Appropriation of Structures

Appropriation of structures is the degree to which the members of the decision-making body agree on what structures should be accepted through adaptive moves as well as their application. Thus, the technology is defined through the use of its features by the organization rather than just its features alone (Reinig & Shin, 2002; Salisbury, Chin, Gopal & Newsted, 2002). This is influenced by the intended purposes and meanings associated with applying the technology. The technology structures can be used directly, related to other structures, replaced by other structures or interpreted as they are applied. Increased agreement on appropriation of structures can lead to greater consistency in the organization's usage patterns of advanced information technology.

Business Processes

Business processes are the actual courses of action that businesses perform in daily operations. Hunt defined business process as "a series of steps designed to produce a product or service" (Hunt, 1996, p. 3). Uses of technology and management of tasks can be in line with the appropriation of structures. As the appropriation of structures vary over time and across adopters, decision processes and technology application outcomes can likewise vary. The business processes determine how the technology can be implemented within the organization. Likewise, the management of the technology can affect implementation of the technology to accommodate business processes.

Technology Process Outcomes

Technology process outcomes are defined as effectiveness and organizational learning (Table 5). Organizational learning may be defined as gaining the necessary knowledge, skills (Attewell, 1992) and expertise (Premkumar & Ramamurthy, 1995) to effectively utilize a technology and apply it to business process. Cooper and Zmud (1990) defined effectiveness as the ability to take full advantage of the information system being implemented. This sub-property examines the fit of the technology as it has been applied to the needs of the organization and its related technologi-

Table 4. Technology application construct definition range

Technology Application	Traditional		Innovative
Appropriation of Structures	Traditional		Innovative
Appropriation moves	Traditional		Innovative
Business Processes	Traditional		Innovative
Task Management	Traditional		Innovative

Table 5. Business process outcomes construct definition range

Decision Outcomes	Low Quality		High Quality
Organizational Learning	Less Successful		Successful
Effectiveness	Less Favorable		Favorable

cal needs. The technology application outcomes are affected by the information gained through the technology application process as well as the implementation of the technology application outcomes. This, in turn, affects technology application processes as well as the medical electronic billing technology structure, external sources of structure and the internal sources of structure.

Research Method

A case study approach was applied to a multi-physician family practice located in the Midwest and identified as "Family Medical." This organization was selected for the study based upon its current level of growth and application of technology to business operations. Family Medical had been formed six years prior to the study when two separate practices, "Practice A" and "Practice B" consolidated their operations into Practice A's larger medical facility. Upon consolidation, Practice B's medical records were manually coded into Practice A's electronic billing system. Over the six year time period, Family Medical had faced tremendous change and technological upheaval as they first combined the operations of two separate facilities and then realized that a new billing application would be necessary to accommodate the aging technology and continuously swelling database. The combined medical practice had grown to provide services to over 22,000 patients and as Practice B's medical records were gradually added to the database, the efficiency of the system slowly declined.

The director of MIS and operations and a billing clerk were interviewed using a focused interview technique. The flexibility of the open-ended questions was supportive of the exploratory nature of the study and allowed for both the collection of facts as well as opinions. Through the utilization of multiple interviews, a more thorough clinic perspective was provided via observation through multiple viewpoints contributed by each medical office interviewee (Straub, 1998).

Documentation and statistics published by the U.S. Department of Health and Human Services, Healthcare Financing Administration, American Medical Association, and Medicare were reviewed as they related to medical clinic mandates and regulations. Through site visits, direct observations were made of the medical billing technology and billing procedures employed in the medical office. Information regarding processes, environmental conditions and office attitudes and structure were observed.

Results

The application of new technology into the business operations of Family Medical illustrated the complex interactions between advanced information technologies, internal and external sources of structure, the application of technology to business processes and, ultimately, the outcomes of the application of the technology to business processes.

The main contact person at Family Medical was "Steve," the business manager. He was in charge of overseeing several aspects of business operations including, accounting, billing operations and information systems. Although Steve recognized the benefits and necessity of technology in the medical office setting, he was still recovering from the stressful toll placed on his company by the latest technology overhaul and regretted losing the stability of the former system.

The previous system was a fairly fail-safe system. Employees just typed into dumb terminals on a Unix platform. It was very easy to use and there was little margin for the user error. The old application caused very few organizational problems unlike the new software. Actually, our old software matched the practice more so than the new software that we purchased.

The decision to purchase the new billing technology arose after the two practices joined forces and realized that they needed to update their outdated billing technology to accommodate current medical billing trends as well as the heavier usage of the system. Newer systems were capable of providing features such as system integration, graphical user interfaces, statistics and sophisticated charting and reports. Although Steve was more familiar with the managerial side of operations rather than the technical side, the Board of Directors elected him to lead the management team in the search for a medical billing system replacement.

It took 2 years for us to choose our billing software and we still chose a bad system. There were a lot of changes in the medical billing technology industry during the time we were trying to select a new system. It was like trying to hit a moving target. There was an evolution going on in the industry. We would go to one conference and the software and company would be there, then, we would go to another conference and the company would have been bought, sold or absorbed by another company. By the time we had gotten down to the actual selection, there were really only two or three integrated software packages to choose from. This was a bad time to have to be choosing a software package. There was too much volatility.

At the urging of the board of directors, the management team finally settled upon an application to recommend. They gathered their research and formalized a report to present at the next board meeting.

Ultimately, management chose the billing software with approval of the board of directors. The software was chosen based upon the features that it provided, specifically, the electronic medical records module of the medical clinic management features. The organization did not focus upon the features of the billing technology [in the practice management portion] of the application. Ironically, we have never been able to get the medical clinic management features to work correctly and the only part of the application that we utilize is the billing portion. In retrospect, we feel that we should have paid more attention to the practice management portion of the application.

Although the selected package came with numerous bells and whistles, Family Medical failed to focus on the features that most fit the needs of the organization and its application to business processes. Family Medical also failed to involve a contract lawyer in carefully delineating the responsibilities of the vendor and the associated timeline in which all parts of the implementation process were to be fulfilled. Several implementation factors were orally discussed and supposedly settled by representatives from Family Medical and the software vendor. However, as the implementation process unfolded, Family Medical found that several services provided by the vendor such as training, conversion, installation support and post-installation support did not quite meet their expectations.

The conversion and implementation processes were worse than they should have been. The installation team was interested in getting the application installed, but not necessarily right, and then moving on. We had so many problems that it was amazing that anything got done.

The changeover [to the new system] was to take place over a long weekend. Complications arose during the installation process and several of the modules would either not work at all or not interoperate with other modules in the system. ... Half way through the patient record upload, the system froze. The technicians tried repeatedly to upload the patient records, but due to "compatibility" issues between the new server and the data upload module of the application, the records would not upload and had to be entered manually. In the process of uploading the data, they had corrupted both the patient information as well as the old system rendering both systems unusable. On top of that, no backups had been created to use to restore the old system. Once most of the modules of the system appeared to be up and running, the vendor's installation team took off.

We didn't really know what would and wouldn't work until we started trying to use the system. When we started filing claims, we found out a lot of things were not right, we were not getting acknowledgments back and claims were not getting to where they were supposed to go. By that time, it was too late. The installation team had left and when we would call the vendor's support line, they would either not answer the phone or not return our messages. ... It took a whole year to track down every problem one by one and figure out why it happened.

Internal structure: The internal structure of Family Medical experienced tremendous upheaval. Before the new medical software was installed, the organization was functionally oriented around payer source with employees specializing in specific billing areas such as Medicare, Medicaid, big insurance companies, and so forth. In order to keep operations afloat, the formalized organization structure disintegrated and job responsibilities were assigned on an as needed basis. People were shifted from various positions to input records into the system.

At the beginning, it was a matter of trying to stay afloat. After the new technology was implemented, we frantically tried to enter all of the patients into the system and be prepared to bill patients on a daily basis. The most important thing that we had to do was to make sure that the patients that we had that day were in the system, covered and billable. The system was used for very little other than processing the day's billing. During this time period, everyone had to be able to help out in other positions. Except for the phone operators, there was no specialization. We moved toward a system where everyone had to do everything. The organization lost in terms of efficiency and speed. The levels disappeared and it was a matter of the company CEO working directly with the billing clerks in order to get the bills processed. Managers and senior account representatives who had more experience and expertise in terms of handling patients, helped in getting the charges and payments posted because we could not afford to bring in a lot of outside help to get everything entered. Patient demographic data is now being entered by reservationists rather than anyone who can be spared and we hope to go back to being more functionally oriented.

Employee morale and respect for various levels of the organization dwindled as problems continued to surface and blame was cast between departments. Areas throughout the organization were affected by the problems caused by the new system.

We went through a period of time when the clinic (medical side also) was waiting on the billing and insurance office to catch up. Everyone perceived the billing department as being very unfamiliar with medical billing technology as well as technology in general. They took some flack for not being caught up because cash flow was so affected. We did not have enough money to give raises for over a year.

At first, if you would have asked the employees if the managers knew what they were doing, they would have said, "No! They have no clue." We were seen as being pretty incompetent in this system, billing processes as well as other forms of technology. The managers were there on nights and weekends, struggling with the billing clerks to get patient records entered. The employees were influenced by seeing the managers get in there and work side-by-side with the people in the billing department. Now that things are starting to settle down in the billing department with the new technology, the attitude toward the competence of this department is no longer as harsh.

Family Medical utilized both informal and formal communication channels throughout the diffusion process. The organization took the standard training and then modified it and condensed the documentation to make it easier for the average person to read. Before the system was installed, they formally discussed with the employees, the benefits of getting the new system. They also encouraged the employees to be supportive in assisting each other in trying to learn and use the new system. After the system was installed and the clinic started experiencing problems, management held formal meetings to discuss the problems with the employees as well as actions being taken to remedy the situation.

We did a lot of ground work and training to try to prepare the employees for the new system. We presented the system to them as being an opportunity to receive training that they would never get anywhere else. We tried to let them know that they were being trained so that they could become familiar with the technology and be able to use any system.... Everyone was willing to share information. What one person learned, that person was ready and willing to share to make everyone's lives easier. ...Management also had to be very upfront and honest with their people and admit to the implementation problems and their level of difficulty. We had many meetings where the problems were discussed and we had to prioritize the issues.

Technology appropriation: Although the system that was purchased had numerous features for both the business and practice sides, Family Medical was unable to utilize its full capabilities. Not only did they have to deal with the installation problems, but they were also faced with the fact that they had purchased the wrong application to fit their business operations. Family Medical was resigned to using the features that they could get to work with minimal to no problems and that fit their operations, ignoring the features that did not fit their organization and continuing to attempt to configure those pieces of the application that they thought would fit their organization but were not yet functional.

The application has a lot of nice features if we could ever learn to use them. It's just too complex. It is more appropriate for a hospital rather than a medical clinic setting. It even has the wrong type of accounting system for what we need in a medical clinic. We purchased the application due to the medical record portion, but we've never been able to get it to work. We decided to leave the medical record portion of the application alone since it would not work. ...We could use some of the information for medical informatics if that part of the system worked. The potential is there, but we just have too many problems to use it.

Application to business processes: As the technology was applied to the business processes, Family Medical realized that they would have to adapt their daily business operations in order keep the business running. Their main concern was processing the patients to be seen that day so that the patient's information would be available when he/she arrived at the clinic and available for bill processing at the end of the day. They focused their energies on using the billing portion of the application and adapted their business processes to accommodate the technology that worked and the resources that were available. Ancillary operations were foregone to accommodate the more pressing business need of bill processing and payment. Without this function, Family Medical would be unable to finance continued operations.

It is difficult to separate where the problems were. There were some problems with the clearinghouse, some problems getting the information from the clearinghouse to the carrier, and some problems with the feedback process in place to make sure that all of the claims were electronically sent and received by the carrier. We have had to alter the way that we did things and our processes, to some extent, to fit the way that the software worked. The billing process changed due to the problems with the technology. We had everyone go through training for using the application for their job and then we had to move people to different positions in order to get jobs done. The management team had to decide what the priorities were and what could be done and what could be let go. There will probably still be things to catch up on a year from now. ...We let a lot of things go that would normally be done on a daily basis just because they were the priorities to keep the business running and to take care of patients. We were too busy trying to deal with the day's patients. ...

External influences: Overcoming internal application appropriation and implementation issues does not define the limits of the issues Family Medical faced in the application of the technology to business processes. There are several external factors that affected the appropriation of the billing technology to business processes. Due to glitches in the software, some of the bills were not being electronically sent to certain insurance carriers. Family Medical did not realize this omission of data until two to three weeks after the bills had been processed. This prompted them to start developing a system of checks and balances to implement in coordination with the insurances companies to insure that bills were being correctly received.

Their business processes were also heavily influenced by their interactions with Medicare as well as customers. As their biggest external business partner, procedural changes in Medicare's electronic claims handling increased delays in claims processing and thus, receipt of payments. Time gaps between the patients' office visits and when they would receive their bills added to the confusion of an already complicated document. In response, Family Medical prepared and trained additional staff to specifically handle customer billing inquiries.

...Some of our bills were not getting processed due to errors in the data tables. We didn't find this out until several weeks had passed. We are in the process of changing the system of checks and balances due to the problems that we have encountered with the new software. ...Most of the issues that arise from external sources are generated by Medicare. They are the most well-established of our external associates. Most of our problems with Medicare arise when they change fiscal mediaries or carriers. This affects the clearinghouse also. It really causes problems with our cash flow because we won't get paid on our processed claims for a while. When Medicare changes to a new carrier, Medicare stops processing claims for about six weeks, thus, this adds to the amount of time that it takes to get the money. Medicare also influences the software developers. They are the ones who have to look at the governmental mandates and write patches to keep their users in compliance.

The customer responses also drive our decisions. The customers are still not happy with the statements that they are getting. This will influence our purchase decision when we replace the current application. There are too many business problems that arise from people not understanding their bills.

Outcomes: Family Medical learned that they had to adapt their use of technology, business processes and organizational structure in order to maintain a minimal level of business operation effectiveness. They continue to wade through the numerous problems created by the implementation of their new medical technology and long for the proficiency of their original system. Although the new system has not been completely installed and configured, they have already begun discussing the possibility of purchasing a replacement system.

The employees liked the previous billing system and its ease of use and navigation. Even though the new system has a graphical interface, after all of the problems we have been through, they still prefer the previous system and would like to go back to it. ... We hope to be using another application in five years.

Discussion

There are several lessons that can be learned from the technology adaptation process experienced by Family Medical regarding choosing a technology, the purchase process and working with vendors and employees.

- **Solicit the input of effected employees in the purchase decision and process.** Family Medical's employees resented having a new technology pushed upon them and especially the fact that they found out about the new technology shortly before the changeover occurred.

- **Match technology features to business needs.** Family Medical chose technology based upon extra features that impressed them rather than the features that would fit the needs of the organization. Once the technology was installed, they found that the features that they needed were not what they had wanted but acceptable and the features that had enticed them to purchase the package were not even functional.

- **Establish priorities and be willing to adapt as needed.** Family Medical was forced to prioritize needs and make immediate and sometimes substantive adaptations in order to keep operations running. Job functions changed across several levels of the organization as the CEO moved from plotting long term strategies to assisting with data entry. The technology implementation goals of the organization changed from implementing an organization-wide comprehensive health information system to getting a few of the integral billing modules operational so the billing office could perform daily functions.

- **Obtain the services of a contract lawyer.** Several of the promises that the vendor had made to Family Medical were not in writing and were forgotten after the software was purchased. Training, documentation, installation, data integration, maintenance, support and updates are some of the factors that need to be determined before a purchase contract is signed.

Conclusion

Examination of the model through case study analysis illustrated the interconnected relationships between advanced information technology, external sources of structure and internal sources of structure on the technology application process. The research found that organizations might adapt any or all of those structures to accommodate the business processes or the appropriation of technology to the business processes. Business processes could also be adapted to accommodate the appropriation of the technology and vice versa.

As illustrated by Family Medical's discontinued use of the medical record module and its continued work with the configuration of the non-working modules, part of the technology appropriation process could be learning what features of the application do not work as well as what to do to accommodate and overcome technical difficulties. The capacity to manage business process tasks might require the organization to focus its energies and resources on one structure or certain aspects of structures and temporarily disregard others. To overcome their numerous technological problems, Family Medical found that it had to prioritize its business operations and focus its energies and resources on those processes that were integral to maintaining daily operations. Auxiliary processes were disregarded until the primary business processes were under control.

The adaptive structuration process is a cyclical process in which the organization continues to adjust to its structures as well as to structural changes. The study found that different iterations of the model could emphasize different characteristics of the variables. When the new technology was first introduced, for the most part, the organization utilized a functionally-oriented internal structure with employees assigned to completing the business processes for a particular payer. Due to the onslaught of problems associated with the introduction of the new system, the internal structure essentially disintegrated as available employees were assigned to work on the highest priority task at hand. As the problems became better controlled, the managers started to return the organizational structure to the functional focus.

One concern regarding previous adaptive structuration theory research was the lack of focus on one level of the organization. While analyzing the case study data and applying the data to the model, it was difficult to focus on only one level of the organization. Elements from the individual, departmental and organizational levels all seemed to provide influence in this analysis of adaptive structuration theory especially as the levels consolidated.

From observations of Family Medical, the researchers found that it is oftentimes best for an organization to delay the purchase of a technology if they are unable to find an appropriate system that provides a good fit with the organization and matches their most significant needs. However, this alternative is only a viable option if the current system is functional and supplementary resources can be used to maintain or achieve the required level of operations. Problems that arise in a system that is poorly matched to the organization will magnify the employees' level of dissatisfaction.

Communication to employees, both implicit and explicit plays a significant role in the diffusion process. In addition to normal information sharing methods, when problems arise during the implementation process, it may be necessary for upper level management to conduct frequent formal meetings to keep employees up-to-date on the status of the situation. As illustrated in the Family Medical case, the employees were greatly affected by the dedication and support management communicated as they worked side-by-side with the billing clerks.

By making adjustments to their internal and external structures, business processes, technology and application of technology, Family Medical was able to persevere through the technology diffusion process. Although several of the results of the diffusion process were rather negative, application of the case to the model verifies the reciprocal relationships between the constructs.

References

Attewell, P. (1992). Technology diffusion and organizational learning: The case of business computing. *Organization Science, 3,* 1-19.

Avolio, B., & Dodge, G. (2001). E-leadership: Implications for theory, research, and practice. *Leadership Quarterly, 11*(4), 615-668.

Bardhan, I. (2007). Toward a theory to study the use of collaborative product commerce for product development. *Information Technology and Management, 8*(2), 167-185.

Barley, S., & Tolbert, P. (1997). Institutionalization and structuration: Studying the links between action and institution. *Organization Studies, 18*(1), 93-117.

Burkhard, R., & Horan, T. (2006). The virtual organization: Evidence of academic structuration in business programs and implications for information science. *Communications of the Association for Information Systems, 17,* 1-37.

Cooper, R., & Zmud, R. (1990). Information technology implementation research: A technological diffusion approach. *Management Science, 36*(2), 123-139.

DeSanctis, G., & Poole, M. (1994). Capturing the complexity in advanced technology use: Adaptive structuration theory. *Organization Science, 5*(2), 121-147.

Furumo, K., & Melcher, A. (2006). The importance of social structure in implementing ERP systems: A case study using adaptive structuration theory. *Journal of Information Technology Case and Application Research, 8*(2), 39-59.

Giddens, A. (1979). *Central problems in social theory: Action, structure and contradiction in social analysis.* Berkley, CA: University of California Press.

Giddens, A. (1984). *The constitution of society: Outline of the theory of structuration.* Cambridge, MA: Polity Press.

Griffith, T. (1999). Technology features as triggers for sensemaking. *Academy of Management Review, 24*(3), 472-488.

Hagland, M. (1998). IT for capitation: Getting the whole picture. *Health Management Technology, 19*(9), 22-26, 45.

Hunt, V. (1996). *Process mapping: How to reengineer your business processes.* New York: John Wiley and Sons, Inc.

Kling, R. (1980). Social analyses of computing: Theoretical perspectives in recent empirical research. *Computing Surveys, 12*(1), 61-110.

Kwon, T., & Zmud, R. (1987). Unifying the fragmented models of information systems implementation. In: J. Boland & R. Hirschheim (Eds.), *Critical issues in information systems research* (pp. 227-251). New York: John Wiley.

LeRouge, C., & Webb, H. (2004). Appropriating enterprise resource planning systems in colleges of business: Extending adaptive structuration theory for testability. *Journal of Information Systems Education, 15*(3), 315-327.

Lucas, H., Jr., & Baroudi, J. (1994). The role of information technology in organization design. *Journal of Management Information Systems, 10*(4), 9-23.

Orlikowski, W. (1992). The duality of technology: Rethinking the concept of technology in organizations. *Organization Science, 3,* 398-427.

Orlikowski, W., & Baroudi, J. (1996). Studying information technology in organizations: Research approaches and assumptions. *Information Systems Research, 2*(1), 1-28.

Peters, L. (2006). Conceptualising computer-mediated communication technology and its use in organizations. *International Journal of Information Management, 26*(2), 142-157.

Premkumar, G., & Ramamurthy, K. (1995). The role of interorganizational and organizational factors on the decision mode for adoption of interorganizational systems. *Decision Sciences, 26*(3), 303-336.

Reinig, B., & Shin, B. (2002). The dynamic effects of group support systems on group meetings. *Journal of Management Information Systems, 19*(2), 303-325.

Salisbury, W., Chin, W., Gopal, A., & Newsted, P. (2002). Research report: Better theory through measurement-developing a scale to capture consensus on appropriation. *Information Systems Research, 13*(1), 91-103.

Straub, K. (1998). Financial systems: The next generation. *Health Management Technology, 19*(7), 12-16.

Thatcher, J., Brower, R., & Mason, R. (2006). Organizational fields and the diffusion of information technologies within and across the nonprofit and public sectors. *American Review of Public Administration, 36*(4), 437-458.

Chapter IX

Understanding Physicians' Acceptance of Computerized Physician Order Entry

Huigang Liang, Temple University, USA

Yajiong Xue, East Carolina University, USA

Xiaocheng Wu, Jiangyin People's Hospital, P.R. China

Abstract

Computerized physician order entry (CPOE) holds potential of reducing medical errors, improving care quality, and cutting healthcare costs. Yet its success depends on physicians' acceptance and usage. We test if TAM can be used to explain physician acceptance of CPOE. A survey study was conducted on physicians who have access to CPOE in a large general hospital in China. Data analyses based on 103 responses support all of the relationships predicted by TAM except the one between perceived ease of use and attitude. With additional data analyses, we find that the PEOU-attitude relationship is negatively moderated by physicians' experience of using CPOE. PEOU does not affect attitude for experienced physicians, whereas when physicians are inexperienced, PEOU has a positive impact on attitude. Our findings suggest that TAM can be applied to explain physicians' acceptance of CPOE, yet its application should be performed with caution.

Introduction

Ample evidence shows that CPOE systems can substantially reduce medication error rates, reduce costs, and improve the quality and efficiency of medication utilization (Bates et al., 1998; 1999; 2001; Kaushal et al., 2003; Kuperman & Gibson, 2003). However, healthcare organizations cannot assume that these benefits will automatically accrue after they implement a CPOE system. This is because IT assimilation is typically influenced by decision processes at two levels: top management decides whether to adopt an IT at the organizational level and employees decide whether and how to integrate the technology into their job routines (Fichman, 2000). It is possible that despite top management's advocacy of CPOE usage, physicians refuse to use the system, leading to project failure. User resistance of IT has long been a problem troubling organizations (Lapointe & Rivard, 2005). Compared to other users, physicians are characterized by a high level of job autonomy (Sharma, 1997) and are less willing to change their behavior to adapt to the usage of IT. Even after CPOE is adopted at the organizational level, physicians may resist it from the beginning or discontinue using it if they perceived the system as problematic (Anderson, 1997). For example, it is reported that during the CPOE implementation at a large healthcare system, some clinicians wanted to go back to manual order entry when they discovered the CPOE's drawbacks (Ahmad et al., 2002). Therefore, physician acceptance is critical to CPOE success. The promised benefits of CPOE cannot be realized unless physicians accept and use the system.

As an important aspect of medical informatics, user acceptance has drawn increasing attention from researchers and practitioners (Lorenzi et al., 1997; Kaplan et al., 2001). It has been recognized that efforts to introduce information systems (IS) into medical practice settings will result in failures and unanticipated consequences if their technical aspects are overemphasized and their social and organizational characteristics are overlooked (Anderson, 1997). The IS discipline has a rich tradition concerning user acceptance of information technology (Davis, 1989; Davis et al., 1989; Moore & Benbasat, 1991; Adams et al., 1992; Agarwal, 1999; Karahanna et al., 1999; Venkatesh, 2000a; 2000b; Venkatesh & Davis, 2000; Venkatesh et al., 2003). The technology acceptance theories applied in the IS field can certainly shed light on user acceptance issues in the medical informatics field given that theory should be generalizable. Among these acceptance theories, technology acceptance model (TAM) is the most widely used, dominant model (Davis, 1989; Davis et al.,

1989; Venkatesh et al., 2007). TAM asserts that users' usage behavior is largely determined by their intention to use the technology. Based on this relationship, TAM explains user acceptance by positing that users' intention to use a certain technology is determined by their attitude, which is shaped by two perceptions: perceived usefulness and perceived ease of use. That is, when users perceive a technology is more useful and easier to use, they will have more positive attitude toward the technology and will have more intention to use the technology. TAM provides an excellent tool to examine user acceptance by focusing on critical subjective predictors. It has been replicated among various types of information systems and in different countries, demonstrating a high level of robustness and generalizability (Venkatesh et al., 2003; Venkatesh et al., 2007). Hence, we contend that TAM is likely to be useful in explaining physicians' acceptance of CPOE.

Our motivation to conduct this research arises from the need of understanding physicians' acceptance of CPOE from a behavioral perspective (Lorenzi et al., 1997; Kuperman & Gibson, 2003) and the awareness that physicians are different from general business IT users due to their special competence in esoteric bodies of medical knowledge (Sharma, 1997). First, behavioral research on physicians' adoption of CPOE is lacking and theory-based research can greatly enhance our knowledge in this uncharted area. Second, it is necessary to test TAM in the context of physician acceptance despite its established legitimacy in the IS discipline. It is possible that the unique attributes of the healthcare context interfere with the relationships predicted by TAM. For example, TAM has been used to explain physician acceptance of telemedicine and it was found that perceived ease of use was not related to user acceptance behavior (Chau, 1996; Chau & Hu, 2001). This is inconsistent with TAM, suggesting that TAM may need to be adapted to account for the specifics of unique contexts.

In this chapter, we report a study that examines whether TAM can be applied to explain physicians' acceptance of a CPOE system. The objective of this study is to test the major relationships suggested by TAM in a large hospital in China and to provide explanations if TAM is supported.

This chapter proceeds as follows. We first describe TAM and develop a series of research hypotheses. Then details of a survey study are provided, following which results of data analyses are reported. After discussing the findings, we conclude the chapter with a short summary.

Technology Acceptance Model

Extant psychology and IS literature suggests that IT acceptance is not only determined by objective technological characteristics, but also, perhaps to a greater extent, by

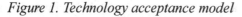

Figure 1. Technology acceptance model

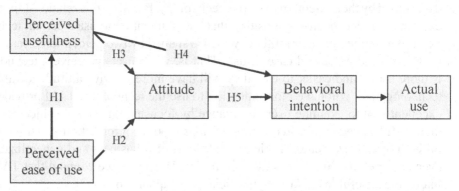

individual beliefs and attitudes toward the technology (Fishbein & Ajzen, 1975; Davis, 1989). In social psychology, theory of reasoned action (TRA) (Fishbein & Ajzen, 1975) is developed to explain how user beliefs and attitudes relate to behavioral intention. According to TRA, attitude toward a behavior is determined by beliefs about the consequences of the behavior. Beliefs reflect an individual's subjective estimate of the probability that performing a given behavior will lead to a given consequence. The causal relationship proposed by TRA is that external stimuli (e.g., technical features of an information system) flow through user perceptions, attitudes, and intentions to affect actual usage behavior. For example, the technical features of a CPOE system influence physicians' acceptance behavior by affecting their perceptions, attitudes, and intentions.

TRA provides a general framework that can be applied to a broad range of acceptance behaviors. Based on TRA, TAM is developed to more accurately delineate technology acceptance behavior (Davis, 1989; Davis et al., 1989). TAM posits that user acceptance is predicted by two beliefs: perceived usefulness (PU) and perceived ease of use (PEOU). PU refers to the degree to which people believe that using a particular system would enhance their job performance, and PEOU is defined as the degree to which people believe that using a particular system would be free of effort. As Figure 1 shows, PU and PEOU determine attitude toward using the system. Attitude leads to behavioral intention to use the system. PU also has a direct effect on behavioral intention. In addition, PEOU influences PU. The interpretation of this link is that given two systems offering identical functionality, a user should find the one that is easier to use to be more useful.

The goal of TAM is to explain information system acceptance and detect design problems (Morris & Dillon, 1997). The IS researchers have developed and validated scales to measure PU, PEOU, attitude toward using, and behavioral intention to use. The literature has shown that these scales are reliable, valid, and generalizable to a variety of information systems (Adams et al., 1992; Taylor & Todd, 1995; Chau,

1996; Straub, 1997; Fenech, 1998). Therefore, these scales can be employed conveniently in the context of CPOE acceptance, thereby avoiding time-consuming and costly effort to develop new measurement instruments.

To understand physicians' acceptance of CPOE, a series of hypotheses were developed based on TAM:

Hypothesis 1: *Physicians' perceived ease of use positively affects their perceived usefulness of the CPOE system.*

Hypothesis 2: *Physicians' perceived ease of use positively affects their attitude toward using the CPOE system.*

Hypothesis 3: *Physicians' perceived usefulness positively affects their attitude toward using the CPOE system.*

Hypothesis 4: *Physicians' perceived usefulness positively affects their behavioral intention to use the CPOE system.*

Hypothesis 5: *Physicians' attitude toward using the CPOE system positively affects their behavioral intention to use the CPOE system.*

Methods

We selected Jiangyin People's Hospital (JPH) as the study site. One of the China's 100 best hospitals, JPH has 1,150 open beds. It has more than 1,304 employees, among which are 429 physicians. To integrate information across departments, JPH implemented a hospital information system purchased from B-soft Group, one of China's largest healthcare information technology vendors. When this study was conducted, JPH installed CPOE systems in its outpatient departments and realized data integration of outpatient departments, pharmacy, and labs. Physicians were able to enter prescriptions or lab orders into computers during patient encounters. After seeing doctors, patients can go directly to the lab or pharmacy without taking paper-based physician orders.

JPH's CPOE is based on Windows operating systems. It provides graphical user interface. Most of tasks can be completed by using a keyboard and a mouse. All the orders must be entered in Chinese. Users have to use a Chinese input method such as Five Stroke or Pin Yin to enter orders. Users can also create order sets for individual use or departmental use. The CPOE supports drug-condition interaction detection.

The Chinese input methods are drastically different from the English input method, since the Chinese language is pictographic. In order to input Chinese into computers, each Chinese character is coded by its pronunciation or structure. The codes are a group of letters, which are similar to English words, but the output is Chinese characters (pictorial symbols), which look dramatically different from the codes. Hence, a mental mapping from coding to characters must be built, posing a challenge to novice users.

A survey method was used to collect data. All the outpatient physicians in JPH were selected as respondents of this study. One of the authors, the IT director of JPH, distributed questionnaires to 200 physicians in 32 outpatient departments. A consent letter was attached at the beginning of the questionnaire to inform respondents that participating in this survey was totally voluntary and the data would be confidential and only used for research purposes.

Questions included in the survey were designed to measure perceptions of physicians about CPOE. The constructs of TAM were considered to be latent variables that cannot be measured directly. Instead, several items were used to assess each latent construct. All the items (see Appendix 1) were adapted from prior research (Venkatesh et al., 2003). Appropriate wording changes were made so that the items fit our research context. For example, the technology of interest in the items was changed to CPOE. Each item is evaluated by a seven-point Likert scale where 1 represents "strongly disagree" and 7 represents "strongly agree."

Results

A total of 103 physicians completed the survey, resulting in a response rate of 51.5%. The average age of these physicians is 37.11 (SD = 8.08) and 68.4% of them are male. The physicians' computer experience is approximately 4.70 (SD = 2.80) months and their CPOE using experience is 3.90 (SD = 4.29) months. The physicians are associated with 20 different specialty departments, suggesting a

Table 1. Respondent characteristics

Variable	Mean	SD
Age	37.11	8.08
Education*	2.89	.49
Computer experience (month)	4.70	2.80
Typing speed (Characters per minute)	37.42	26.15
CPOE experience (month)	3.90	4.29

* Education level: 4 = Graduate degree; 3 = Four-year college degree; 2 = Two-year college degree; 1 = High school or lower.

reasonable representation of the hospital. Table 1 shows the responding physicians' characteristics.

Evaluating Measurements

Validity and reliability of the measurements are assessed by examining factor loadings and reliability coefficients. Cross factor loadings are obtained by performing a confirmatory factor analysis. As shown in Table 2, each item's factor loading on the construct which it is intended to measure (bolded) is greater than 0.70, showing convergent validity (Hair et al., 1998). Besides, each item's loading on its assigned construct is much greater than its loading on other constructs, showing discriminant validity (Gefen et al., 2000). To evaluate reliability of the instruments, Cronbach's alpha coefficients were calculated. The alphas for PU, PEOU, attitude, and behavioral intention are .91, .92, .97, and .84, respectively. All of the coefficients are well above the recommended value of .70 (Nunnally, 1978), indicating that these instruments are highly reliable.

Table 2. Confirmatory factor analysis

Item	Mean	SD	Usefulness	EOU	Attitude	Intention
U1	5.03	1.83	**.88**	.06	.29	.40
U2	4.50	1.92	**.93**	.17	.44	.47
U3	4.49	1.95	**.94**	.31	.39	.31
U4	3.92	1.71	**.79**	.25	.33	.48
EOU1	5.94	1.19	.21	**.82**	.10	.22
EOU2	5.65	1.33	.24	**.88**	.07	.19
EOU3	5.80	1.26	.20	**.90**	.12	.23
EOU4	5.89	1.21	.16	**.94**	.13	.23
A1	5.25	1.74	.46	.08	**.94**	.38
A2	4.97	1.76	.50	.11	**.97**	.29
A3	4.92	1.72	.49	.12	**.96**	.27
A4	5.02	1.74	.49	.12	**.94**	.28
INT1	5.59	1.64	.26	.14	.19	**.90**
INT2	5.51	1.72	.41	.05	.29	**.95**

Table 3. Hypotheses testing results

Hypothesis	Relationship[a]	B	F	R^2	Result
H1	PEOU→PU	.26**	7.07**	.07	Supported
H2	PEOU→A	.06	78.78**	.62	Not supported
H3	PU→A	.77**			Supported
H4	PU→BI	.22*	72.27**	.60	Supported
H5	A→BI	.59**			Supported

[a]   *A: attitude; BI: behavioral intention*

*   *p < .05*

** *p < .01*

Testing Hypotheses

Three linear regression analyses were conducted by using SPSS 11.5 to test the hypotheses. Average scores were computed for each construct so that a single value could be used in the regression equation. In the first regression analysis, H1 was tested by regressing EOU on usefulness. In the second analysis, EOU and usefulness were entered into the regression model as independent variables and attitude as the dependent variable. Similarly, the final regression analysis took usefulness and attitude as independent variables and behavioral intention as the dependent variable. As Tables 3 shows, except H2, all of the hypotheses were supported.

The data analysis results suggest that TAM is partially supported. While most relationships hypothesized based on TAM are confirmed, the PEOU–A relationship is not significant. This finding is quite surprising. PEOU, often in other terms such as usability and user-friendliness, has been found to be highly correlated with satisfaction of CPOE (Lee et al., 1996). It is widely acknowledged that healthcare information systems should be easy to learn and easy to use so that physicians who usually have an extremely busy schedule are willing to use them. Our finding about the role of PEOU in physician acceptance of CPOE seems to contradict this traditional wisdom. To explore why the data analysis shows that PEOU cannot affect physicians' attitude toward CPOE, we performed additional data analyses to examine the interaction between PEOU and CPOE experience.

Supplementary Analyses

Prior research finds that user experience has an impact on the importance of factors influencing IT acceptance (Taylor, 1995). It is possible that PEOU fails to affect attitude due to the moderating effect of physicians' CPOE experience. That is, PEOU's effect on attitude is contingent on the level of physician's CPOE experience. Physicians with more CPOE experience are likely to discount PEOU since they already know how to use the system, while physicians who have little CPOE experience tend to regard PEOU as an important factor when they evaluate a CPOE system. To verify this speculation, we conducted a hierarchical regression analysis to test the moderator effect of CPOE experience on the PEOU-attitude relationship. The multiplicative term of PEOU and CPOE experience was calculated to represent their interaction, as recommended by Baron and Kenny (1986). Change in the amount of variance explained ($\Delta R2$) is the most appropriate test of the significance of an interaction term (Cohen & Cohen, 1983). If entering the interaction term into the regression leads to a significant $\Delta R2$, we can conclude that the moderation effect exists.

The hierarchical regression consisted of three steps with attitude set as the dependent variable. In the first step, PU was entered into the regression equation as a control variable. PEOU and CPOE experience were entered into the equation in the second step. In the third step, the interaction term was entered. To include PU as a control variable is necessary to detect the true moderation effect. If usefulness is excluded, the regression coefficient of the interaction term may be inflated, leading to a type I error for the interaction term.

Table 4 shows the testing results of the moderator effect of CPOE experience on the PEOU-attitude relationship. PU accounts for 62% of variance in attitude. When PEOU and CPOE experience were added to the equation, there was no significant R2 change. Adding the interaction term did lead to a small but significant R2 change ($\Delta R2 = .03$, $p < .01$). The regression coefficient of the interaction term is negative. This suggests that CPOE experience negatively moderates the EOU-attitude relationship, meaning that when physicians have less CPOE experiences, their perceived ease of use has a stronger positive relationship with attitude, and when physicians

Table 4. The moderator effect of CPOE experience on the EOU-attitude relationship

Steps	β	F	R2	ΔR2	VIF
Step 1					
Usefulness	.79**	155.25**	.62	.62**	1.20
Step 2					
CPOE experience	-.07	52.49**	.63	.01	1.26
Ease of use	.08				1.13
Step 3					
EOU*CPOE Experience	-.20**	45.09**	.66	.03**	1.26

** $p < .01$

Figure 2. The moderating effect of CPOE experience on the PEOU-attitude relationship

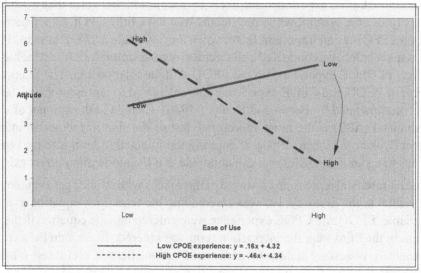

have more CPOE experiences, the strength of this positive relationship will diminish, disappear, or become negative.

In addition, the interaction between PEOU and CPOE experience was plotted. As recommended by Aiken and West (1991), two separate equations were derived for the high and low conditions (one standard deviation above and below the mean) of CPOE experience. As shown in Figure 2, when CPOE experience is low, the PEOU-attitude relationship is positive, whereas when CPOE experience is higher, the magnitude of the relationship decreases and finally the relationship can even become negative.

From the interaction plot, it is difficult to see which condition results in a significant PEOU-attitude relationship. The magnitude of the regression coefficients of the two equations might be deceiving. Therefore, more regression analyses were carried out on split data sets. We split the data into two sets according to the physicians' average CPOE experience (3.9 month): one set with 3.9 months or more CPOE experience, another with less than 3.9 months CPOE experience. Two identical regression analyses were conducted on these data sets by regressing PEOU and PU on attitude. The results indicate that when physicians have high CPOE experience, PEOU has a negative relationship with attitude, but this relationship is insignificant ($\beta=-.11$, $p=.45$). When physicians have low CPOE experience, PEOU has a significant impact on attitude ($\beta=.174$, $p<.05$).

Table 5. Regression analysis on split data sets

CPOE Experience	Hypothesis	Relationship	β	F	R^2
High (>= 3.90)	H2	EOU→A	-.11	15.27**	.58
	H3	U→A	.76**		
Low (< 3.90)	H2	EOU→A	.17*	71.92**	.68
	H3	U→A	.74**		

* $p < .05$

** $p < .01$

Discussion

TAM offers a parsimonious method for evaluating CPOE systems in use or under development (Morris & Dillon, 1997). Physician perceptions mediate technical characteristics of CPOE systems and offer an easy way to assess system acceptance. Developers can more accurately assess whether a system will ultimately be accepted by physicians by gathering physician perceptions of the system. As our data analyses show, 66% of variance of attitude and 60% of variance of behavioral intention are accounted for by the model, which verifies that TAM is a powerful tool in explaining physicians' acceptance of CPOE.

TAM can be used at various stage of the system development lifecycle of a CPOE system. System developers could easily use a questionnaire to gather user data concerning perceptions and attitudes about the target system. Potential acceptance of a system could be predicted at the design stage by surveying physicians about a prototype of the system. TAM could also be used to compare several designs in light of physician perceptions and attitudes. For example, several prototypes based on different designs may be developed and demonstrated to physicians. Then the physicians' perceptions of these prototypes can be compared to select the best design.

TAM can also be used to identify system design problems. For example, TAM might predict that a CPOE system is unlikely to be used because physicians believe the system would not be very useful. However, TAM cannot inform designers specific design problems and how to increase user perceptions of usefulness. The importance of TAM is that it could tell something is wrong with the system. This information is valuable because it alerts designers to examine the system design and ensure that the system sufficiently addresses key aspects of its intended users.

While we confirm the validity of TAM in explaining physicians' acceptance of CPOE, it is worth noting that user experience cannot be neglected when applying TAM. An important contribution of this study is that we identify the moderator effect of CPOE experience on the PEOU-attitude relationship. This finding helps explain the inconsistent effects of PEOU in previous studies.

PEOU has been found to both significantly determines healthcare professionals' acceptance of personal digital assistants (Liang et al., 2003) and have no relationship with physicians' acceptance of telemedicine (Chau, 1996; Chau & Hu, 2001). This inconsistency can be easily reconciled if experience is known as a moderator. The respondents in Liang et al.'s study are likely to be new to personal digital assistants, whereas those in Chau's and Chau and Hu's studies are likely to be experienced with telemedicine.

When physicians become more experienced with CPOE, they tend to put less weight on PEOU when they evaluate the system. Hence, ease of use is a significant factor influencing attitude of beginners, but the significance decreases and disappears as experience grows. This finding has implications for CPOE design and implementations. If we do not differentiate users according to their experiences, PEOU appears to be dominated by PU when users shape their attitude toward system use. This creates a false impression that ease of use is not important for CPOE. Guided by this false impression, CPOE designers may overly emphasize usefulness of CPOE systems by adding numerous complicated functions and underestimate the essential role of usability issue. Such systems are likely to encounter great acceptance problems since new users who have little experience with CPOE tend to resist using systems that are difficult to use.

A limitation of this study is that the respondents are from a Chinese hospital. It needs to be careful to generalize our findings to other hospital contexts due to differences in culture, norm, and healthcare settings. For example, hospital IT infrastructure and legal support for using health information systems are lacking in China (Liang et al., 2004). The efforts required to use COPE for Chinese physicians are different from those for American physicians. For example, entering Chinese characters into computers is dramatically more difficult than English data entry. These characteristics of the IT context in China undermine the generalizability of our findings. Nonetheless, we argue that, regardless of their nationality, medical professionals receive similar medical training and share some common characteristics such as professional autonomy and intellectual superiority which tend to transcend geographical and cultural boundaries. The commonality of the healthcare profession is likely to mitigate the generalizability concern. Another limitation of this study is the utilization of self-report to collect data. Common method variance (Podsakoff & Organ, 1986; Podsakoff et al., 2003) might be present in the data and lead to biased conclusions.

While TAM provides a parsimonious explanation of IT acceptance, it is also criticized for being too parsimonious and excluding important contextual factors (Bagozzi, 2007). This study can be extended by taking into account contextual factors such as social influences from physician clans, coercive pressures from the organization, and legal influences from the government. In addition, it is interesting to examine factors impeding CPOE adoption. For example, the impact of anxiety on physicians' acceptance of CPOE can be examined to generate insights.

Conclusion

This chapter describes an empirical study which finds that TAM can be applied to explain physicians' acceptance of CPOE. A considerable amount of variance of behavioral intention to use CPOE is explained by TAM. In addition, the study yields an important finding regarding the role of PEOU. It is found that physicians' experience of CPOE negatively moderates the effect of PEOU on attitude. This suggests that PEOU is a significant predictor of CPOE acceptance before physicians get substantial system usage experience. When physicians become experienced users, they are unlikely to perceive ease of use as an important factor.

References

Adams, D., Nelson, R., & Todd, P. (1992). Perceived usefulness, ease of use, and usage of information technology: A replication. *MIS Quarterly, 16*(2), 227-247.

Agarwal, R. (1999). Are individual differences germane to the acceptance of new information technologies?. *Decision Sciences, 30*(2), 361.

Ahmad, A., Teater, P., Bentley, T., Kuehn, L., Kumar, R., Thomas, A., & Mekhjian, H. (2002). Key attributes of a successful physician order entry system implementation in a multi-hospital environment. *J Am Med Inform Assoc, 9*(1), 16-24.

Aiken, L., & West, S. (1991). *Multiple regression: Testing and interpreting interactions*. Newbury Park, CA: Sage.

Anderson, J. (1997). Clearing the way for physicians' use of clinical information systems. *Communications of the ACM, 40*(8), 83-90.

Bagozzi, R. (2007). The legacy of the technology acceptance model and a proposal for a paradigm shift. *Journal of the Association for Information Systems, 8*(4), 244-254.

Baron, R., & Kenny, D. (1986). The moderator-mediator variable distinction in social psychological research: Conceptual, strategic, and statistical considerations. *J Person Soc Psych, 51*(6), 1173-1182.

Bates, D., Cohen, M., Leape, L., Overhage, J., Shabot, M., & Sheridan, T. (2001). Reducing the frequency of errors in medicine using information technology. *J Am Med Inform Assoc, 8*(4), 299-308.

Bates, D., Leape, L., Cullen, D., Laird, N., Petersen, L., Teich, J., et al. (1998). Effect of computerized physician order entry and a team intervention on prevention of serious medication errors. *JAMA, 280*(15), 1311-1316.

Bates, D., Teich, J., Lee, J., Seger, D., Kuperman, G., Ma'Luf, N., et al. (1999). The impact of computerized physician order entry on medication error prevention. *J Am Med Inform Assoc, 6*(4), 313-321.

Chau, P. (1996). An empirical assessment of a modified technology acceptance model. *Journal of Management Information Systems, 13*(2), 185.

Chau, P., & Hu, P. (2001). Information technology acceptance by individual professionals: A model comparison approach. *Decision Sciences, 32*(4), 699-719.

Cohen, J., & Cohen, P. (1983). *Applied multiple regression/correlation analysis for the behavioral sciences,* (2nd ed.). Hillsdale, NJ: Erlbaum.

Davis, F. (1989). Perceived usefulness, perceived ease of use, and user acceptance of information technology. *MIS Quarterly, 13*(3), 319-338.

Davis, F., Bagozzi, R., & Warshaw, P. (1989). User acceptance of computer technology: A comparison of two theoretical models. *Management Science, 35*(8), 982-1003.

Fenech, T. (1998). Using perceived ease of use and perceived usefulness to predict acceptance of the World Wide Web. *Computer Networks & ISDN Systems, 30*(1-7), 629.

Fichman, R. (2000). The diffusion and assimilation of information technology innovations. In: R. Zmud (Ed.), *Framing the domains of IT research: Glimpsing the future through the past* (pp. 105-127). Cincinnati, OH: Pinnaflex Educational Resources, Inc.

Fishbein, M., & Ajzen, I. (1975). *Belief, attitude, intention and behavior: An introduction to theory and research.* Reading, MA: Addison-Wesley.

Gefen, D., Straub, D., & Boudreau, M.-C. (2000). Structural equation modeling and regression: Guidelines for research practice. *Communications of the AIS, 4*(7).

Hair, J., Anderson, R., Tatham, R., & Black, W. (1998). *Multivariate data analysis,* (5th ed.). Englewood Cliffs, NJ: Prentice Hall.

Kaplan, B., Brennan, P., Dowling, A., Friedman, C., & Peel, V. (2001). Toward an informatics research agenda: Key people and organizational issues. *J Am Med Inform Assoc, 8*(3), 235-241.

Karahanna, E., Straub, D., & Chervany, N. (1999). Information technology adoption across time: A cross-sectional comparison of pre-adoption and post-adoption beliefs. *MIS Quarterly, 23*(2), 183-213.

Kaushal, R., Shojania, K., & Bates, D. (2003). Effects of computerized physician order entry and clinical decision support systems on medication safety: A systematic review. *Arch Intern Med, 163*(12), 1409-1416.

Kuperman, G., & Gibson, R. (2003). Computer physician order entry: Benefits, costs, and issues. *Ann Intern Med, 139*(1), 31-39.

Lapointe, L., & Rivard, S. (2005). A multilevel model of resistance to information technology implementation. *MIS Quarterly, 29*(3), 461-491.

Lee, F., Teich, J., Spurr, C., & Bates, D. (1996). Implementation of physician order entry: User satisfaction and self-reported usage patterns. *J Am Med Inform Assoc, 3*(1), 42-55.

Liang, H., Xue, Y., & Byrd, T. (2003). PDA usage in healthcare professionals: Testing an extended technology acceptance model. *International Journal of Mobile Communications, 1*(4), 372-3389.

Liang, H., Xue, Y., Byrd, T., & Rainer, K. (2004). EDI usage in China's healthcare organizations: the case of Beijing's hospitals. *International Journal of Information Management, 24*(6), 507-522.

Lorenzi, N., Riley, R., Blyth, A., Southon, G., & Dixon, B. (1997). Antecedents of the people and organizational aspects of medical informatics: Review of the literature. *J Am Med Inform Assoc, 4*(2), 79-93.

Moore, G., & Benbasat, I. (1991). Development of an instrument to measure the perceptions of adopting an information technology innovation. *Information Systems Research, 2*(3), 192-239.

Morris, M., & Dillon, A. (1997). How user perceptions influence software use. *IEEE Software, 14*(4), 58-65.

Nunnally, J. (1978). *Psychometric theory,* (2nd ed.). New York, NY: McGraw-Hill.

Podsakoff, P., MacKenzie, S., Lee, J., & Podsakoff, N. (2003). Common method biases in behavioral research: A critical review of the literature and recommended remedies. *Journal of Applied Psychology, 88*(5), 879-903.

Podsakoff, P., & Organ, D. (1986). Self-reports in organizational research: Problems and prospects. *Journal of Management, 12*(4), 531-544.

Sharma, A. (1997). Professionals as agent: Knowledge asymmetry in agency exchanges. *Academy of Management Review, 22*(3), 758-798.

Straub, D. (1997). Testing the technology acceptance model across cultures: A three country study. *Information & Management, 33*(1), 1.

Taylor, S. (1995). Assessing IT usage: The role of prior experience. *MIS Quarterly, 19*(4), 561-570.

Taylor, S., & Todd, P. (1995). Understanding information technology usage: A test of competing models. *Information Systems Research, 6*(2), 144-177.

Venkatesh, V. (2000a). Determinants of perceived ease of use: Integrating control, intrinsic motivation, and emotion into the technology acceptance model. *Information Systems Research, 11*(4), 342-365.

Venkatesh, V. (2000b). Why don't men ever stop to ask for directions? Gender, social influence, and their role in technology acceptance and usage behavior. *MIS Quarterly, 24*(1), 115-137.

Venkatesh, V., & Davis, F. (2000). A theoretical extension of the technology acceptance model: Four longitudinal field studies. *Management Science, 46*(2), 186-204.

Venkatesh, V., Davis, F., & Morris, M. (2007). Dead or alive? The development, trajectory and future of technology adoption research. *Journal of the Association for Information Systems, 8*(4), 267-286.

Venkatesh, V., Morris, M., Davis, G., & Davis, F. (2003). User acceptance of information technology: Toward a unified view. *MIS Quarterly, 27*(3), 425-478.

Appendix 1. Measurement Instruments

Usefulness (r = .92)

U1: *I would find the CPOE useful in my job.*

U2: *Using the CPOE enables me to accomplish tasks more quickly.*

U3: *Using the CPOE increases my productivity.*

U4: *Using the CPOE increases quality of care I provide.*

Ease of Use (r = .91)

EOU1: *My interaction with the CPOE would be clear and understandable.*

EOU2: *It would be easy for me to become skillful at using the CPOE.*

EOU3: *I would find the CPOE easy to use.*

EOU4: *Learning to operate the CPOE is easy for me.*

Attitude (r = .97)

A1: *Using the CPOE is a good idea.*

A2: *The CPOE makes work more interesting.*

A3: *Working with the CPOE is fun.*

A4: *I like working with the CPOE.*

Intention to Use (r = .84)

INT1: *Assuming I have access to the CPOE, I would use it.*

INT2: *Given that I have access to the CPOE, I predict that I would use it.*

Chapter X

Entrepreneurial IT Governance in a Rural Family Practice Residency Program

Carla Wiggins, Idaho State University, USA

John C. Beachboard, Idaho State University, USA

Kenneth Trimmer, Idaho State University, USA

Lela "Kitty" Pumphrey, Zayad University – Abu Dhabi, UAE

Abstract

This study describes and assesses the evolution of IT governance practices in a rural family practice residency program. The need to establish IT governance was driven by the practice's desire to implement electronic medical records capability. The authors employed a prominent information technology (IT) governance framework to conduct this assessment and exposed significant strengths and weaknesses in terms of the suitability of the IT gover-

nance framework within the rural healthcare setting as described. Given the relatively slow adoption rates within the healthcare industry in general, and among rural health providers more specifically, we present local knowledge (Geertz, 1985). In doing so, we provide an additional perspective for those seeking to construct theoretical bases for the formulation of health policy intended to promote the adoption of IT as a means of improving healthcare in the rural United States. In addition, this chapter describes the role of IT in enabling the residency practice to embrace current practice improvement initiatives.

Introduction

Healthcare is arguably the most transaction-intense industry in our society. Yet compared to other industries, healthcare has significantly underinvested in information technology (IT). Even today the vast majority of healthcare transactions occur via telephone, fax, paper, and electronic data interface (EDI). The result of this archaic information communication system is that much data is not captured, is captured incorrectly or inefficiently, and is difficult to retrieve and use (Barber, Caillouet, Ciotti & Lohman, 1994; Wager, Lee & Glaser, 2005).

Health information is typically spread throughout the healthcare organization and held in incompatible legacy systems with little or no interconnectivity or interoperability (Pendharkar, Khosrowpour & Rodger, 2001). These disparate systems need to be tied together. Healthcare executives are focused on improving the quality, reducing the cost, and expanding access to healthcare, but cannot improve what cannot be measured and cannot measure inconsistently captured or inaccessible information that is reported and held in non-compatible home-grown systems and databases.

In an industry where the paper medical record has been considered the "gold standard," electronic medical record systems (EMR), by capturing complete patient information, are believed to be an increasingly vital facet for improving: patient safety and quality of care, operational efficiency, and compliance with regulations while reducing medical errors and decreasing the risk of law suits. Still, an EMR is perceived by many to be a money pit rather than a source of efficiency, income, and enhanced quality of care.

United States healthcare is struggling with decision making, implementation, standardization, and connectivity surrounding the EMR. This is indicative of the unsystematic and independent nature of healthcare organizations in the United States. Fewer than 1 in 5 hospital information technology (IT) executives report that their organizations have a fully operational EMR. In fact, the number of healthcare organizations reporting a functional EMR actually decreased from 19% in 2004 to 18% in 2005 (Lawrence, 2005). Only 8% of physicians report using computerized order entry systems (CPOE) and only about ⅓ of U.S. hospital emergency and outpatient departments use EMR (Study shows limited use of electronic medical records, 2005).

Perhaps no single industry is as complex and convoluted in its structure, process, and "product" as the U.S. healthcare industry. It is constituted from a tremendously diverse set of public, private, and quasi-public organizations and agencies ranging in size from very small (i.e., solo physician offices) to very large (i.e., integrated health systems such as Kaiser Permanente and Hospital Corporation of America), cost reimbursement governmental programs (Medicare and Medicaid) and private organizations (Blue Cross/Blue Shield, and other private insurers). Additionally, it is often said that only the nuclear power industry is more heavily regulated than U.S. healthcare. In this schizophrenic environment, other healthcare organizations are both partners and competitors. Yet, within this complicated and multifaceted industry, organizations strive to meet their missions and serve their patients, constituents, and communities. How are decisions made in such an environment? More specifically, given the expected benefits of modernizing healthcare with information technology, how are IT governance decisions made in what is often referred to as a constant state of chaos?

This manuscript tells a revelatory story of a rural family practice residency program that implemented an EMR. The residency program, which trains primary care physicians and provides primary care services to widely disbursed rural communities, received a federal grant for the acquisition and implementation of the EMR, with the simple initial goal of enhancing the practice's clinical research capabilities. As the purchase and implementation of the EMR progressed, however, the practice's simple research goal mutated and morphed into a much larger goal of extending the system throughout rural clinics and providers in the region.

IT Governance in Healthcare

Traditionally, governance is "defining and realizing missions and goals, establishing strategic direction, policies and objectives to that end, and monitoring implementation" (McNally, 2003). Governance commonly concerns the patterns of authority that determine the use of organization resources and the integration of differences among organizational interests (Daily, Dalton & Cannella, 2003; Sundaramurthy & Lewis, 2003).

Viewed as a set of formal authority relationships, an organization's board of directors or trustees governs through its relationship with top management, and in turn, top management governs departments through its relationships among various subunits. IT governance parallels corporate governance in that it refers specifically to the patterns of authority over IT resources and the means for integrating IT interests.

IT governance decisions determine the design of the technical infrastructure, the form of application management, and the alignment of the organization's corporate strategy and integrated information practices (Sambamurthy & Zmud, 1999).

Weill and Ross (2004) define IT governance as "specifying the decision rights and accountability framework to encourage desirable behavior in using information technology" (Weill & Ross, 2004, p. 2). Furthermore, although the terms are often used interchangeably, IT governance and IT management are related, yet separate, endeavors.

Whereas the domain of IT management focuses on the efficient and effective supply of IT services and products, and on the management of IT operations, IT governance faces the dual demand of (1) contributing to present business operations and performance, and (2) transforming and positioning IT for meeting future business challenges (Peterson, 2004, p. 44).

Perhaps the trickiest aspect of IT governance is leaping that fence that divides the technical from the managerial world. While IT professionals certainly must go a long way toward being able to positively communicate with business process owners, functional managers need to invest a similar effort in understanding the terminology used within IT with a goal of recognizing how some seemingly technically-focused decisions have real business consequences.

Weill and Ross (2004) regard the establishment of IT principles as the most fundamental governance decision an organization must make regarding the employment of information technology. IT principles embody executive-level attitudes regarding the role information technology is to play in supporting the organization's mission and strategy. For example, while some healthcare professionals may view IT as a "necessary but evil" expense, other healthcare professionals may view information technology as providing a strategic investment that cannot only reduce the cost of providing healthcare but also ultimately improve the quality of healthcare provided. These attitudes are directly reflected in the organization's IT governance principles and policies and establish a basis for the identification of applications that the enterprise desires to implement. In the healthcare industry, applications directly contribute to patient care as well as support the organization's administrative functions. Decisions concerning IT principles and application needs drive the technical decisions concerning the organization's IT architecture and IT infrastructure.

Finally, the organization must make IT investment and prioritization decisions. Not only must management decide which software applications will best serve their organization's needs, but they must also determine how much to invest in the IT infrastructure.

These five areas (establishment of IT principles, identification of applications, IT architecture, IT infrastructure, and IT investment and prioritization) are the most important decisions made under the conceptualization of IT governance employed in this chapter. While architecture and infrastructure decisions may be quite technical, organizations with well-designed IT governance mechanisms ensure that the IT principles and application needs drive design and infrastructure investment.

It is important to note that Weill and Ross (2004) are less concerned with what decisions are made than with ensuring that organizations have effective mechanisms in place to make these decisions. In their study of IT governance processes at 256 enterprises, they found the ability of senior management to accurately describe how these decisions were made proved to be the best predictor of high governance performance (Weill, 2004).

The ability of management to describe decision-making processes is similar to the McGinnis et al. (2004) argument that traditional control theories of governance applied to IT may not apply in rural healthcare settings. Rather, these authors posit that governance is a pattern of social relations integrating organizational activities. Contrary to the dominant paradigms of hierarchy, power, and resource based governance, coordination and communication appear to provide the most effective mechanism for IT governance for at least some healthcare organizations.

IT governance processes largely determine the extent and effectiveness with which organizations adopt and use information technology. Healthcare organizations face uniquely challenging circumstances in establishing effective IT governance mechanisms required for the infusion of information technology into the day-to-day provision of medical services. Cost remains an almost insurmountable barrier to IT adoption, particularly in medical groups; many practices simply cannot afford the upfront costs. Medical practices also face physician and staff resistance to the use of EMR systems (Darr, Harrison, Shakked & Shalom, 2003). EMRs "have been over-engineered and are not intuitive, forcing physicians to spend more time clicking through screens and menus to get their work done" (Brown, 2005, p. 48).

While healthcare lags other U.S. industries in IT adoption, IT is increasingly vital to healthcare's efforts to fulfill its missions and reach performance and productivity goals (Goldsmith, Blumenthal & Rishel, 2003). The provision of high-quality care can be enhanced and better monitored by the effective and appropriate use of IT (Zabada, Singh & Munchus, 2001) According to the Institute of Medicine (1998), safety, effectiveness, patient centeredness, timeliness, efficiency, and equitability are the characteristics necessary for delivering excellent patient care. Each of these vital characteristics can be enhanced, monitored, and improved by the appropriate use of IT via effective governance.

Within the context of IT, an entity must continuously adjust to a rapidly changing environment or risk falling behind the competition. Healthcare entities have turned to, and have become increasingly dependent upon, IT as a means of creating efficiencies and providing more effective service.

Methodology: An Interpretivist Case Study Design

This study employs a single-site case study design to provide a fine-grained examination of the creation and operation of an EMR system in a university affiliated medical practice providing healthcare services to a rural population.

The research takes an interpretive philosophical approach illustrated by an analogy developed by Slife and Williams (1995). In describing interpretive ways of knowing, they ask the reader to consider the difference between a map of a city and an informal account of that city provided by a resident. The map, while admittedly an interpretation, represents an abstraction of an objective reality, depicting "only those features of the place that would remain unchanged *if no one lived there* (e.g., patterns of streets, layouts of buildings)." The informal account from the city resident is quite different although ultimately as informative, perhaps more so. While "necessarily personal, incomplete and biased…" the personal account might describe the best places to eat or sections of towns to avoid. By providing such description, the informal account "gives *meaning* to the town, from a native's point of view." Certainly, it is not the only description or possible interpretation but it is legitimate nonetheless.

As are many scholars, we are interested in understanding impediments to the adoption of information technology within the healthcare industry and the identification of viable strategies for surmounting those impediments. The selection of a single-site case study is particularly appropriate when investigating complex social phenomena where establishing appropriate boundary conditions between the phenomenon of interest and its environment is problematic (March, Sproull & Tamuz, 1991; Stake, 1994; Yin, 1994). The selection of a single-site case study was further warranted given the family practice residency's status as an early adopter of technology within its segment of the healthcare industry.

Research activities and processes included in this study can be grouped into the following categories:

- **Data collection.** While documentary evidence was examined, the primary data sources were 14 face-to-face interviews with seven key informants at the practice. The selection of participants was purposive, and snowball techniques identified additional informants. Key informants are listed in Table 1. Interviews were organized around the research question but were conducted using the "active interview" approach (Fontana & Frey, 1994; Holstein & Gubrium, 1994).

- **Data analysis.** Analysis consisted primarily of the creation of a case narrative that seeks to accurately reflect interviewee perceptions. The objective was to develop an accurate and rich description of a phenomenon as seen through the eyes of the study participants. Related literature is referenced to provide useful context.

- **Validity and reliability assessments.** The authors used the results of the unstructured interviews to develop narrative themes representing participants' varied perspectives. Where possible, we used participant checks to test whether our interpretation of interview data fairly represents participant views (Altheide & Johnson, 1994; Miles & Huberman, 1994; Patton, 2002).

Rather than conducting some variation of discourse analysis typically associated with interpretive studies, that authors' construction of the case narrative presented in the next section should be read as a case history and section "Impact on Clinical Functions" as historical interpretation or analysis consistent with a historical and ante-narrative method recommended by Dalcher (2004) as being particularly appropriate for the study of information system failures. While we do not perceive the subject implementation effort as a failure, the knowledge as it concerns IT governance practices is "fragmented, distributed and hidden with the context" (Dalcher, 2004, p. 306). Dalcher argued that traditional research methods are unsuitable for studying information system failures because of the emergent properties inherent in such failures and an inability to "clearly delineate causes and effects" (Dalcher, 2004, p. 306). We simply are extending Dalcher's methodological recommendation to include a wider variety of IS implementation experiences.

These procedures demonstrate the authors' commitment to employing disciplined data elicitation and analysis techniques consistent with recommendations of leading qualitative researchers and methodologists.

Table 1. List of key informants

Informant	Position
Joseph (Joe) Clark, M.D.	Director of FM
Robert (Bob) Wood, M.D.	Associate Director of FM
Rita Ford, Pharm D.	Director of Grants, Research and Information Systems
Anne Wright	Director of Information Technology
John (Jack) Hopkins, M.D.	Third-Year Resident Physician
James (Jim) Wilson, M.D.	First-Year Resident Physician
Mary Miller	Accounts Receivable Manager

* *Fictitious names used to preserve participant's anonymity.*

Family Medicine

Family Medicine (FM) is a health provider in the intermountain region of the Rocky Mountains that also serves as a residency program (RP). RPs for family medical practice typically require three years of post-doctoral experience as physician to completes their training. FM's RP is a department in the College of Health Professions at the regional university. FM is located in a city of 55,000, a regional hub for farming and ranching communities. In addition to providing family medicine, the residency physicians also participate in outreach to rural healthcare clinics within the region, rotating within the five rural clinics managed by another partner, Healthy West (HW). The residency program at FM is also part of the demonstration: assistance in rural training (DART) project, a regional funding program for residency rotation in the rural environment.

FM is managed by a Director, Joe Clark, M.D. who is on the faculty of the university and on the staff of physicians at the Regional Medical Center (RMC). All physicians and residents at FM are on both the university faculty and hospital staff.

There are two additional upper management positions at FM. Bob Wood, M.D., is associate director and Rita Ford, Pharm D. is director of Grants, Research, and Information Systems. Wood and Ford had been pursuing acquisition of an electronic medical record (EMR) system with numerous unsuccessful grants. A principal jus-

Figure 1. Family medicine relationships

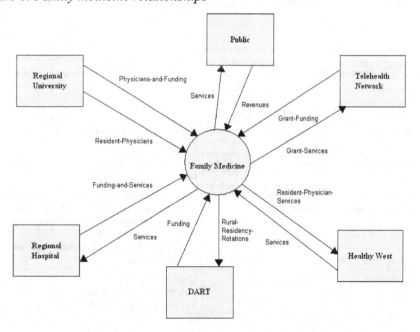

tification for the EMR was quality data for research purposes. An opportunity arose for FM to address its EMR needs by participating in a grant request by the Telehealth Network (TLN) of the university, as TLN also shared in the rural healthcare mission. The environment that FM operates within is represented in Figure 1.

An in-depth discussion of the project to acquire and implement the EMR is discussed elsewhere (Dalcher, 2004). A timeline of the events involved in the selection and implementation of the system is represented in Table 2. A brief discussion follows.

After receiving the grant, Clark initiated an investigation into EMR systems. Clark consulted with colleagues regarding the feasibility of an EMR. A committee of physicians experienced with EMR evaluated a number of systems, narrowing them to three viable, wireless-enabled, EMR systems.

Following system selection, Clark hired Anne Wright who designed, acquired, and built the wireless network that would serve as the system's backbone. Next, a third-year resident, Dr. Jack Hopkins, spent a week at a medical practice that had recently implemented the selected system, General Electric's Centricity.

After Hopkins' return, Wright planned the implementation of the EMR. First, she began to build interfaces with the hospital system to enable Mary Miller, accounts receivable manager, to phase in the billing system. Miller spent approximately three months making certain that charges generated by both FM and the hospital for FM patient services were accurately captured and billed. At the end of this reconciliation period, FM began to invoice patients and insurance providers and maintain their accounts receivable independent of the hospital billing system. Next, Wright began to build interfaces between the hospital's laboratory, radiology, and pharmacy to

Table 2. Sequential events in electronic medical record implementation at Family Medicine

Event	FM Participants in study	Actions
Grant Process	Wood, Ford	Grant received for systems in both statewide Residency Programs.
System Selection	Clark	Advising group formed, EMRs assessed, EMR software selected; IT Director hired.
System Implementation	Wright, Hopkins, Miller, Wilson, Clark	Hardware selected, visits made, system installed, users trained, data input, system maintained, common system configuration implemented, chart room eliminated, transcription eliminated Advising group formed for system implementation conflict resolution.
Implementation Follow-up	Wood, Wright, Wilson	Quality of data source, addition of information technology assistant, benefits of broad system availability, additional time for file maintenance

provide the systems charting functions with supporting data. Third, patient data was input as data entry personnel were being trained on the system. Finally, Hopkins assisted in providing training on using the EMR to FM's other physicians.

As the initial EMR implementation at FM was commencing, Wright began to extend the system to the residencies of physicians and residents. For example, first-year resident Jim Wilson received training in the EMR at the clinic from Hopkins, and had his home system configured for terminal server services by Wright. Wilson, a native of the region, will have received almost all of his residency training with an EMR, and can do his paperwork and patient research from his home as well as the clinic.

An overriding strategy for systems implementation governance was initiated by Clark. The advisors from system selection had warned Clark about conflicts that frequently arose during the implementation of EMRs. To alleviate this, Clark formed an implementation advisory committee which consisted of community members, hospital representatives, and a network of associates who had been 'down the path' of EMR implementation. This committee enabled Wright to mitigate opposition to specific system implementation issues by providing firm guidance in areas of physician and staff systems conflict.

The chart system was eliminated from FM six months after the initiation of system conversion. One year after the initiation of the conversion, Wood noted that a major benefit of the system was chart availability. The EMR enabled the physician to access a patient's data anywhere in the FM complex and on the hospital campus, no longer did physical charts need to be located. A downside to this, mitigated by the elimination of the transcription department, was the time it took to input the results and assessment of patient visits. Wood also commented that the conversion from the paper system to the EMR made them aware of inaccuracies in the previous chart system.

Twelve months after initiating the system conversion, Wright saw herself in an enhanced role. The remaining funding from the grant was being used to implement a similar system in the state's other residency program. Wright found herself as a consultant for this project in addition to supervising an IT support person at FM.

Discussion

While this study was originally conceived of as a traditional IS implementation case, the authors' attention gradually was drawn to the ad hoc, almost serendipitous, manner in which the EMR project was conceived, developed and implemented. Having a general familiarity with the IT governance literature briefly discussed in section IT Governance in Healthcare as well as recognizing the common perception that the health industry has been slow in its adoption of information technology, we refocused our analysis and conducted follow-up interviews to obtain a better understanding of the influence of formal and informal IT governance mechanisms on the formulation and execution of the EMR initiative. In this section, we extend our discussion of relevant IT governance literature and applicable U.S. healthcare policy to further lay the groundwork for our identification and analysis of four issues to be addressed in the development of IT governance mechanisms particularly relevant to the diffusion of IT-enabled healthcare services in the rural United States.

The benefits expected to be derived from information technology are so significant that in 1996 the U.S. government enacted the Health Insurance Portability and Accountability Act (HIPAA). The act directed U.S. Department of Health and Human Services to provide a set of rules governing health information. The rules have been created to standardize the communication of electronic health information between and among healthcare providers to protect and secure private individually identifiable health information. Notably, the legislation does recognize potential risks associated with establishing an EMR system, nor does it include significant provisions intended to safeguard patient privacy (Fedorowicz & Ray, 2004).

Despite perceived benefits and the legislative mandate of HIPAA rules, progress in the implementation of EMR capabilities has been slow (Lawrence, 2005) and resistance exists to the use of EMR systems, particularly on the part of physicians (Darr, Harrison, Shakked & Shalom, 2003). Furthermore, studies exist indicating that practicing physicians and other healthcare professionals have reason to be cautious concerning much of the hyperbole expounding the cost savings and healthcare benefits to be derived from EMR systems. In a seminal article, Eric Brynjolfsson failed to find any significant correlation between increased IT investments and multiple measures of financial success indicating that IT investments do not always deliver the anticipated benefits (Brynjolfsson, 1994). While there have been many explanations offered for his unexpected and counter-intuitive finding, the conclusion that must be drawn is that organizations are capable of making good and not so good investments in information technology.

The research on IT governance has provided important insights into an organization's ability to effectively translate IT investment into desired outcomes. Weill and Ross declared "IT value depends on more than good technology" and suggested "when senior management abdicate to IT executives' responsibility for IT success, disaster often ensues" (Weill & Ross, 2004, p. 17). Based on their extensive research, they have concluded "effective IT governance is the single most important predictor of the value an organization generates from IT" (Weill & Ross, 2004, p. 3-4). Accordingly, an examination of the IT governance function associated with the implementation of EMR at FM practice should prove useful.

As discussed above, Weill and Ross (2004) identify key IT governance decisions: IT principles, IT architecture, IT infrastructure, business application needs, and

IT investment priorities. Then they propose alternative arrangements that can be employed by organizations for making these decisions.

Without intending criticism of Weill and Ross's work, the FM case does not easily conform to the models depicted in their governance arrangement matrix. An analysis of this lack of fit provides insight into the unique challenges faced within the healthcare industry and suggests a need for further elaboration of IT governance theory to better accommodate the needs of enterprises operating in complex inter-organizational environments.

To explore this issue further within the context of our case study, we focus our discussion on four important areas: defining the enterprise, scale and resources, social governance, and cautionary observations.

Defining the enterprise. While not discounting the emergence of complex inter-organizational relationships emerging in many commercial industries, establishing or defining pragmatic organizational boundaries within the health industry is uniquely difficult. As outlined above, FM is a cooperative venture jointly supported by a public university and locally (county) owned regional medical center. Furthermore, FM, by hosting general residences, must maintain a relationship with and support the standards of the broader medical education community and the DART regional medical consortium.

The governance models proposed by Ross and Weill apply to a more cohesive organizational form where enterprise boundaries, while complex, are still generally identifiable. The governance models then apply within the context of these relatively well- defined organizational boundaries. The quasi-public and heavily regulated organizational environment in which FM operates simultaneously permits a degree of independence and entrepreneurship with respect to FM internal operations and initiatives yet FM remains answerable to and under the jurisdiction of two much larger and independent institutions, that is, the regional medical center and the local university. This was particularly evidenced by the State's delay in purchasing the selected EMR product based on a prior contractual relationship with another EMR provider.

Despite the complex set of inter-relationships, FM was able to act in an entrepreneurial manner in initiating this EMR project. Lacking many of the formal policies and decision-making mechanisms associated with larger enterprises, FM established an advisory committee to participate in making substantive project decisions. The use of this ad hoc advisory committee additionally served to promote the active cooperation of its larger governing institutions.

As enterprises increasingly cooperate in the development of standardized IT-enabled processes, IT governance models will likely require elaboration to reflect the external entities (e.g., industry standards organizations) that may strongly influence application and infrastructure development dictating the magnitude and allocation of IT resources. We do not mean to imply that organizational management will be able to abrogate its IT governance responsibilities. On the contrary, greater effort will be required to monitor and perhaps attempt to influence external developments so that organizational needs can be met. While much of this effort will necessarily lie within the technical domain, the significant intertwining of technology and business (healthcare) processes will necessitate the involvement of medical and administrative professionals.

Scale and resources. Despite its close association with two multi-million dollar enterprises, FM is a relatively small, independent organization that, on a general scale and scope, resembles many private physician practices. On average, FM sees 60 patients per day with an average of 15,660 patient visits per year. FM's current practice size is 12,000 patients.

There are 14 resident physicians at FM, whose salaries are funded by the University and RMC, as is Clark's salary. Three residents graduated in 2005, bringing the number of program graduates to 50, half of whom are practicing in rural communities. Presently, there are 17 physicians in the residency program. The remaining staff of 20 employees is funded by RMC. FM contributes positive cash flows to RMC.

Without the availability of the TLN grant, this initiative could not have been undertaken. There was no anticipated financial return on EMR investment for the FM. Certainly, there are various financial savings resulting from reducing some of the labor-intensive administrative processes, for example, transcription of physician notes and maintaining paper medical records. However, these savings were not expected to cover the full cost of the software application and expanded IT infrastructure.

In addition to supporting FM's somewhat unique research mission, the benefits of EMR are expected to accrue over time in the form of improved healthcare for patients for a variety of reasons more fully described in other literature (see for example Amatayakul, 2001; Chung, Choi & Moon, 2003; Stausberg, Koch, Ingenerf & Betzler, 2003; Rosenbloom, Grande, Geissbuhler & Miller, 2004; Brown, 2005; Hough, Chen & Lin, 2005; Snyder, Paulson & McGrath, 2005).

The expected quality of healthcare benefits is certainly non-trivial. However, the extent and timing of improved healthcare are not known with certainty and have not been quantified. Furthermore, given the structure and rigidity of Medicare, Medicaid, and third-party reimbursement policies, the cost of improving healthcare cannot be passed on to the majority of FM's patients.

In short, it is difficult for small and independent practices to justify making investments in EMR particularly until the full costs of implementing and operating an IT infrastructure with requisite degrees of performance, reliability and security are truly understood. The Weill and Ross IT governance model primarily reflect the profit-making motivation of modern commercial enterprises in their discussion of establishing principles. Given the diverse participants, in both size and profit motivation, and given the public good anticipated to result from more effective IT employment within the health services industry, the establishment of effective IT principles becomes paramount. Healthcare participation in the development of IT principles will likely be expanded beyond the decision archetypes identified.

Social governance. FM faces complex governance challenges. It operates under the supervision of two significant yet independent institutions: the University and the Regional Medical Center. It is obliged to support the disparate needs of these two institutions, yet operates largely as an independent practice. The convoluted governance structure has contributed to the evolution of socially constructed collaborative governance processes focused on identification and accomplishment of jointly held objectives in a manner that virtually defies clear explanation. The social collaborative processes conducted among members of these distinct institutions and within the FM practice provided the basis for the entrepreneurial approach observed in the launching and execution of the EMR project.

The initial motivating idea for launching the EMR project at FM was straightforward and needs-driven. A practicing physician with research and educational responsibilities desired a better way to analyze data generated by the FM practice. Lacking resources, a search for grant funds resulted. In seeking the grant funds, the researcher's needs were aligned with state and federal initiatives to improve rural healthcare, which legitimately related to the mission of the practice. In evolving its project goals to meet this broader objective, FM management displayed flexibility and opportunism reminiscent of the "garbage can" model of decision making described by Cohen, March and Olsen (1972).

The social collaborative culture of the enterprise was further demonstrated by the ad hoc creation of the advisory board that assisted in the refinement of technical and functional requirements, evaluated alternatives and recommended the product that was finally purchased. In addition, a separate ad hoc group was utilized to assist in the actual system implementation. As internal participants negotiated the configuration and use of the application, a group of physician practitioners experienced in using EMR was recruited. This second committee counseled the practice concerning implementation and use of specific features and provided an independent third party to deflect, depersonalize, and resolve conflicts among the practice's staff.

The pattern of decision making appears to fit with the McGinnis et al. (2004) work specific to the healthcare industry. In that study of rural healthcare providers, the authors posited that the overall institutional governance reflected a pattern of social relations employed to integrate organizational activities. Both cases emphasize the importance of informal organizational mechanisms and are consistent with other research investigating strategic IT alignment (Chan, 2002). The importance of emergent social relationships contrasts with the structural determinants typically described in governance research. Tellingly, Weill and Ross concluded that the specific pattern of IT governance mattered less than the ability of study participants to accurately describe the governance processes used within their respective organizations (Weill & Ross, 2004). While not explicitly addressing the issue of informal organizational relationships, their findings appear to indicate that a strong degree of "transparency" within the governance processes is indicative of more effective IT governance. It becomes a question for future research as to whether such transparency is associated with the development of strong social relationships identified by McGinnis, et al. (2004).

Cautionary notes. Thus far we have focused on the positive aspects of the FM's EMR initiative. Yet the ad hoc approach to the formulation of this initiative has engendered risks as well.

The two physicians most responsible for the initiation of this effort, Clark and Wood, confess to having a relatively limited knowledge of information technology. While this undermines any argument that technology is being chased for technology's sake, there was a risk that the resource and management commitments required to maintain reliable and secure services, once implemented, would not be fully understood.

A technical lead was not hired until after the grant had been awarded. Fortunately, FM was able to bring on an exceptionally talented individual. Admittedly, the previous statement smacks of hyperbole, but we shall explain. One person assumed overall technical responsibility for:

- Design, specification and implementation of required IT infrastructure
- Installation, configuration and customization of EMR applications and supporting data base management systems (DBMS)
- Complete oversight of the execution of migration from paper to electronic records
- Coordination and development of customized interfaces with regional medical center applications, for example, billing, scheduling and laboratory applications
- Development and implementation of security architecture including compliance with HIPAA guidelines and regulations
- Provision of user training and being FM's help desk

Essentially, one individual is serving as strategic IT planner, systems (including servers, desktops, tablet PCs, network, DBMS and applications) architect, project manager, systems administrator (for all systems identified above), trainer and help desk.

Therein lies a serious problem. Beyond the apparent difficulty in identifying an individual possessing requisite technical and managerial knowledge and skills to accomplish these tasks, there is an important contingency that a single individual is unable to address. That is, Anne Wright, even with an assistant, constitutes a single and absolutely critical point of failure. While this type of problem is not unheard of even in very large enterprises, it far too common in small healthcare practices. This "single point of failure" structure is evidence of weaknesses in the IT governance processes in this study and has significant implications for the healthcare community as discussed below.

Impact on Clinical Functions

Subsequent to the implementation of the EMR, FM has been able to assess the impact of the EMR on clinical functions. This section briefly summarizes the initial justification for the EMR and presents an update of the current state of clinical functions due to the EMR at FM.

While the impact of the electronic health record on clinic operations at the FM has been qualitatively pervasive and profound, the objective measurement of this impact is complex. The EMR implementation was funded largely by a federal line item appropriation. The primary objective of this funding was to transform the clinical records at FM into a searchable electronic clinical database for research and quality assurance purposes. The advent of the EMR has augmented the Department's academic functions and has been critical in efforts to access external funding. The database has been searched on multiple occasions for potential subjects who meet eligibility criteria for clinical research study protocols, resulting in improved efficiency and increased research productivity. The EMR has resulted in a set of initiatives that will be discussed within the context of the four important areas outlined in our discussion

Defining the enterprise. The Department's current Health Resources and Services Administration Title VII project, "Quality as Culture: Teaching the New Model of Practice," is designed to improve quality of patient care while implementing components of the American Academy of Family Physician's Future of Family Medicine (FFM) initiative (American Academy of Family Physicians, n.d.). EMR implementation is central to the FFM. FFM recommendations promote practice measurement for quality outcomes and patient safety as well as implementation of the multidisciplinary chronic care model. The project also includes a transition of care program that is dependent on remote access to the electronic clinical database. Availability of the existing EMR clearly improved the likelihood of project approval in an increasingly competitive grant funding environment.

The EMR is available at both FM and the local hospital. In addition to laboratory reports performed at the hospital, the residents and other physicians at FM now have access to the radiology system. Furthermore, prescriptions can now be entered electronically and filled online at local pharmacies.

Scale and resources. The EMR has allowed the Department to participate in efforts at the state and federal level to document adherence to best practices and thereby enhance reimbursement. The State Medicaid Office has used the clinic as a test site for their new pay-for-performance program. The clinic has also led the community in participation in Medicare's Physician Quality Reporting Initiative. The Family Medicine Center did experience a 9.9% reduction in total clinic visits in the year of EMR implementation (2004-2005). This has been followed by increases above the 2003-2004 baseline of 7.6% in 2005-2006 and 16.3% in 2006-2007. Total clinic visits reached 17,800 for the fiscal year ending June 30, 2007, which is an increase of approximately 2,400 patients per year. Because of a number of coincidental changes in provider staffing levels and clinic processes, neither the initial decrease nor the subsequent increases in annual visit numbers can be fully accredited to the impact of the EMR implementation. However, it is clear to management that the EMR did not handicap FM in increasing their patient visits. In addition, the EMR has enabled FM to refine their clinical process workflow.

Social governance. As previously discussed, FM has two major constituents, the state university and local hospital. The EMR has facilitated academic and grant-oriented initiatives at the university. FM's EMR is available for all FM residents and physicians while at the hospital, and provides a seamless interface between patient health records residing at either the hospital or FM.

In addition, with the last class of residents graduating that had spent all but the first six months of their residency with the EMR, the education of residents at FM is extending the use of EMR to additional health providers. One of the former residents will work for Healthy West while remaining a preceptor at FM. It should be noted that Healthy West is currently in the process of assessing EMRs. This formal resident is a strong proponent of EMRs.

An additional resident from this class has joined a family medicine practice in a nearby community in the same geographic region. This practice is co-located with a variety of other healthcare providers within the same physical facility. This entire group of healthcare providers is currently in the process of implementing an EMR.

In addition, the former resident has brought the family medicine practice in this area together with the Department of Family Medicine to provide an additional rotation facility for the residents at FM. Further evidence of the role of social governance is demonstrated in the support function that the IT staff at FM is providing to this EMR implementation.

Cautionary notes. Efficiencies provided by the EMR due to more accurate patient billings has enabled FM to hire an assistant to Anne Wright. The assistant provides more of operational support. This helps mitigate the reliance on Anne pointed out previously. The assistant also provides FM with the ability to maintain the EMR at all times. Furthermore, the increase in IT staff has enabled FM to establish support relationships with other local healthcare providers. The availability of technical support and resulting IT infrastructure has enabled FM to create resources that are scalable, in that they not only enable internal efficiencies at FM, but also allow them to extend their resources to the wider regional healthcare environment, thus extending their social governance.

An additional example of social governance is the addressing of the overall shortage of qualified IT personnel in health professions. The University, through the College of Business, College of Health Professions, and Department of Family Medicine, will offer an undergraduate degree focusing on business, information, operations, and healthcare topics. As a culmination to this program, graduates will be required to serve a practicum with FM and the EMR.

Conclusion and Limitations

In summary, governance serves to coordinate organization decisions and activities both vertically from top to bottom and laterally across organization functions and departments. Thus, governance is the mechanism that assures that strategy formulation and implementation produce desired organizational performance. However, in the chaotic U.S. healthcare environment, where local and regional health organizations are both competitors and partners, we suggest that IT governance theory should be extended to explicitly address the implications of evolving industry technology standards and practices.

Furthermore, governance theory must also recognize the "public good" nature of health services and the impact of government legislation and regulation on the development and evolution of enterprise IT principles. Finally, even within the context of strong industry and legislative influence, governance theory should recognize that an entrepreneurial style of governance exists among and between organizations.

Further research is needed to determine whether this governance approach is suited to other U.S. healthcare organizations or other nations. It is generally accepted that the U.S. healthcare system differs from that of almost all other industrialized nations in that the rest of the industrialized world has socialized healthcare or socialized insurance. However, the lessons learned regarding the strategies employed by the Family Medicine residency program in IT governance may fit other rural healthcare organizations.

The exploratory nature of this work is a limitation. This is a preliminary assessment of IT governance in one specialized setting—a family practice residency program associated with a state university. Using qualitative date from a descriptive case study means care must be taken in generalizing our findings and conclusions to other rural healthcare facilities. However, this preliminary work will pave the way for other studies of IT governance in rural healthcare. Using a variety of qualitative and quantitative techniques, researchers may wish to further examine issues of leadership, decision making, coordination, and entrepreneurship in governance. In addition, this study extends the role of IT governance as an enabler of improved relationships (more patients) due to increased performance measurements (more patient visits) (Banker, Kalvenes & Patterson, n.d.).

The literature discussing EMR identifies significant potential benefits to be derived from effective EMR implementation. IT governance research strongly suggests that a lack of executive involvement in IT governance decisions, that is, deferring too many decisions to the IT staff, significantly increases the risk of not deriving expected value from IT investments. Healthcare professionals expend tremendous time and energy in developing the knowledge base required to provide healthcare services. There is an understandable reluctance on the part of many such professionals to invest even more time and effort in learning the capabilities and limitations of information technology. However, as information technology becomes increasingly embedded in the day-to-day processes of providing health services, such an investment will be required. The fact is that not only does information technology have the potential to significantly improve patient care; misuse can be expensive, dangerous and potentially deadly.

Because FM is undergoing a number of practice improvement initiatives, identifying any one of them as the primary driver for the increase in clinical visits is far beyond the scope of this research. However, it is clear that the EMR has provided a required base for the initiatives, and is therefore an enabler of practice governance through IT.

The impact of this governance strategy on other rural healthcare providers in the region needs to be assessed in the future. Perspectives on improved patient healthcare provided by the EMR should be assessed from the physician, professional/non-clinical staff, and patients involved in the rural environment.

References

Altheide, D., & Johnson, J. (1994). Criteria for assessing interpretive validity in qualitative research. In: N. Denzin & Y. Lincoln (Eds.), *Handbook of qualitative research*, (pp. 485-499). Thousand Oaks, CA: Sage.

Amatayakul, M. (2001). EMR: The coming of age. *IT Healthcare Strategist, 3*(10), 1-4.

American Academy of Family Physicians. (n.d.). *Future of family medicine project.* Retrieved July 20, 2007 from http://www.futurefamilymed.org/x13525.html

Banker, R., Kalvenes, J., & Patterson, R. (n.d.). Information technology, contract completeness, and buyer-supplier relationships. *Information Systems Research, 17*(2), 180-193.

Barber, N., Caillouet, L., Ciotti, V., & Lohman, P. (1994). Experts debate the future of healthcare computing. *Healthcare Financial Management, 48,* 66-74.

Brown, N. (2005). Driving EMR adoptions: Making EMRs a sustainable, profitable investment. *Health Management Technology, 26*(5), 48-49.

Brynjolfsson, E. (1994). The productivity paradox of information technology. *Communications of the ACM, 36*(12), 67-77.

Chan, Y. (2002). Why haven't we mastered alignment? The importance of informal organizational structure. *MIS Quarterly Executive, 1*(2), 97-112.

Cohen, M., March, J., & Olsen, J. (1972). A garbage can model of organizational choice. *Administrative Science Quarterly, 17*(1), 1-25.

Chung, K., Choi, Y., & Moon, S. (2003). Toward efficient medication error reductions: Error-reducing information management systems. *Journal of Medical Systems, 27*(6), 553-561.

Daily, C., Dalton, D., & Cannella, A. (2003). Corporate governance: Decades of dialogue and data. *Academy of Management Review, 28*(3), 371-382.

Dalcher, D. (2004). Stories and histories: Case study research (and beyond) in information systems failures. In: M. Whitman & A. Woszczynski (Eds.), *The handbook of information systems research,* (pp. 305-322). Hershey, PA: Idea Group Publishing.

Darr, A., Harrison, M., Shakked, L., & Shalom, N. (2003). Physicians' and nurses' reactions to electronic medical records: Managerial and occupational implications. *Journal of Health Organization and Management, 17*(5), 349-359.

Fontana, A., & Frey, J. (1994). Interviewing: The art of science. In: N. Denzin & Y. Lincoln (Eds.), *Handbook of qualitative research,* (pp. 262-272). Thousand Oaks, CA: Sage.

Fedorowicz, J., & Ray, A. (2004). Impact of HIPAA on the integrity of healthcare information. *International Journal of Healthcare Technology and Management, 6*(2), 142-157.

Geertz, C. (1985). *Knowledge: Further essays in interpretive anthropology.* New York, NY: Basic Books.

Goldsmith, J., Blumenthal, D., & Rishel, W. (2003). Federal health information Policy: A case of arrested development. *Health Affairs, 22,* 44-55.

Holstein, J., & Gubrium, J. (1994). Phenomenology, ethnomethodology, and interpretive practice. In: N. Denzin & Y. Lincoln (Eds.), *Handbook of qualitative research,* (pp. 262-272). Thousand Oaks, CA: Sage.

Hough, C., Chen, J., & Lin, B. (2005). Virtual health/electronic medical record: Current status and perspective. *International Journal of Healthcare Technology and Management, 6*(3), 257-275.

Lawrence, S. (2005). Portable EMRs are still to Come. Eweek.com/print_article2/0,2533,a=147019.

March, J., Sproull, L., & Tamuz, M. (1991). Learning from samples of one or fewer. *Organization Science, 2*(1), 1-13.

McGinnis, S., Pumphrey, L., Trimmer, K., & Wiggins, C. (2004). Sustaining and extending organization strategy via information technology governance. *Hawaii International Conference on System Sciences 37*. Hawaii.

McNally, D. (2003). The board: The roles and responsibilities of nonprofit board membership. *Pennsylvania CPA Journal, 73*(4), 46-49.

Miles, M., & Huberman, A. (1994). *Qualitative data analysis: An expanded sourcebook.* Thousand Oaks, CA: *Sage.*

Patton, M. (2002). *Qualitative research & evaluation methods,* (3rd ed.). Thousand Oaks, CA: Sage.

Pendharkar, P., Khosrowpour, M., & Rodger, J. (2001). Development and testing of an instrument for measuring the user evaluations of information technology in healthcare. *Journal of Computer Information Systems, 41*(4), 84-90.

Peterson, R. (2004). Integration strategies and tactics for information technology governance. In: W. Van Grembergen (Ed.), *Strategies for information technology governance* (pp. 37-80). Hershey, PA: Idea Group Publishing.

Rosenbloom, S., Grande, J., Geissbuhler, A., & Miller, R. (2004). Experience in implementing impatient clinical note capture via a provider order entry system. *Journal of American Medical Information Association, 11*(4), 310-315.

Sambamurthy, V., & Zmud, R. (1999). Arrangements for information technology governance: A theory of multiple contingencies. *MIS Quarterly, 23*(2), 261-290.

Slife, B., & Williams, R. (1995). *What's behind the research? Discovering hidden assumptions in the behavioural sciences.* Thousand Oaks, CA: Sage.

Snyder, K., Paulson, P., & McGrath, P. (2005). Improving processes in a small healthcare network: A value-mapping case study. *Business Process Management Journal, 11*(1), 87-99.

Stake, R. (1994). Case studies. In: N. Denzin & Y. Lincoln (Eds.), *Handbook of qualitative research,* (pp. 236-247). Thousand Oaks, CA: Sage.

Stausberg, J., Koch, D., Ingenerf, J., & Betzler, M. (2003). Comparing aper-based with electronic patient records: Lessons learned during a study on diagnosis and procedure codes. *Journal of American Medical Information Association, 10*(5), 470-477.

Study shows limited use of electronic medical records. (n.d.). *Healthcare Financial Management, 59*(5), 27.

Sundaramurthy, D., & Lewis, M. (2003). Control and collaboration: Paradoxes of governance. *Academy of Management Review, 28*(3), 397-415.

Wager, K., Lee, F., & Glaser, J. (2005). *Managing healthcare information systems.* San Francisco, CA: Jossey-Bass.

Weill, P. (2004). Don't just lead, govern: How top-performing firms govern IT. *MIS Quarterly Executive, 3*(1), 1-17.

Weill, P., & Ross, J. (2004). *IT governance: How top performers manage IT decision rights for superior results.* Boston, MA: Harvard Business School Press.

Wiggins, C., Pumphrey, L., Beachboard, J., & Trimmer, K. (2006). Entrepreneurial governance in a rural family practice residency program. *Hawaii International Conference on System Sciences 39.* Kauai, Hawaii.

Yin, R. (1994). *Case study research: Design and methods,* (2nd ed.). Thousand Oaks, CA: Sage.

Zabada, D., Singh, S., & Munchus, G. (2001). The role of information technology in enhancing patient satisfaction. *The British Journal of Clinical Governance, 6*(1), 9-16.

Chapter XI

Telehealth Organizational Implementation Guideline Issues:
A Canadian Perspective

Maryann Yeo, University of Calgary, Canada

Penny A. Jennett, University of Calgary, Canada

Abstract

The current status of policies, guidelines and standards related to the organizational context of clinical telehealth practice were investigated. The directions these should take to meet the healthcare needs of Canadians also were outlined. An environmental scan approach was employed, consisting of a literature review, stakeholder survey questionnaire, and 12 key informant interviews. The literature review resulted in 260 sources related to organizational leadership issues, of which 176 were abstracted. The stakeholder survey questionnaire response rate was 64% (156/245), with 55% (84/154) completing the organizational context section. All (100%) key informants who were selected for interviews participated. Findings were categorized into four key organizational themes: organizational readiness, quality assurance, account-ability, and continuity. Organizations need to review existing policies, standards, and guidelines in order to determine whether telehealth is covered and, if not, revise them or develop new telehealth-specific policies. Telehealth policies and procedures should be integrated with those in existence for face-to-face services.

Introduction

In Canada, there are 14 health jurisdictions; all are engaged in deploying telehealth applications. Telehealth, as defined in this project, is "the use of information and communications technology to deliver health and healthcare services and information over large and small distances" (Picot, 1998). Clinical telehealth applications are now operational in tertiary and community healthcare settings. As the number of telehealth projects, programs, and services has increased steadily, greater attention is being focused on policy and quality issues related to the delivery of telehealth services. There is increasing interest among healthcare professionals and administrators, healthcare institutions, organizations, businesses, government agencies, and regulatory bodies to develop and adopt policies, procedures, guidelines, and standards for use within provinces across Canada.

The National Initiative for Telehealth Guidelines (NIFTE) was established in order to develop consensus on a national, interdisciplinary framework of guidelines for use by health-sector organizations (National Initiative for Telehealth Guidelines, 2003). The guidelines were designed by telehealth providers for use by health professionals in developing their specific standards and as benchmarks for standards of service and by accrediting agencies in developing accreditation criteria. A major activity of the project was an Environmental Scan designed to examine four content areas related to telehealth: Organizational Context, Technology and Equipment, Clinical Standards and Outcomes, and Human Resources (National Initiative for Telehealth Guidelines Research Consortium, 2003).

The organizational context team investigated the status of policies, guidelines, and standards as they related to the organizational or administrative context of clinical telehealth practice in Canada. In addition, this component also explored the directions that telehealth administrative policies, guidelines, and standards should take in order to meet the healthcare needs of Canadians. The purpose of this article is to synthesize the findings of the environmental scan and to summarize the organizational issues and recommendations related to clinical telehealth implementation within organizations.

Literature Review

There is a recognized need for national standards for healthcare professionals and guidelines for the accreditation of healthcare organizations and facilities that provide telehealth services. This lack of standards and guidelines has been considered to be a barrier to the successful integration of telehealth into healthcare facilities. Standards are requirements that an organization must meet in order to earn accreditation and are important, because they provide a benchmark for measuring quality. At present, there are no existing Canadian telehealth accreditation standards. A variety of policies and guidelines were found in the literature review. Although many published papers, reports, and documents were reviewed, few provided insight into organizational policies, standards, or guidelines with respect to the provision of telehealth services nationally or internationally. The majority of the documents reviewed on the subject of organizational policies, guidelines, and standards for telehealth and telemedicine tended to focus on technical aspects. Standards need to be established for the administrative management of telehealth services. In addition, national standards need to be established for the management of privacy, confidentiality, and security, as well as for the documentation of policies and procedures.

The Advisory Committee on Health Infostructure (2001) asserted that several ingredients must be in place if the national health infostructure is to be implemented in an effective manner, including strong leadership; a clear and comprehensive strategy and detailed plan; and a common understanding of federal, provincial, and territorial initiatives. Jennett and Andruchuk (2001) stated that the successful implementation of telehealth services in Canada depends on several key factors: (1) the readiness of the environment; (2) systematic needs analyses, strategic business plans, and diverse, collaborative partnerships; (3) adequate equipment and IT vendors; (4) staged implementation; and (5) evaluation. Jennett and Siedlecki (2001), in a paper looking at the issue of policy development in telehealth, concluded the following:

The success of the telehealth venture is contingent on the development of policy to support and enable the use of technology in delivering quality care and equal access to stakeholders. A successful system is seamless, ubiquitous, and integrated. It supports a single point of access to stakeholders and incorporates clinical, administrative, educational, and transactional functions. The policy enabling this success ensures that privacy, confidentiality, and security are ensured; equality of appropriate access is provided; jurisdictional boundaries are not an impediment to optimal care; cultural diversity and human dignity are respected; stakeholder needs are met; and the telehealth service is timely, cost-effective, and patient-centered.(Jennett & Siedlecki, 2001, p.57–58)

There is a recognized need to develop telehealth policies, guidelines, and standards, but few policies, guidelines, or standards actually were found to exist in practice within Canada. Those policies, guidelines, and standards that do exist are specific to a particular organization, program, or project and are not integrated.

Research Methodology

An environmental scan approach was used to address the following research questions: (1) What is the status of policies, guidelines, and standards as they relate to the organizational or administrative context of clinical telehealth practice in Canada? (2) What direction should telehealth administrative policies, guidelines, and standards take to meet the healthcare needs of Canadians? As illustrated in Figure 1, the organizational context environmental scan framework methods included a literature review, stakeholder survey questionnaire, and key informant interviews.

Literature Review

The purpose of the literature review was to (1) identify key issues that need to be explored in the stakeholder survey, specific to the organizational context; (2) help

Figure 1. Organizational context environmental scan framework

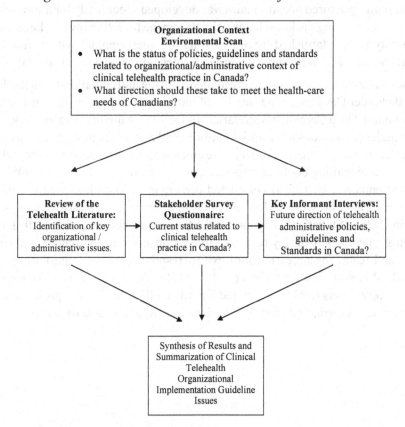

to formulate the survey questions. The literature search was limited to English only, with an emphasis on Canada. The search of articles explicitly dealing with the organizational context (and similar keywords) of telehealth and policy issues, such as standards, guidelines, and protocols, resulted in 260 papers and documents being obtained and reviewed. Of these, 176 references met the review criteria (dealing with organizational context of telehealth and policy issues, such as standards, guidelines, and protocols) and were abstracted. The number of articles explicitly dealing with the organizational context of telehealth and policy issues was minimal. The majority of the literature obtained was related to the topics of organizational readiness, accountability, quality assurance, and continuity within the context of telehealth and/or health technology.

Stakeholder Survey Questionnaire

A mailed survey questionnaire was used to collect the more structured and quantitative information about the organizational context from telehealth stakeholders. Questions were asked about readiness for telehealth, leadership of telehealth programs, quality assurance, policies, processes, accessibility, and coordination of services. The semi-structured questionnaire was developed specifically for the environmental scan survey, using the knowledge gained from the literature review. Face and content validity were established by pilot testing the questionnaire with a sample of nine stakeholders that were representative of telehealth practice in Canada.

A total of 245 questionnaires were mailed to all the individuals listed in the Telehealth Stakeholder Database, a mailing list of individuals and organizations compiled and maintained by a Canadian Secretariat. To facilitate a quality response rate, an e-mail reminder (two weeks after initial mailing) and a second questionnaire mailing (two weeks after the e-mail reminder) were employed. Questionnaires were coded so that the second mailing could be targeted to non-responders. Of the 156 (64%) returned questionnaires, 84 (55%) completed the organizational leadership section of the survey. These 84 were coded and analyzed. Descriptive statistics were calculated using SPSS (Statistical Program for the Social Sciences) Version 11.0. The respondents' open-ended survey responses were transcribed and content analyzed by the research team. The largest portion (36%) of respondents completing the organizational leadership section were nurses (n=30), while administrators (n=18) accounted for 21%, physicians (n=11) accounted for 13%, allied healthcare professionals (n=6) accounted for 9%, and other professions (n=18) accounted for 21%.

Key Informant Interviews

The specific objectives of the 12 key informant interviews were to determine directions that telehealth polices, guidelines, and standards should take, and how they should evolve in order to meet the healthcare needs of Canadians. Organizational key informants were defined as individuals who frequently used telehealth (delivering or receiving telehealth services) within an organization in order to provide care or information related to care and who held management or administrative leadership positions within their organizations. The organizational key informants were selected by the researchers from individuals listed in the Telehealth Stakeholder Database to be representative of organizations offering clinical telehealth services across all Canadian provinces and territories. All (100%) key informants selected for interviews participated. Six physicians, three nurses, two administrators, and one psychologist participated in the interviews.

Semi-structured, open-ended questions were developed and asked during a telephone interview. The interviews were tape recorded with key informants' consents. The key informants were asked to provide their thoughts and opinions about what key organizational factors should be in place for the successful implementation of clinical telehealth services. The tape-recorded interviews were transcribed. The transcriptions and handwritten notes were summarized and analyzed independently by two researchers. Analysis was a multi-step process involving each researcher independently reviewing the transcriptions; becoming familiar with the content; and extracting significant comments, themes, phrases, or ideas. The researchers then met and discussed the independently reviewed transcripts in order to reach consensus on the common themes, phrases, or ideas.

Results

The following summaries synthesize and describe the four key organizational themes identified during the environmental scan: Organizational Telehealth Readiness, Accountability, Quality Assurance, and Continuity.

Organizational Telehealth Readiness

The need to systematically assess an organization's readiness to use telehealth technology was identified. Overall, the survey findings and key informants' responses support the literature, stressing the importance of organizational readiness in ensuring the long-term success of telehealth programs and services. Organizational readiness for telehealth is a multi-faceted concept consisting of planning, workplace environment, healthcare systems, and technical readiness.

Planning Readiness

An important component of an organization's telehealth readiness is planning readiness (Advisory Committee on Health Infostructure, 2001; Jennett & Andruchuk, 2001). Planning readiness involves organizations being able to demonstrate that the organizational leadership has completed required upfront work in terms of planning for the implementation and sustainability of telehealth (Alliance for Building Capacity, 2002). Planning readiness includes (1) a telehealth strategic plan, including a needs assessment and analysis, business plan, marketing plan (internal and external), communication plan, and evaluation plan; and (2) leadership, including program champions and collaborative partnerships. The dynamics of the planning process and order in which the steps in the planning process are conducted are very important. A phased approach to implementing the strategic plan was identified as important by the key informants.

A needs assessment and analysis was identified as an important factor in the successful implementation of telehealth. The majority (73%) of survey respondents reported that their healthcare organization or facility had conducted a needs assessment for its telehealth services. All 12 key informants (100%) noted that a needs analysis is a critical component of a healthcare organization's telehealth readiness and that there are several components to a needs analysis, including an assessment of community readiness and provider readiness. The rapidly changing status of telehealth services suggests that an almost ongoing approach to needs assessment should be in place. Organizational policies and guidelines should reflect this unique aspect of telehealth. A strategic business plan is an important component of organizational telehealth readiness. Indeed, the majority (83%) of survey respondents reported that their telehealth services were part of their organizational business plan, or that the business plan was in development. These findings are an indication that telehealth services are becoming recognized as a part of routine healthcare services. A telehealth strategic business plan needs to take into account research and evaluation of telehealth as an innovation. Given the rapidly changing nature of telehealth, the needs assessment and business plan must remain open to change and revision on a regular basis. Two subthemes—cost-benefit/cost effectiveness and financial readiness for sustainability—were identified. An indicator of sustainable funding would be that new investment dollars are put forth by the organization in order to address service gaps that use telehealth.

The survey findings indicated that the marketing of telehealth services is in an evolving phase. Only three of the 84 respondents reported that their organizations had a marketing plan in place or in development. Healthcare organizations currently are marketing primarily internally among healthcare providers within their institution or region or to their partners rather than to external audiences. A need was recognized for an open communication plan and for all stakeholders to be kept informed during the planning and implementation stages. It was felt to be critical for achieving buy-in and support for the planned programs, facilitating the change process, and team building. Since telehealth involves communication between organizations, a good working relationship between them is needed, as well as a sense that the receiving organization is a trusted authority.

Leadership Readiness

One of the key informants used the term *leadership readiness* to refer to the need to have program champions and collaborative partnerships in place and informed prior to beginning a telehealth program (Ash, 1997). Survey respondents (36%) indicated that there is a move toward the involvement of multiple advocates in senior positions or telehealth committees. Different types and levels of program champions and/or primary advocates are needed, based on their ability to influence. Within organizations, two types are needed: a clinical or provider champion and a senior-level administrative champion. At the community level, someone from within the community is required to promote what telehealth can provide (Alliance for Building Capacity, 2002). Senior management support is critical for the success and sustainability of telehealth services in healthcare organizations. All 12 key informants (100%) indicated that collaborative partnerships are an important component of organizational readiness. These partnerships should be in place before beginning and should include a variety of partnerships with different groups. The types of partnerships developed depend on the scope and application of the telehealth services. Partnerships need to be revised over time. Collaborative partnerships demonstrate that an organization has the ability to partner.

Workplace Environment Readiness

Findings also noted that organizations need to take into account the impact that telehealth services have on the workplace environment and work routines (Aas, 1999). The workplace environment should be ready to implement telehealth services (Aas, 2001). The identified components of workplace environment readiness include awareness of legislation; professional, and regulatory requirements; structural readiness; administrative support for telehealth; along with change management, human resources, healthcare system, and technical readiness. Healthcare organizations ready to use telehealth technology are aware of all legislation and professional regulations that may impact the delivery of telehealth services (e.g., health information protection laws that mandate policies and procedures to be in place in order to protect the privacy and confidentiality of sensitive information) as well as regulatory specific policies to determine telehealth coverage.

The workplace environment must be ready for the required telehealth technology and equipment (Kaplan, 1997). An organization with structure, capacity, means, and resources to implement telehealth is required because of the large amount of coordination needed to deliver and to receive requests for services. The workplace setting should have telehealth equipment in locations where it is convenient for providers and where it can facilitate the delivery of patient care (i.e., structural readiness). Support needs to be established for clinical decision making, functioning, and the process of using the telehealth system. These administrative support policies and procedures include mechanisms for the transfer of patients; a standardized, well-defined, easy-to use referral system; a standard and consistent method of recordkeeping at both the receiving and referring sites; and definitions for who gets privileges to use telehealth both at the receiving and referring sites. The introduction of telehealth services into an organization is often disruptive to the work environment (Aas, 1999; Ash, 1997). Readiness also means that the organization's leadership understands this impact and has a change management plan in place (Garside, 1998; Southon, Sauer & Dampney, 1997).

Human Resources Readiness

Human resources readiness involves having adequate and dedicated human resources in order to implement the strategic plan. Clarification of roles and responsibilities provides the required policies and procedures that are related to user characteristics, such as training and specialty. Six key informants (50%) stressed that an organization that is ready to use telehealth technology would have an education or learning plan in place for those individuals who provide care via telehealth.

Healthcare System Readiness

Healthcare system readiness for telehealth involves the healthcare system being ready in terms of providing strategic support and expertise and having policies, guidelines, and procedures in place at provincial/territorial and/or national ministry levels related to the required infrastructures, funding, remuneration, support for innovation, and diffusion processes (Olsson & Calltorp. 1998-1999).

Technical Readiness

Four key informants (33%) stated that the technical requirements and feasibility of providing telehealth services were essential components of organizational readiness with respect to such things as network and local site technical readiness and interoperability, technical feasibility, bandwidth, verification of fidelity of data transmission, and procedures to make sure that it is checked regularly. Technical support must be in place. Two key informants (17%) representing rural and remote telehealth services stressed that the technology support aspect of telehealth equipment requires consideration, particularly related to the maintaining of equipment in communities that do not have easy access to technology support services.

Quality Assurance

The literature review indicated a need to determine whether or not telehealth does improve the quality and accessibility of care (Jennett, Gao, Hebert & Hailey, 2000; Kangarloo, Dionisio, Sinha, Johnson, & Taira, 1999; Office of Health and the Information Highway, 2000; Yawn, 2000). All 12 key informants (100%) and survey respondents reported that telehealth quality assurance is important. Nearly all respondents (83%) indicated that their organizations were collecting some data or had such activities in development. Telehealth services evaluation is evolving; however, there is still a lack of sophistication in data collection. Evaluation of telehealth services currently focuses on the collection of system utilization, technical performance data, patient/client satisfaction, and provider satisfaction data. The more challenging areas related to the provision of telehealth services, such as access to care/services (Jennett, Person, Watson, & Watanabe, 2000), patient/client outcomes, cost-benefit/cost effectiveness, the impact on workflow, team relationships, provider roles, and responsibilities need to be evaluated more frequently. In addition, all aspects of the telehealth encounter should be evaluated, including a patient's physical and psychological comfort, technical quality of the service, quality of communication between caregivers and patients, duration of the consultation, timeliness of the care delivery, degree of confidentiality, and the costs (Hailey & Jennett, 2004; Sisk & Sanders, 1998). Informed, evidence-based evaluation of quality of care and cost effectiveness is still mainly in an early stage. However, the need to have baseline data to show that quality of care and patient safety are at least equal to face-to-face encounters is becoming recognized. The collection of both qualitative and quantitative data to evaluate telehealth services is needed (Lee, 1997). Four key informants (33%) indicated that telehealth services should be evaluated in a continuous and ongoing process. All key informants (100%) expressed that regular review of telehealth services should be part of an organization's overall evaluation process. It was suggested that they be done quarterly for the first year and then semi-annually.

The survey findings indicated that a wide range of organization or program-specific indicators and measures are being used to evaluate telehealth services. Standardization of data collection tools, common measures, and key indicators for telehealth applications are needed. Key performance indicators for telehealth should be defined in order to ensure consistency in how they are monitored, reported, and evaluated. Four key informants (33%) responded that standardized quality indicators, defined at both the program level and the organizational level, are needed related to system utilization, patient and provider satisfaction, and technical performance.

At the organizational level, a condition of accountability is the requirement of monitoring what is occurring through the development of an ongoing evaluation plan. Part of this accountability for quality assurance involves organizations having mechanisms in place in order to make the necessary adjustments to services, based on evaluation results.

Accountability

For each accountability issue, strengths and areas for improvement were identified. Key informants indicated that strengths can be demonstrated by the policies and procedures that organizations have in place and by the accountability mechanisms and structures present to address key requirements. Eight topics were identified: governance framework; privacy, confidentiality, security, and ethics; cultural awareness; document and storage of patient/client telehealth records; liability and risk management; licensure; cross-jurisdictional services and other liability issues; and remuneration/reimbursement.

Governance Framework

Organizations need to develop a governance framework that focuses on the roles and responsibilities of all individuals involved in telehealth activities (Industry Canada, 2001). Two issues related to the governance structure of the organization were identified:

1.   Where telehealth is positioned in the organizational structure as well as the lines of accountability for telehealth services were reported to be important by both key informants and survey respondents. The person to whom telehealth is accountable should be at a high senior administrative level and positioned in the organization to make a strategic impact.

2.   Administrative processes should be in place in order to support the governance structures and to help those individuals responsible for telehealth to assume accountability. Telehealth services ultimately should be accountable to a board or some other body that would provide governance with the appropriate administrative steps to support that structure: technical, personnel, supervisory,

and managerial. To whom and for what telehealth is accountable needs to be defined and documented in writing. There are three levels of accountability: the health system itself, including health regions; the organization (administrative and clinical accountability); and the Privacy Commission (consent, confidentiality, and privacy).

Privacy, Confidentiality, Security, and Ethics

The literature indicated that privacy, confidentiality, and security must be considered when implementing telehealth services (Committee on Maintaining Privacy and Security in Health Care Applications of the National Information Infrastructure, 1997; Privacy Working Group, 2000). The practice of telehealth does not appear to raise any new policy issues regarding confidentiality. Traditional confidentiality policies should be applied in this new context with consideration for the specific technical issues involved in applying these polices for telehealth applications. In 2001, COACH, Canada's Health Informatics Association, published Guidelines for the Protection of Health Information (Canada's Health Informatics Association, 1997) as a framework to assist health organizations in the development and implementation of comprehensive privacy and security programs.

Protection of privacy requires organizational-level policies (Committee on Maintaining Privacy and Security in Health Care Applications of the National Information Infrastructure, 1997; Privacy Working Group, 2000). Most organizations have corporate privacy policies, and thus, 70% of questionnaire respondents and all key informants (100%) felt that a separate privacy policy specific to telehealth was not needed. However, existing privacy policies will have to accommodate the crossing of organizational and facility boundaries and the sharing of highly personal information. Organizational policies are required to govern who can be present during a videoconferencing session and who must declare themselves.

Confidentiality is an important issue that requires organizational-level policies around the protection of health information and the consenting process (American Medical Association, 1996; Privacy Working Group, 2000). Confidentiality is protected under the Health Information Act or similar provincial legislation, and the principles must be reflected in writing in the organization's policies (Canada's Health Informatics Association, 1997). The policies must reflect the impact of the human, organizational, and technical aspects of telehealth.

All key informants (100%) identified security as an important organizational policy issue, an area in which additional policies and standards related to telehealth were needed. Telehealth has some unique aspects that require special mention in the organization's security policies, guidelines, and procedures (Canada's Health Informatics Association, 1997). These policy and procedures issues are similar to those around electronic health records, and key informants believed that in the near future, these would be integrated. In addition, two informants (17%) stated that there should be an educational component in order to deal with the security issues related to human behavior. This was felt to be of particular importance in the remote regions of Canada due to the use of lay healthcare providers and lay telehealth coordinators.

The majority of survey respondents (65%) stated that their organizations did not have telehealth-specific codes of ethics and appeared to rely on their organizations' existing codes of ethics and/or legal guidelines. However, there are several ethical aspects related to telehealth concerning informed consent, protection of confidentiality, privacy and security, handling of confidential electronic information, and so forth that are unique to this method of delivering health services (Iserson, 2000). Respondents' suggestions on what should be included in a telehealth code of ethics support the need to review existing codes of ethics to determine if they include telehealth-specific ethical considerations. All 12 key informants and 13% of questionnaire respondents believed that the same ethical principles that apply in face-to-face care should be applied to telehealth encounters. Existing provincial/territorial policies, standards, guidelines, and procedures should be used. The issue of consent for healthcare via telehealth is one area that was identified as needing special consideration (Joint Interdisciplinary Telehealth Standards Working Group. 1998; Stanberry, 1998). Organizations should have procedures in place to have patients/clients give informed consent before they agree to the telehealth consultation. In addition, policies need to be in place that outline what information needs to be given to patients/clients for informed consent. Two key informants (17%) reported that special ethical needs must be taken into consideration in policies, standards, guidelines, and procedures when providing telehealth services to First Nations and Inuit communities in the more isolated and remote areas of Canada.

Documentation and Storage of Patient/Client Telehealth Record

Although 56% of survey respondents reported that there was a protocol in place in their organizations or facilities for the documenting and storing of patient information for telehealth, the wide range of survey responses to the location of the patients' medical records (18% referring site; 18% consulting site; 24% copies at both sites; 12% other) indicated that there were no uniform standards that everyone could follow. Recordkeeping and documentation for telehealth care was identified as another accountability issue that requires organizational policies to be in place so that what is going on can be tracked and so that two institutions can generate a record for the same patient and same encounter (Huston, 1999). With the coming age of the electronic health record, three key informants (25%) felt that standards should be developed in keeping with the total electronic communication environment.

Liability and Risk Management

The literature review indicated that there are several types of liability relating to the health professionals involved, the technology, the organization or institution, the human resources and training, and the telehealth application (Canadian Nurses Association, 2000; Saltzman, 1998). Organizations should have a written policy statement regarding whether healthcare providers need to be certified or not in order to potentially cover liability issues related to credentialing and privileging. It is recommended that established risk management policies be followed and that new telehealth-specific policies be created for anything not covered under existing policies (Switzer, 2001).

Licensure, Cross-Jurisdictional Services, and Other Liability Issues

Licensure was felt to be an important policy issue (Blum, 2000; Jacobson & Selvin, 2000). However, there was lack of agreement among the survey respondents and key informants as to whether or not it was necessary to require health professionals to be licensed in order to practice telehealth.

A number of policy issues need to be resolved with respect to the provision of cross-jurisdictional telehealth services (Pendrak & Ericson, 1996). Four key informants (33%) and 39% of survey respondents indicated that a common Canada-wide level of agreement should be in place with respect to cross-jurisdictional services. Also, policies regarding other cross-border liability issues need to be established at the national level by professional associations or regulatory bodies before healthcare organizations can put in place their organizational policies and procedures. Until national policies are developed, interim policies and agreements are required in order to address these issues.

Remuneration/Reimbursement

The issue of reimbursement, as it relates to physicians and other healthcare professionals in private practice, is unique to telehealth due to its borderless and cross-jurisdictional nature (Hogenbirk, Pong & Liboiron, 2001; Pong & Hogenbirk, 2000). All key informants (100%) felt that the development of policies in order to address reimbursement for health professionals paid on a fee-for-service basis is not an organizational-level issue and would have to be handled at the provincial level.

Continuity

Overall, the findings indicated that organizational leaders are just beginning to integrate telehealth into healthcare organizations and facilities as a service.

Integrated Telehealth Delivery Model

Organizations have to ensure that they do not develop policies and procedures that are different from existing policies and procedures for a regular visit. An integrated telehealth delivery model should be developed that positions telehealth as a strategic resource, which makes it possible to continuously improve the organization's capacity to deliver services and information across distances. One key informant indicated that a high accreditation rating should be given to an organization in which healthcare providers, during the course of the day, move easily from one medium to another as seamlessly as talking on the phone, going to a meeting, or sending an e-mail.

Administrative Interoperability

Telehealth services should be integrated into existing administrative policies, guidelines, and procedures. There are clearly the following well defined policies and guidelines that need to be in place for telehealth: technical interoperability; clinical practice, including liability; protection of privacy; freedom of information; and financial issues (Jennett & Siedlecki, 2001; Lemaire, 1998-2000). An integrated system of information and communication technologies rather than a focus on just videoconferencing is required in order to enable continuity of care, particularly in the remote areas of Canada. Scheduling of telehealth services is a unique administrative interoperability issue that requires standardization. Two key informants indicated that administrative policies should be put in place that allow all providers access to information about teleconsultations. As telehealth applications become more complex (e.g., homecare, preoperative care at a distance, regionalization of health facilities), some central coordination of telehealth communications will be required. A standard for coordination and linkages should be developed along with administrative structures to facilitate these standards. How do we make it work in a practical sense? How much is centralized? How much is a function of existing administrative structures, and how much needs to be new? Telehealth can provide coordination and linkages to facilitate the continuity of care without physically having to move patients. Telehealth can facilitate a different way of linking together virtually rather than physically, but the coordination has to come from the providers or organizations.

Coordination of Multiple Telehealth Services

Key informants suggested that organizations should look at how they currently deliver several services and deliver multiple telehealth services in the same manner and try as much as possible to integrate into routines that are already in place. The organization of outpatient services was proposed by one key informant as a useful model. A small-core telehealth group is needed to look after and manage the equipment and physical space. Macro-level organizational policies should be in place that are relevant to all telehealth applications (e.g., what has to happen in the event of a failure; maintenance standards; how booking is done; considerations of privacy, ethics, and informed consent). Coordination of multiple telehealth services should be the responsibility of a telehealth management committee, with site coordinators or network coordinators responsible for day-to-day operations. Setting priority criteria and guidelines for use of the services would be an administrative responsibility. The site coordinators would be coordinating the clinical services, using the developed criteria and guidelines.

Strategies and Policies to Ensure Sustainability

Business plans, regular reviews, and reliable, long-term funding strategies were identified as mechanisms around which policies and guidelines should be developed in order to ensure accountability and sustainability of telehealth services within organizations. One key informant stated that the extent to which an organization has demonstrated continuity would be evident by how much telehealth is in place. The majority of survey respondents (83%) and all 12 key informants (100%) recognized the importance of long-range business plans in terms of sustainability of telehealth services within an organization. However, they tended to believe that five years was too long of a period for a telehealth business plan to be in place, as it is difficult to do a long-range business plan with such a vibrant, growing technology. Program-related infrastructure supports need to be developed in order to ensure sustainability (e.g., bridging, scheduling, information repositories, telehealth information repositories, and directories). The budget for telehealth should be an integrated part of the complete budget, not an add-on. Long-term funding was identified by all key informants (100%) as being critical to the sustainability of telehealth services. A sustainability policy with funding to sustain it needs to be in place across Canada.

Discussion and Conclusion

This organizational environmental scan established that there are a number of organizational-level items that require consideration when developing policies, standards, and guidelines for telehealth services (see Table 1). These include the human, physical, and environmental infrastructures required for telehealth; organizational telehealth readiness; the business case specific to telehealth services; the governance

Table 1. Summary of clinical telehealth organizational implementation guideline issues

Key Themes	Issues
General Organizational Issues	Concept of a Virtual Organization Integration of Telehealth Policies Telehealth-Specific Policy Issues Flexibility and Sensitivity to Innovation Multiple Types of Clinical Telehealth Applications and Technologies
Organizational Telehealth Readiness	Planning Readiness • Telehealth Strategic Plan • Needs Assessment and Analysis • Strategic Business Plan • Leadership Readiness • Evaluation Plan • Dynamics of Planning Workplace Environment Readiness • Awareness of Legislation, Professional and Regulatory Requirements • Structural Readiness • Administrative Support for Telehealth • Communication Plan • Change Management Readiness • Human Resources Readiness HealthCare System Readiness Technical Readiness
Quality Assurance	Ongoing Evaluation for Quality Assurance Key Performance Indicators
Accountability	Governance Framework Privacy, Confidentiality, Security, and Ethics Documentation and Storage of Patient/ Client Telehealth Records Liability and Risk Management Licensure Cross-Jurisdictional Services Remuneration/Reimbursement
Continuity	Integrated Telehealth Delivery Model Administrative Interoperability Coordination of Multiple Telehealth Services Strategies and Policies to Ensure Sustainability

framework for telehealth; provincial, territorial, national, and international policy-related activities; different policies, guidelines, and procedures for different types of telehealth activities; quality assurance, including safety and required processes and indicators; and the integration of telehealth services with existing non-telehealth services. In addition, telehealth quality assurance, accountability, and continuity policies, standards, guidelines, and procedures should be integrated as much as possible with those in existence for face-to-face services.

These findings are a demonstration of the current status of telehealth in Canada and are reflective of the organizational implementation issues related to clinical applications in 2003.

The pan-Canadian funding and jurisdictional priorities and envelopes at the time of this work focused considerable attention on telehealth readiness and evaluation. Thus, it is not surprising that the majority of the findings relate to the areas of organizational readiness and accountability. Attention had not yet been directed to telehealth clinical outcomes, quality of care, or patient safety at the time of this study. This may be why less input was provided in these areas.

Telehealth is an innovation with rapidly changing characteristics and is a new alternative way of providing services. Therefore, organizations must move beyond site-specific focus to network considerations. The recommendations arising from these findings provided the groundwork for the development of the Organizational Context sections of the NIFTE framework of guidelines (National Initiative for Telehealth Guidelines, 2003). These sections are Organizational Readiness, Overarching Organizational Leadership Issues, Accountability, Quality Assurance, and Continuity. These are now being operationalized and considered in the organizational hospital accreditation processes.

Acknowledgment

The Health Telematics Unit (HTU) expresses its gratitude to the Richard Ivey Foundation for funding. The HTU researchers appreciate the collaborative insights and efforts of the NIFTE Research Consortium members, the NIFTE Secretariat, and the NIFTE Advisory and Steering Committees. Appreciation is expressed to all stakeholders who participated in the survey questionnaire and key informant interviews. The research team also would also like to thank the HTU staff, researchers and student research assistants for their work on this project.

References

Aas, I.H.M. (1999). Telemedicine and the organization of the health sector. *Journal of Telemedicine and Telecare, 5*(S1), 26–28.

Aas, I.H.M. (2001). A qualitative study of the organizational consequence of telemedicine. *Journal of Telemedicine and Telecare, 7*(1), 18–26.

Advisory Committee on Health Infostructure. (2001). *Tactical plan for a pan-Canadian health infostructure: 2001 update. Office of health and the information highway.* Ottawa: Health Canada. Retrieved August 17, 2005, from http://www. hc-sc.gc.ca/ohih-bsi/pubs/2001_plan/plan_e.html

Alliance for Building Capacity. (2002). *Framework for rural and remote readiness in Telehealth.* Calgary: University of Calgary.

American Medical Association. (1996). *The promotion of quality telemedicine, Part II. CME resource guide.* Chicago: American Medical Association.

Ash, J. (1997). Organizational factors that influence information technology diffusion in academic health science centers. *Journal of the American Medical Informatics Association, 4*(2), 102–109.

Blum, J.D. (2000, March). Telemedicine: The cyber physician and credentialing. *Health Care Law Monthly, 2,* 3–12.

Canada's Health Informatics Association. (1997). *Guidelines for the protection of health information.* Toronto: COACH.

Canadian Nurses Association. (2000). Telehealth: Great potential or risky terrain? *Nursing Now, 9,* 1–4.

Committee on Maintaining Privacy and Security in Health Care Applications of the National Information Infrastructure. (1997). *For the record: Protecting electronic health information.* Washington, DC: National Academy Press.

Garside, P. (1998). Organizational context for quality: Lessons from the fields of organizational development and change management. *Quality in Health Care, 7*(supp.), 8–15.

Hailey, D., & Jennett, P. (2004). The need for economic evaluation of telemedicine to evolve: The experience in Alberta, Canada. *Telemedicine Journal and e-Health, 10*(1), 71–76.

Hogenbirk, J.C., Pong, R.W., & Liboiron, L.J. (2001). *Fee-for-service reimbursement of telemedicine services in Canada, 1999/2000* (Report prepared for the Office of Health and the Information Highway, Health Canada). Sudbury, Ontario: Laurentian University.

Huston, J.L. (1999). Telemedical record documentation. *Topics in Health Information Management, 19,* 59–65.

Industry Canada. (2001). *Medical imaging technology. WG 5-Final Working Group Report. Ethical issues related to telehealth.* Ottawa: Industry Canada.

Iserson, K.V. (2000). Telemedicine: A proposal for an ethical code. *Cambridge Quarterly in Healthcare Ethics, 9*(3), 404–406.

Jacobson, P.D., & Selvin, E. (2000). Licensing telemedicine: The need for a national system. *Telemedicine Journal and e-Health, 6*(4), 429–439.

Jennett, P., & Siedlecki, B. (2001). Telehealth policy: Building a functional system. *Telehealth Law, 1*(4), 53–58.

Jennett, P.A., & Andruchuk, K. (2001). Telehealth: "Real life" implementation issues. *Computer Methods and Programs in Biomedicine, 64*(3), 169–174.

Jennett, P.A., Gao, M., Hebert, M.A., & Hailey, D. (2000). Cost-benefit evaluation of telehealth implementation implications for regions and communities. In *Proceedings of the 2000 International Conference on Information Technology in Community Health*, Victoria, British Columbia, Canada (pp. 146–153).

Jennett, P.A., Person, V.L., Watson, M., & Watanabe, M. (2000). Canadian experiences in telehealth: Equalizing access to quality care. *Telemedicine Journal and e-Health, 6*(3), 367–371.

Joint Interdisciplinary Telehealth Standards Working Group. (1998). *Telemedicine creating virtual certainty out of remote possibilities* (Report of the Interdisciplinary Telehealth Standards Working Group for the Department of Human Services [State of Victoria]). Retrieved August 17, 2005, from http:www.dhs.vic.gov.au/ahs/archive/telemed/execsum.htm

Kangarloo, H., Dionisio, J.D.N., Sinha, U., Johnson, D., & Taira, R.K. (1999). Process models for telehealth: An industrial approach to quality management of distant medical practice. In *Proceedings of the 1999 American Medical Informatics Association Annual Symposium*, Los Angeles, California, USA.

Kaplan, B. (1997). Addressing organizational issues into the evaluation of medical systems. *Journal of the American Medical Informatics Association, 4*(2), 94–101.

Lee, M. (1997). *Telehealth in Canada: Clinical networking, eliminating distances.* Ottawa: CANARIE.

Lemaire, E. (1998-2000). *Using communication technology to enhance rehabilitation services. A solution oriented manual.* Ottawa: Institute for Rehabilitation Research and Development.

National Initiative for Telehealth Guidelines. (2003). National Initiative for Telehealth (NIFTE) framework of guidelines. Ottawa: NIFTE. Retrieved August 17, 2005, from http://www.cst-sct.org/resources/FrameworkofGuidelines2003eng.pdf

National Initiative for Telehealth Guidelines Research Consortium. (2003). *Final report of the national initiative for telehealth (NIFTE) guidelines—Environ-*

mental scan of organizational, technology, clinical and human resources issues. Ottawa: NIFTE.

Office of Health and the Information Highway. (2000). *Evaluating telehealth "solutions": A review and synthesis of the telehealth evaluation literature*. Ottawa: Health Canada.

Olsson, S., & Calltorp, J. (1998/1999). *Telemedicine: A tool for organizational and structural change in healthcare*. London: Kensington Publications.

Pendrak, R.F., & Ericson, R.P. (1996, December). Telemedicine and the law. *Healthcare Financial Management Magazine, 50*, 46–49.

Picot, J. (1998). *Sector competitiveness frameworks series: Telehealth industry part 1—Overview and prospects*. Ottawa, Canada: Industry Canada.

Pong, R.W., & Hogenbirk, J.C. (2000). Reimbursing physicians for telehealth practice: Issues and policy options. *Health Law Review, 9*(1), 3–12.

Privacy Working Group. (2000). *Principles for the privacy protection of personal health information in Canada*. Retrieved August 17, 2005, from http://www.cna-nurses.ca/CNA/documents/pdf/publications

Saltzman, K.M. (1998). Health care technology and the law. *Medical Group Management Journal, 45*(4), 68–74.

Sisk, J.E., & Sanders, J.H. (1998). A proposed framework for economic evaluation of telemedicine. *Telemedicine Journal, 4*(1), 31–37.

Southon, F.C., Sauer, C., & Dampney, C.N.G. (1997). Information technology in complex health services: Organizational impediments to successful technology transfer and diffusion. *Journal of the American Medical Informatics Association, 4*(2), 112–124.

Stanberry, B. (1998). The legal and ethical aspects of telemedicine 4: Product liability and jurisdictional problems. *Journal of Telemedicine and Telecare, 4*(3), 132–139.

Switzer, D.P. (2001). Network liability: A new frontier for healthcare risk management. *Journal of Healthcare Risk Management, 21*(2), 3–13.

Yawn, B.P. (2000). Telemedicine: A new framework for evaluation. *Telemedicine Journal, 6*(1), 55–61.

Appendix A. Organizational Focus Survey Questionnaire

The questions in this section ask about your organization's or facility's readiness for telehealth, leadership for your telehealth program, quality assurance, policies, processes, accessibility, and coordination of services.

1. Did your organization/facility conduct a needs assessment for its telehealth services?

❏ Yes

❏ No

❏ Uncertain (*Please explain*):

2. *If yes,* when was this needs assessment done?

❏ Less than one year ago

❏ Between 1 year and 2 years

❏ Between 2 years and 3 years

❏ Greater than 3 years ago

3. Are your telehealth services a part of your organization's overall business plan?

❏ Yes

❏ To be considered in the near future

❏ No

❏ Uncertain (*Please explain*):

4. Do your telehealth services operate on a remuneration basis (e.g., cost-recovery or fee-for-service basis)?

❏ Yes — ALL

❏ Yes — PARTIALLY (*Please explain*):

   What is?

   What is not?

❏   No

❏   Uncertain (*Please explain*):

5. Do you market your telehealth services?

❏   Yes

❏   No

❏   Uncertain (*Please explain*):

6. What is the location of your telehealth services (e.g., large hospital, small hospital, walk-in clinic, physician's office)?

❏   On-site location (*Please specify*):

❏   Off-site location (*Please specify*):

❏   Other (*Please specify*):

7. Do your telehealth services have a program champion (i.e., primary advocate)?

❏   Yes   ➔ **Go to question 8**

❏   No   ➔ **Go to question 9**

❏   Uncertain (*Please explain*):

8. *If yes,* who acts as the telehealth program's primary advocate? What position does he or she hold in your organization/facility (e.g., physician, administrator, etc.)?

Please specify:

9. Do you collect data to evaluate your telehealth services?

❏   Yes — all services ➔ **Go to question 10**

❏   Yes — some services

❏   No   ➔ **Go to question 11**

❏   Uncertain (*Please explain*):

10. *If yes,* how do you evaluate your telehealth services?

Please specify:

10a. Does your organization/facility collect data to determine the impact that tele-health services have on the following?

	Yes	In Dev.	No	Uncertain
The quality of care/service	❏	❏	❏	❏
System utilization	❏	❏	❏	❏
Patient/client outcomes	❏	❏	❏	❏
Cost of care/service vs. its benefit	❏	❏	❏	❏
Patient/client access to care/service	❏	❏	❏	❏
Provider's satisfaction with care/service	❏	❏	❏	❏
Patient's/client's satisfaction with care/service	❏	❏	❏	❏
Technical performance	❏	❏	❏	❏
System integration with established services	❏	❏	❏	❏
Workflow	❏	❏	❏	❏
Health team relationship	❏	❏	❏	❏
Provider roles and responsibilities	❏	❏	❏	❏
Other (*Please specify*):	❏	❏	❏	❏
_____	❏	❏	❏	❏

11. Are there baseline data available so that the impact of telehealth services can be compared to data prior to telehealth?

❏   Yes

❏   No

❏   Uncertain (*Please explain*):

12. The following are some telehealth policy issues that have been identified in the literature. Does your organization/facility have written policies in place for the following areas as they relate to telehealth? *Please check yes, no, or uncertain for each.*

	Yes	In Dev.	No	Uncertain
a) Reimbursement	❏	❏	❏	❏
b) Security	❏	❏	❏	❏
c) Privacy	❏	❏	❏	❏
d) Confidentiality	❏	❏	❏	❏
e) Liability	❏	❏	❏	❏

f) Cross-Jurisdictional Services   ☐   ☐   ☐   ☐

g) Ethics   ☐   ☐   ☐   ☐

h) Other (*Please specify*):

_____   ☐   ☐   ☐   ☐

13. Does your organization/facility or province/territory have a policy developed for dealing with cross-border licensure and other liability issues?

☐   Yes

☐   In development

☐   No

☐   Uncertain (*Please explain*):

Ethics, Privacy, Confidentiality and Security

15. In your organization, is there a telehealth-specific code of ethics for telehealth personnel?

☐   Yes

☐   In development

☐   No

☐   Uncertain (*Please explain*):

16. What telehealth-specific items would you suggest for inclusion in a code of ethics for telehealth personnel? (*Please specify*)

17. Are there policies regarding the role of non-clinical staff during confidential telehealth activities within your organization? For example, do you have a policy that requires non-medical staff to sign non-disclosure agreements?

☐   Yes

☐   No

☐   In Development

☐   Uncertain (*Please explain*):

18. Does your organization/facility conduct security assessments/audits of its tele-health services?

❑ Yes

❑ No

❑ Uncertain (*Please explain*):

19. Does your organization/facility have procedures in place for dealing with breaches of client/patient privacy or confidentiality?

❑ Yes

❑ In Development

❑ No

❑ Uncertain (*Please explain*):

20. Does your organization/facility have a risk management strategy in place for its telehealth services?

❑ Yes

❑ No

❑ Uncertain (*Please explain*):

21. In your organization, which of the following methods are used to ensure patient confidentiality for a telehealth encounter (*Choose as many as apply*):

❑ Physical security measures (e.g., locking away equipment when not in use)

❑ Confidentiality clauses in employees' contracts

❑ Training of employees regarding confidentiality

❑ Secure storage of telehealth medical records (e.g., passwords, encryption, etc.)

❑ Following the standards for health information privacy developed by the Canadian

Institute for Health Information for maintaining patient confidentiality

❑ No protocols/procedures to ensure confidentiality for telehealth encounters

❑ Other (*Please specify*):

22. In your organization/practice, when is it necessary to obtain consent (verbal or written) for a telehealth encounter?

❑   Consent is implied by the patient arriving and participating in a telehealth encounter → *Go to question 26*

❑   Consent is necessary for all telehealth encounters

❑   Consent is necessary only under certain conditions

23. In your organization what type of consent is required for the following telehealth parameters? *(choose one of the following options for each parameter by placing a check mark (,) in the box)*

Telehealth Parameter	Verbal Consent Required	Written Consent Required	No Consent Required	N/A	Uncertain
Telehealth as a medium for service delivery					
Diagnosis and treatment recommended					
A permanent videotape is to be kept					
There is a surgical procedure involved					
The patient is part of a research study					

24. In your organization, what information is included in a written informed consent form? *(Choose as many as apply)*

❑   Potential risks, consequences, and benefits

❑   Description of procedures that will be followed

❑   Who has case responsibility and their obligations

❑   Who has access to patient information (privacy and security measures)

❑   Where patient health record will reside

❑   How and what information will be transmitted

❑   Whether session is to be photographed or videotaped

❑   No written consent form is obtained

❑   Other (*Please specify*):

25. In your organization, please indicate who is responsible for obtaining consent (verbal or written) for each of the following telehealth parameters. (*choose one of the following options for each parameter by placing a check mark (,) in the box*)

Telehealth Parameter	Telehealth Coordinator	Referring Physician/ Health Professional	Consulting Physician/ Health Professional	Both Physician/ Health Professional	Other Staff	No Consent Required	N/A	Uncertain
Telehealth as a medium for service delivery								
Diagnosis and treatment recommended								
A permanent videotape is to be kept								
Surgical procedure is involved								
The patient is part of a research study								

26. In your organization, is there a protocol for documenting and storing patient information for telehealth?

❑   Yes

❑   No   ➔ **Go to question 28**

❑   In development

❑   Uncertain ➔ **Go to question 28**

27. In your organization, where is the patient's medical record stored, or where will it be stored for a telehealth encounter? (*Choose one*)

❑   The referring site (i.e., where the patient is located)

❑   The consulting site (i.e., where the consultant is located)

❑   Copies of the patient's medical record should be stored at both sites

❑   Other (*Please specify*):

28. Do you have additional observations and/or comments regarding the standards and/or guidelines pertaining to the organizational/leadership component of telehealth?

Thank you for your participation!

Appendix B. Organizational Focus
Key Informant Interview Questions

We are interested in your thoughts and opinions about what the key organizational factors are for the successful implementation of telehealth services. We will be addressing four content areas: (1) Organizational Readiness; (2) Accountability; (3) Quality Assurance; and (4) Continuity.

Organizational Readiness

➢ **Telehealth readiness is defined as "the degree to which users, health-care organizations, and the health system itself are prepared to participate and succeed with telehealth implementation" (The Alliance for Building Capacity, 2002, p. 2).**

1.   In your view, what policy and procedures need to be in place to be able to say that an organization is **ready to use telehealth technology**?
2.   What do you view to be **key components** of administrative or organizational leadership readiness?

Accountability

➢ **Being accountable is defined as being "responsible; required to answer for conduct, tasks, or activities. This responsibility may not be delegated" (Canadian Council on Health Services Accreditation, 2001, Glossary, p. 1).**

➢ **A number of content areas come under the Accountability heading, including liability and risk management; credentialing and privileging; ethics, governance, and leadership; privacy, confidentiality, and security.**

3.   From your perspective, what **written policies/standards/protocols/guidelines** need to be in place in order to ensure accountability in an organization providing telehealth services?
4.   What written policies **should be** in place for telehealth?

Quality Assurance

➢   Quality is defined as "the degree of excellence; the extent to which an organization meets clients' needs and exceeds their expectations" (Canadian Council on Health Services Accreditation, 2001, Glossary, p. 15).

➢ Quality Assurance is defined as "strategies to verify that a product, process, or service conforms to and meets specifications or requirements" (Canadian Council on Health Services Accreditation, 2001, Glossary, p. 16).

5.   In your opinion, what policies and procedures specific to quality assurance are needed for organizations that are providing telehealth services?

6.   What are various **components of quality assurance** that would **require policies and procedures** (e.g., ongoing data collection)?

7.   If yes, **what type of telehealth data** should be collected?

Continuity (coordination, linkages, and administrative interoperability)

➢   Continuity is defined as "the provision of unbroken services that are coordinated within and across programs and organizations, as well as during the transition between levels of services, across the continuum, over time" (Canadian Council on Health Services Accreditation, 2001, Glossary, p. 5).

➢   The continuum is defined as "an integrated and seamless system of settings, services, service providers, and service levels to meet the needs of clients or defined populations" (Canadian Council on Health Services Accreditation, 2001, Glossary, p. 5).

8.   In your opinion, what are the **policies, guidelines, and procedures** that need to be in place in order **to enable coordination** of an organization's telehealth services?

9.   If an organization offers **more than one telehealth service** (e.g., telepsychiatry, telehomecare, telelearning), **how should they be coordinated**?

10. In your opinion, what strategies, policies, or procedures need to be in place in order to ensure the **accountability and sustainability** of telehealth services within an organization?

Conclusion

That's all the questions I have for you today. Is there anything else that you would like to comment upon with respect to telehealth organizational issues and the development of standards, guidelines, and accreditation?

Thank you for your time.

This work was previously published in International Journal of Healthcare Information Systems and Informatics, Vol. 1, Issue 3, edited by J. Tan, pp. 24-46, copyright 2006 by IGI Publishing, formerly known as Idea Group Publishing (an imprint of IGI Global).

Chapter XII

Computer Usage by U.S. Group Medical Practices 1994 vs. 2003 and Type of Usage Comparison to IT Practices in Taiwan

Marion Sobol, Southern Methodist University, USA

Edmund Prater, University of Texas at Arlington, USA

Abstract

Research on the use of information technology in healthcare has focused on hospitals and health maintenance organizations (HMOs). However little has been done to study the use of IT in group medical practices. In 1994, we conducted a pilot study of group medical practices and then repeated this pilot study in 2003 to obtain a longitudinal picture of the IT services used by these private practices. Researchers can use this to form ideas of the important issues and changes involved in IT usage in group medical practices over the past decade, thus providing a needed benchmark to fill a gap in the existing literature and that can be used to compare domestic as well as international practices. For example, an expanded form of this study was conducted in Taiwan showing some differences in IT integration abroad. Brief analyses of some of these initial findings are presented at the end of the chapter.

Introduction

Healthcare is an information industry. Information technology (IT) is used to capture, organize and distribute data and information to healthcare providers. The efficiency and timeliness of that data affects the outcome of care. Thus it would seem to be a given that the various agents in the health industry (i.e., hospitals and private practices) would leverage IT to a high degree. However, despite rapidly evolving technologies, the healthcare systems in most countries have been slow to adopt these innovations. In the U.S., the healthcare industry lags behind other industries in IT adoption to support daily and strategic supply chain operations. Why is this the case? What barriers do medical professionals face in implementing IT and how has that changed over time? These are some of the issues that need to be better understood.

Studies of the introduction of computer technology in medical settings in the United States have focused on hospitals (Sobol, Humphrey, & Jones, 1992; Griffith & Sobol, 2000; Sobol & Smith, 2001) and more recently on health maintenance organizations (HMOs). In these papers such issues as barriers to the introduction of technology in hospitals, returns to adoption of technology and the market status of the adoption of different technologies have been studied. It was found that there are many barriers to the adoption in hospitals. The longitudinal issues of what the changes have been in the last decade have been studied with the results that certainly there has been an increase in adoptions over the past decade. These increases have occurred in both transactional, informational and strategic uses of technology (Sobol & Woods, 2000) . This trend is expected to increase. A survey in 2002 by Sheldon I. Dorenfest & Associates of Chicago indicated that IT spending on healthcare in 2002 would be $21.6 billion (Dorenfest, 2002).

While the focus has been hospitals and HMOs, very little has been done to study the use of IT in group medical practices both small and large. This is the case even though researchers have for years trumpeted the impact of IT on physicians' practice (Rodger, Pendharkar, & Paper, 1996; Shine, 1996). In 1994, we conducted an initial study of group medical practices of three or more doctors; we completed a later study in 2003 to obtain a longitudinal picture of the IT services used by these private practices. While this is not yet the definitive study of IT in group medical practices, it can be used to form ideas of the important issues and changes involved in IT usage in the smaller group medical practices over the past decade, thus providing a needed benchmark to fill a gap in the existing literature and to start an intensive investigation of changes in IT usage.

In this chapter we look at the differences in computer usage, computer facilities, sources of computer information, and the satisfaction with computer usage in group medical practices from 1994 to 2003. We compare these characteristics and the amount of time spent on business issues by size of practice and years in practice for group medical practices studied in 1994 and 2003. We also take a brief look at some differences in types of usage in Taiwan versus the United States at the beginning of the 21st century, to give some idea of where the IT usage in medical practice in the U.S. stands with regard to the rest of the world.

Background

There has been a great deal of research on IT as well as healthcare. Unfortunately, much of this has been of limited use to practicing physicians. From the computer science side of research, most work has been done on theoretical computing structures. This includes work such as neural net applications of drug/plasma levels (Tolle, Chen, & Chow, 2000) or parsing methods for biomedical texts (Leroy, Chen, & Martinez, 2003). When trying to overlap IT and near term healthcare concerns, the research has tended to focus on public policy (Magruder, Burke, Hann & Ludovic, 2005) or on hospitals. This includes work done on hospitals and adoption of computer based IT (Sobol et al., 1992; Sobol & Woods, 2000), as well as the impact of IT use on hospital staffing and payroll (Sobol & Smith, 2001). Other work has focused on the barriers to IT adoption within healthcare (Sobol, Alverson & Lei, 1999).

On the other end of the spectrum, some research has been conducted on issues surrounding IT in private practices. This research has tended to be very specific in nature, however. This includes whether or not medical practices should hire an IT person or outsource (Lowes, 2005) or the use the use of electronic billing systems by private practices (Burt, 2005). Other research tends to focus on a hot technology that is currently being embraced such as electronic medical records (Miller & Sim, 2004; Palattao, 2004). What is lacking is an overall benchmark or "snapshot" of overall IT use by private practice physicians. That is the goal of this research.

Methodology

In the summer of 1994, a mail survey was sent to a sample of 270 multiple physician groups within Maricopa County, Arizona, who were chosen from lists of a value-added reseller. These practices were medical groups containing three or more physicians. A total of 65, or a response rate of 24% of usable replies were received. This is a good response for a mail survey. In the summer of 2003, 54 physicians were surveyed in group practices of three or more in the Arlington/Mansfield area of Tarrant County, Texas. The surveys were given to the business managers' offices and were returned by mail. Thus, in essence both were mail surveys utilizing the same questionnaire. Both counties (Maricopa and Tarrant) included large metropolitan areas (Phoenix and Fort Worth), were 71-77% white and had median per capita income of approximately $22,250-$22,500. In both counties 65-69% of the people were in the labor force. These statistics show both interview sites to be similar Southwestern areas. The group practices in Tarrant County were randomly chosen from a list of 525 physicians in group practices and provided a sampling rate of 10%. The size of the practices and the years in practice in both surveys were well distributed over a wide spectrum of sizes and age of practice. In the following paragraphs, we will look at the use of computers in group medical practice with the primary perspective of assessing how this usage has changed over the last decade.

First, we will use rank order correlation to determine if the orders of importance for various technologies (hardware and applications) have remained the same over the decade. Spearmans' rho was chosen for this because it makes no assumptions about the shape of the relationship between variables. Secondly, we will employ tests of the differences in proportions for software and hardware adoptions, important types of technology and applications, time spent on business applications and sources of computer information, comparing 1994 and 2003. These tests will be developed for the whole groups and will also focus on differences by the size of the practice (number of doctors) and the number of years in practice. Finally, some comparisons to IT adoptions in Taiwan, as an example of how other countries' medical professionals are using IT applications will be offered. The Taiwan questionnaire was sent to business managers in 2003 and a total of 77 practices responded.

Survey Results

Characteristics of the Samples

The practices in the 1994 sample tended to be larger in terms of the number of physicians than the 2003 sample. As we can see from Table 1A, about one quarter of the group practices in 1994 were less than five while 60.4% of those in 2003 were less than five, and if we look at practices of less than 10, 50% of the 1994 sample as compared to 75% of the 2003 group. Why this disparity? There are many different factors. For example, the Arlington area is a fast growth area and new start-up practices are forming. However, these are not just new physicians but include older practices that are moving to the faster growing areas. In addition, during the past ten years, many practices have become part of hospital-based groups in order to save on costs. This leveraging of resources among a large hospital network has meant that there is less of a need to have larger individual practices in order to distribute costs. There may be other factors but these are hard to delineate. Because of this,

Table 1. Characteristics of samples, 1994 vs. 2003, U.S.

A. Number of Physicians In Practice	1994 (U.S.)	2003 (U.S.)	2003 (Taiwan)
Less than 5	24.1%	60.4%	82.0%
6-10	25.9	15.7	3.8
10-24	31.6	15.7	2.6
25+	18.4	8.2	--
Not answered	--	--	12.8
	100.0%	100.0%	100.0%
B. Years in practice			
0-5	23.1	23.1	21.8
6-10	16.8	16.8	23.1
11-15	8.5	8.5	24.3
16-20	12.3	12.3	14.1
21+	27.7	27.7	16.7
No answer	1.5	1.5	--
	100.0%	100.0%	100.0%

for the studies in this chapter, we will look at the variables by practice size so we can study small versus large practices.

In terms of years in practice, the samples are similar. In Table 1B we see that in 1994 about 23.1% of the practices had been in business five years or less while 17.3% of the 2003 practices had been in practice 5 years or less. If we look at 6-10 years in practice, 16.9% of the 1994 group as opposed to 11.5% had been in practice 6-10 years. Adding these groups to form groups in practice 0-10 years we get 40% for 1994 and 27.8% for 2003. Thus the 2003 practices tended to be smaller and somewhat older. To account for these differences, we will separate a number of our analyses by practice size and years in practice.

We can see from Table 1 that the practices in Taiwan tended to be smaller than in the United States. Years in practice were similar for the two groups except that the U.S. tended to have a larger percentage of practices that were more than 10 years old.

Current Computer Systems

The computer systems used have changed over the last decade. We can see from Table 2 that in 1994, 15.4% used individual PCs (non-connected, in even a local area

Table 2. Current computer systems, 1994 vs. 2003, U.S.

System	1994	2003
Individual PCs (not connected)	15.4%	17.5%
Network connected PCs	35.4	61.4*
Midrange or Mini Computer	16.9	8.8
Mainframe Computer	13.8	3.5*
Network PCs & Mainframe	3.1**	--
Network PCs & Mini	4.6**	--
Service Bureau	--	8.8**
Don't Know	10.8	--
	100%	100%

* Indicates that the differences are significant at the .05 level using a paired t-test, two tail

** Reflects differences in available services.

network) while 17.5% in 2003 used individual PCs (non-connected). This remained about the same. However, there has been a big move to network connected PCs.

Types of Business Applications Used

We have examined the types of computer equipment in group practice offices; we now turn to the types of applications used by these offices. This is important because when the doctors were asked if they were satisfied that the applications met their business requirements, 86.7% of doctors in 1993 were. In 2003, the level of satisfaction had risen slightly to 91.0%. So while there have been complaints that physicians are not open to using information technology in hospital settings (Florien, 2003), physicians apparently are satisfied using IT in their own practices. Table 3 indicates the types of uses of computer applications for the 1994 and 2003 samples. The rank order of overall uses in 2003 is highly correlated with uses in 1994.

Table 3. Applications used in group medical practice, 1994 vs. 2003, U.S.

	Percent Who Used Application	
Applications	1994	2003
Personnel Scheduling	48.3%	26.9%*
Facility Scheduling	21.7	28.8
Patient Scheduling	51.7	55.8
Insurance Billing	95.0	86.5
Practice Billing	85.0	80.8
Business Record Keeping	78.3	65.4
Patient Record Keeping	53.8	46.7
Using Networking Software	51.9	30.0***
Using Hospital Network Software	32.7	11.7***
Vendor Networking	10.0	9.6
Expert Systems	10.0	11.5
Imaging Technology	--	11.5**
Voice Recognition	0	7.7**
† Spearman's Rank Order Correlation Coefficient rho = .949, p = .00001		

* *Significant at .05 level.*

** *Reflects differences in available services.*

*** *Reflects the fact that practices were automatically networked.*

† There were at least three possible ways to compare the percentages: Spearmans' rho, Kendall's tau and gamma. Since the questions were the same but the samples were not paired, Spearman's rho was chosen.

Since the earlier sample contained a larger number of larger medical practices we will separate the study by group size to make the statistics more comparable. (See Table 4). Generally, the order of importance of the usage of applications has remained the same (r = .949). This should come as no surprise since the basic business aspects of managing a medical business/practice have not changed. In 1995, a survey of physician managers found that the key issues they needed support in were personnel management, computing, budgeting and financial management issues. (Cordes, Rea, Rea, & Vuturo, 1995)

Practice networking is higher for large groups and seems to have risen for all groups since 1994. Hospital networking by computer for groups of less than 10 physicians has risen considerably from 3.8% to 46.7%. Vendor networking seems to have stayed the same.

We now consider the relationship between years in practice and usage of different computer applications (Table 5). We used rank order correlation to compare the relative amount of use of each of these applications by years in practice (Table 5) and the rankings have remained similar over the decade. However, different applications show differing amounts of use.

Table 4. Application used by group practice size, 1994 vs. 2003, U.S.

Applications	Groups Less Than 10		Groups 10 or Greater	
	1993	2004	1993	2004
Personnel Scheduling	42.3%	13.3%	48.0%	32.4%
Facility Scheduling	15.4	33.3	28.0	27.0
Patient Scheduling	53.8	53.3	50.0	56.8
Insurance Billings	100.0	100.0	92.0	81.1
Practice Billing	84.6	73.3	80.0	83.8
Business Record Keeping	80.8	53.3	80.0	70.3
Patient Record Keeping	34.6	66.7	52.0	48.6
Practice Networking	19.2	33.3	36.0	59.5
Hospital Networking	3.8	46.7	24.0	27.0
Vendor Networking	7.7	6.7	12.0	10.8
Use of Expert System	3.8	20.0	16.0	8.1
Imaging Technology	3.8	13.3	28.0	10.8
Voice Recognition	0	6.7	0	0

$rho = .767$ $rho = .925$

$p = .002$ $p = .00006$

Table 5. Applications used by years in practice 1994 vs. 2003, U.S.

Applications	Years in Practice					
	0 - 10		11 - 20		21 Plus	
	1994	2003	1994	2003	1994	2003
Personnel Scheduling	71.4%	13.3%	38.9%	38.9%	35.3%	26.3%
Facility Scheduling	33.3	33.3	11.1	33.4	17.6	21.1
Patient Scheduling	60.9	53.3	50.0	61.1	35.3	52.6
Insurance Billings	95.8	100.0	94.4	83.4	94.1	78.9
Practice Billing	87.5	73.3	77.8	83.4	88.2	84.2
Business Record Keeping	83.3	53.3	66.7	88.9	77.8	52.6
Patient Record Keeping	54.2	66.6	27.8	66.7	42.9	31.6
Practice Networking	37.5	40.0	27.8	72.3	17.6	47.4
Hospital Networking	8.3	46.7	11.1	38.9	17.7	15.8
Vendor Networking	12.5	6.7	11.1	11.1	5.8	10.5
Use of Expert Systems	0	20.0	16.7	11.1	17.7	10.5
Imaging Technology	16.7	13.3	16.7	5.6	17.6	15.8
Voice Recognition	4.2	0	0	16.7	0	5.3

$rho = .719$ $rho = .771$ $rho = .828$

$p = .00561$ $p = .003$ $p = .00048$

Importance of Different Types of Savings with Respect to Business Aspects of the Medical Practice

We then looked at the overall rankings of the importance of different types of savings or improvements to business practice that could be achieved by utilizing computers (columns 5 & 6, Table 6). We asked respondents to rank the importance of different types of savings from computer adoptions on a scale from 1 to 5 (with 5 being very important). In more recent years (2003), respondents have been inclined to say that different savings are very important. On every one of thirteen categories in Table 6 (columns 5 and 6), the 2003 sample is 15% to 35% higher than their counterparts were in 1994. In both years, improving insurance claim processing was ranked as most important. In 1994, 70.2% said this but by 2003, 85.8% found this type of savings most important. Other important savings issues in 2003, with 70% or more ranking them as important, were improving patient record keeping, access to patient or hospital information, increasing cash flow and reducing administrative overhead.

The next area was the comparison of the importance of different types of savings by the age of the practice (Table 7). These could be cost reduction or quality improvements. In Table 6, we have classified the savings. Overall, the three groups (0-10, 11-20, 21+) order of importance (by use) of the applications was the same although the individual usage percentages differed widely.

Time Spent on Business Aspects of Practice

A very striking difference in the decade was the increased amount of time being spent by doctors on the business aspects of their practices. In 1994, 64.6% of the doctors said that they spent less than 10% of their time on business aspects while in 2003, only 23.1% spent less than 10% on business; indeed they spent far more time on these aspects. About a quarter of the doctors in 1994 said they spent up to 25% of their time on business and 21.2% of the 2003 sample recorded this answer. The striking difference was that in 2003, 55.7% of the doctors spent *more than 25%* of their time on business as compared to only 9.2% of the doctors in 1993, reporting that they spent more than 25% of their time on business issues (see Table 8).

Table 9 shows the importance of different types of savings by time spent on business aspects. One of the key changes from 1994 to 2003 was that in 1994 both groups cited insurance claims processing as most important. On the other hand, in 2003 access to patient and hospital information had become most important, thus reflecting a key shift in focus.

Table 6. Importance of different types of savings from computer adoptions, 1994 vs. 2003, U.S., by number of people in the group

		Less than 10		10 or More		All	
		1994	2003	1994	2003	1994	2003
CR	Reducing administrative overhead	59.3%	66.7%	44.0%	80.6%	54.0%	70.3%
CR	Improving insurance claim processing	70.4	86.7	68.0	83.3	70.2	85.8
QI	Improving patient record keeping	37.0	80.0	52.0	77.8	45.9	79.4
QI	Access to patient or hospital information	26.9	80.0	52.0	63.9	38.4	75.8
CR	Increasing cash flow	55.6	66.7	52.0	88.9	55.9	72.5
QI	Use of computer technology	22.2	66.7	33.3	66.7	23.4	66.7
QI	Use of image storage of patient records	14.8	60.0	8.0	52.8	13.3	58.1
CR	Reduce service bureau costs	28.0	33.3	21.4	50.8	24.5	37.8
QI	Enhance professional image	37.0	46.7	40.0	77.8	39.3	54.8
QI	Business training for support or staff	11.1	46.7	24.0	61.1	19.6	50.4
QI	Business management of practice	33.3	66.7	37.5	66.7	35.0	66.7
CR	Financial performance/ controls	44.4	66.7	52.0	72.2	47.5	68.1
QI	Business planning	22.2	60.0	36.0	69.4	27.5	62.4

$$rho = .440 \qquad rho = .775 \qquad rho = .746$$
$$p = .133 \qquad p = .002 \qquad p = .003$$

CR = cost reduction   QI = quality improvements

Sources of Information on Running Business Aspects of Their Practice

The doctors in both surveys were asked, "Where do you get the information you need to run the business aspects of your practice?" This question suggested sources and allowed doctors to fill in blank lines. Also, it allowed respondents to check many answers. We will compare overall answers for the two surveys (Table 10). The ranking stayed approximately the same for 2003 as it had been in 1994 (rho = .813, p = .04). However in 2003, there was more reliance on associations and

Table 7. Importance of different types of savings from computer adoptions, 1994 vs. 2003, U.S., by years in practice

	0 – 10 Years		11 – 20		21+	
	1994	2003	1994	2003	1994	2003
Reducing administrative overhead	54.0%	66.7%	70.6%	88.2%	37.5%	73.7%
Improving insurance claim processing	66.7	88.7	76.5	88.9	68.8	78.9
Improving patient record keeping	42.3	80.0	47.4	94.5	41.2	63.2
Access to patient or hospital information	28.0	80.0	31.6	82.7	58.9	47.4
Increasing cash flow	48.0	66.7	52.6	88.9	70.6	89.5
Use of computer technology	12.0	66.6	26.3	76.4	41.2	57.9
Use of image storage of patient records	8.0	60.0	15.8	58.4	17.7	47.4
Reduce service bureau costs	13.0	33.3	25.0	47.2	41.2	52.6
Enhance professional image	32.0	46.7	31.6	82.7	52.9	73.7
Business training for support or staff	12.0	46.7	21.1	58.4	29.4	63.2
Business management of practice	25.0	66.7	31.6	53.5	47.1	78.9
Financial performance/ controls	40.0	66.7	47.4	66.0	58.9	78.9
Business planning	16.0	60.0	36.8	66.7	35.3	73.7

$$rho = .688 \qquad rho = .672 \qquad rho = .554$$
$$p = .009 \qquad p = .004 \qquad p = .049$$

Table 8. Percent of doctor's time spent on the business aspects of their practice, 1994 vs. 2003, U.S.

Percent of Time Spent in Business Aspects of Practice	1994	2003
Less than 10%	64.6%	23.1*
10% up to 25%	24.6	21.2
More than 25%	9.2	55.7*
No Answer	1.6	--
	100%	100%

* Difference (1994 to 2003) is significant at the .05 level, using a paired t-test, two tailed.

Table 9. High importance of different types of savings from computer adoptions, 1994 vs. 2003 by time spent on business aspects

	Time Spent by Doctors on Business Aspects of Their Practice			
	Less Than 10 Percent		More Than 10%	
	1994	2003	1994	2003
Reducing administrative overhead	53.8%	16.7%	54.5%	27.5%
Improving insurance claim processing	64.1	25.0	81.8	27.9
Improving patient record keeping	46.1	50.0	45.5	64.9
Access to patient or hospital information	39.5	100.0	36.4	82.7
Increasing cash flow	59.0	83.3	50.0	80.2
Use of computer technology	23.8	50.0	22.7	70.3
Use of image storage of patient records	17.8	41.7	4.5	55.0
Reduce service bureau costs	31.5	41.7	11.1	55.0
Enhance professional image	38.5	41.7	40.9	35.0
Business training for support or staff	17.9	8.3	22.7	7.6
Business management of practice	34.2	0.0	36.4	12.6
Financial performance/controls	46.2	8.3	50.0	7.6
Business planning	20.5	8.3	40.9	9.9

rho = .198   *rho = -.163*
p = .518   *p = .594*

Correlating 1994 (<10% vs. 10%+), rho = .884, p = .000006
Correlating 2003 (<10% vs. 10%+), rho = .957, p = .0000003

professional meetings and on professional journals. Use of consultants had tapered off but vendors were more likely to be relied upon for information.

Discussion

In viewing Table 2, we see that in 1994, 35.4% of the offices had network-con-nected PCs while in 2003, 61.4% had network-connected PCs. In 1994, 16.9% of the offices had mid-range or mini computers while in 2003 only 8.8% had these large computers. No doubt this is due to the enhanced capacities of today's PCs. No one in 2003 reported a network of PCs and mainframes, while in 1994 about 7.7% used these facilities. The past decade has also shown a difference between the computing services that are available for physicians to use. For example, in 2003,

Table 10. Sources of information to run business

Sources	Percent Who Checked Answers 1994	2003
Colleagues	55.4%	53.1%
Associations/Professional Meetings	46.2	67.3*
Professional Journals	46.2	59.2*
Business Publications/Newspapers	7.7	10.2
Consultants	55.4	34.7*
Universities	3.1	14.3
Vendors	21.5	38.8*
Other (CPAs, Billing Companies, Business Managers)	13.8	10.2
	rho = .813	
	p = .040	

* Difference (1994-2003) is significant at the .05 level, using a paired t-test, two tailed.

8.8% of the practices reported that they used outside service bureaus to handle their computer needs. Application service providers (ASPs) were not commonly available in 1994.

Table 3 shows that in general the rank orders for application usage by practice size has remained the same in the last decade (rho = .767 and .925 respectively). Personnel scheduling by computer is done more often on the computer by large firms, but has gone down over the decade. Facility scheduling has gone up and patient scheduling has stayed the same or increased slightly. It seems that insurance billings for large firms using computers have decreased somewhat but for smaller firms 100% of insurance billing is done by computer. This difference may be due to age differences of physicians (older physicians tending to be in larger groups). We will assess the impact of age on IT usage later.

Looking at Table 4, we see the use of expert systems has gone up considerably in small practices from 3.8% to 20%. This is due to the fact that decision support systems have played an increasingly widespread role as the healthcare industry has embraced managed care (Dutta & Heda, 2000). This was predicted by McCauley and Ala (1992). One other area that has seen change is that of imaging technology. This may be due to the impact of telemedicine. In the early 1990's imaging technology was very expensive and only large groups and hospitals could afford it. Today, there is a minimal cost associated with it and new applications such as remote or telemedicine have attracted new physicians (Prater & Roth, 2003).

If we look at Table 5, we see that different applications have grown and fallen in importance depending on the age of the practice. The younger practices (0-10 years in practice) were more likely to use hospital networking, patient record keeping and expert systems than their counterparts were in 1994 and 2003. They were less likely to use the computer for personnel scheduling, probably because they were in smaller practices. If we look at the middle group 11-20 years in practice, they were more likely to do patient scheduling, patient record keeping and practice networking than were their counterparts in 1994. So relatively new (10 years or less) and intermediate aged practices (11-20 years) were more likely to use computers than the older practices (21 years plus). In most other areas, the applications listed were utilized by the same percentage or less for each of the years in practice groups in 2003 as compared to 1994.

Table 6 shows that except for access to patient or hospital information, the same issues were very important in 1994 as in 2003 but not at the 70% level. No doubt because there was relatively little networking capacity in 1994, this issue was only ranked as very important by 38.4% of the sample. Assessing the importance of savings with relation to practice size (Table 6, columns 1-4), the three most important issues for smaller practices (less than 10 physicians) in 2003 are improving insurance claims processing, improving patient record keeping and access to patient hospital information. In 1994, the smaller practices chose improving insurance claims processing, increasing cash flow and financial performance controls. So they were stressing the importance of the computer for billing and financial purposes. The smaller practices were not as likely to rank order these types of savings in the same orders in 1994 as they did in 2003 (rho = .44, p = .133). For the larger practices (10 or more physicians), in 2003 the most important savings were increasing cash flow, improving insurance claims processing and reducing administrative overhead. For 1994, the top importance (for large practices) was for improving insurance claims processing. There were four other savings that tied for second place, improving patient record keeping, access to patient and hospital information, increasing cash flow and financial performance controls. Uses devoted to quality improvements (QI) almost doubled in importance from 1994 to 2003. On the other hand, uses aimed at cost reduction increased in importance by 15 to 20 percentage points. Thus, it seems that early computer introductions were primarily devoted to cost reductions while later introductions may be more focused on quality improvements such as enhancing professional image, access to patient hospital information and improving patient record keeping. Looking at the younger practices (0-10 years), we see that here again improving insurance claims processing was the most important issue in 1994 and 2003. Reducing administrative overhead was next in importance in 1994 and then increasing cash flow ranked third. In 2003, improved patient record keeping and access to patient and hospital information tied for second place. Thus in 2003, the informational and strategic uses of IT (such as long term planning and marketing improvement) are becoming as important as transactional uses. However the top uses were mainly those that led to cost reductions rather than quality improvements.

Using Table 7, and looking at the mid-term practices (11 to 20 years), again insurance claims processing was most important in both years, reduction of administrative overhead came in second in 1994 and third in 2003. Tying for first in 2003 was increased cash flow, and improving insurance claim processing. Tying for third in 2003 was a new variable enhanced professional image, and access to patient or hospital information. Here we see the older doctors starting to focus on quality improvements. Finally, when we look at the older practices (21 years or more), increased cash flow comes out first for 2003 with improving claims processing, business management of the practice and business training for support or staff and financial controls vying for second place. Evidently, the older firms were sensing the need for updates and for more training and better business management practices. In 1994, the older practices ranked increasing cash flow first and improving insurance claims processing second. So over the years, the older practices have sensed the need for better business management and quality improvements. This need has probably been instrumental in the encouragement of the recent developments in management training and executive education for doctors and dentists (Glasser, 1997; Lazarus, 1999; Lipson, 1997).

With respect to the data from Table 8, we see that in 1994, 65% of the doctors spent less than 10% of their time on the business aspects of their practice. By 2003, 55.7% of the doctors reported that they spent more than 25% of their time on business aspects. With all of the different, current issues such as HMOs, health insurance, Medicare, and Medicaid, doctors must personally make more decisions and consult with third parties to justify the use of medical techniques and billing. So we see that a decade ago, "physician" and "administrator" referred to two different people. Today physicians realize that they have to embrace both titles, and their separate (and sometimes opposing) strategies (Lipson, 1997; Lazarus, 1999).

When we look at the importance of savings from computer adoptions and compare doctors who spend less than 10% of their time on the business aspects of their practice, we find that there is no correlation between the importance of various types of usage in the 1994 versus 2003 (Table 9). In 1994, the three most important savings were improving insurance claims processing, increasing cash flow and reducing administrative overhead. In 2003, access to patient hospital information, increasing cash flow and improved patient record keeping and use of computer technology was the highest. Thus, the doctors in 2003 who spent little time on business stressed the patient information and record keeping. When we look at the doctors spending more than 10% of their time on business aspects in 1994 and 2003, we also find little correlation between the various types of usage. In fact, a somewhat negative correlation is what they found as the most important savings.

In 1994, improving insurance claim processing, reducing administrative overhead, increasing cash flow and financial performance controls were most important. In 2003, access to hospital patient hospital information and increasing cash flow were first and second in importance and use of computer technology came in third. These doctors in 2003 were also interested in reducing service bureau costs and image storing of patient records which were not concerns for their counterparts in 1994, since image storage was not common in the early 1990s. Moreover, patient record keeping has grown tremendously in importance, probably due to the new HIPPA legislation (Jonietz, 2003).

If we compare the two groups (under 10% and 10% plus) for 2003, there is a very high correlation (rho = .957 and p = .0000003, bottom of Table 9). Thus for each year, separately, the time spent by doctors on business matters does not seem related to the importance they accord to different business aspects. However, over the decade, different business aspects have become more important.

This last assessment seems to be the overarching theme of the data. The changes that have occurred in IT usage during the last decade have been in response to physicians trying to adapt to greater business demands on them. Physicians are becoming more aware of this with new programs in medical schools that focus on business. Texas Tech, for example, has instituted a combined M.D. and MBA program. As physicians become business people as well as healers, they have had to embrace information technology in different ways. Apparently, the profession as a whole is adapting to this change. This is seen in Table 10, where the amount of business information provided by associations/professional meetings, professional journals and vendors has increased statistically by a significant amount from 1994. On the other hand, the use of consultants has decreased significantly from 1994 where it was the number one source of information. This shows that physicians no longer have to pay experts to provide business information to them but are being supported by their profession.

A Brief Comparison to Taiwan

The U.S. is considered to have the most advanced medical research in the world; unfortunately, it is very behind in terms of IT. Taiwan is a small island nation with 24 million people and it is famous for its IT industry. In terms of overall health expenditures as a percentage of GDP, Taiwan spends about ⅓ of the U.S. amount (5.7% to the U.S., 13.9% from 1997 to 2001). However, Taiwan has implemented national electronic medical records (EMRs) and smart cards. While Taiwan spends less on healthcare overall, it is more advanced in terms of EMR usage.

With the implementation of the BNHI in 1995, the Taiwanese citizens obtained comprehensive medical care such as health prevention, clinical care, hospitalization, resident care and social rehabilitation. Starting from the year 2000, the BNHI was committed towards establishing a proactive management-style for the National Health Insurance Program. This included a great deal of IT usage. While the U.S. is still trying to develop a standardized health record system, Taiwan phased out the paper-based NHI Card on January 1, 2004 and substituted the NHI-integrated circuit smart card as the only valid healthcare card. This is a smart card containing the entire data set for the patient. With the adoption of the NHI Card, and its attendant electronic medical record (EMR), all medical examination record information can be identified in real time by any healthcare professional.

This national smart card component seems to have had a direct impact on operations in Taiwan. When comparing technologies used by physicians in Taiwan and the U.S., there was alignment except for the use of EMRs, which the Taiwanese use to a much greater extent than U.S. physicians. We showed previously that patient record keeping has grown tremendously in importance in the U.S., probably due to the new HIPPA legislation (Jonietz, 2003). However, that same HIPPA privacy legislation about keeping paper records has slowed down the adoption of the digitized medical record. This comparison deserves more research because "many other countries like Brazil, Denmark, and Canada have achieved modest success in automating patient records" (Sukel, 2007).

When we compared U.S. group medical practices to those in Taiwan, we found that in terms of barriers to the adoption of IT, difficulty in terms of deciding on potential costs was a problem in considering IT adoption for 50% of U.S. practices as apposed to 24% of Taiwanese practices. However, in both countries, doctors were very concerned with return on investment, while Taiwanese doctors thought that patient tracking was the most important use of IT. In the U.S., cash management and billing follow-up was the most important use. Having an IT champion was more important to explaining extensive IT usage in the U.S. than in Taiwan. Taiwanese doctors were most likely to emphasize the need for training although they were more computer literate than American doctors. Thus in Taiwan, the computer was used for more informational and strategic uses than in the U.S. As we have seen in this study, American practices over the last decade have moved toward adoption of more informational and transactional uses, but they are still behind these practices in Taiwan.

Conclusion

Since the 1970s, researchers and practitioners have attempted to apply IT to the practice of medicine in order to increase efficiencies and decrease costs; the work is far from over, however. Technological leaps such as the Internet and World Wide Web have been born and begun to impact medicine (Prater & Roth, 2002). The medical industry still has no clear common goals for IT and very few universally accepted standards. More than 90% of the $30 billion in health transactions are carried on via phone, fax or paper (Shine, 1996). As an example, in only 22% of clinics in North America can a clinician call up a medical record, input information and enter orders (MRI, 2002). To quote Tommy Thompson, the former U.S. Secretary of Health and Human Services, "Some grocery stores have better technology than our hospitals and clinics" (Turner, 2004). Other researchers have argued that we are beginning to see the first-level benefits of digitization such as increases in speed, control, account-ability, and cost containment (Flower, 2003). This line of thinking is supported by the new Federal 10-year initiative to "use Medicare as a vehicle for pilot programs ranging from handling prescriptions electronically to moving patient records online so that caregivers—and patients—can refer to them regardless of time or place" (Turner, 2004). This chapter shows that physicians have, in increasing numbers, embraced the use of IT in these areas. Thus, one of the benefits of this chapter is to show the growth and trend lines of the various types of IT use by physicians for the past decade. We have also noted the move from primarily transactional uses of IT to informational and strategic uses.

Also, we have been able to look at the changes in infrastructure for group medi-cal practices over the past decade. We have compared the different applications used over the decade by different sized practices and by relatively new versus old practices. We have also measured the importance of different types of savings from computer adoptions and shown that especially for small practices, the importance of these types of savings have changed significantly. Finally, we have shown the tremendous increase in time that physicians must devote to the business aspects of their practices.

We see a trend from the use of IT in transactional uses such as billing and insur-ance company dealings to more informational uses as patient record and contact with hospitals (Dutta & Heda, 2000). There has also been an increase in strategic emphasis of IT. This would include such uses as enhancing professional image use of expert systems and business planning, which have significantly increased in im-portance over the decade (Tables 3, 6). As we have observed before, U.S. practices were still behind practices in Taiwan, for example. Moreover, we see big changes in infrastructure as discussed by Weill and Broadbent (1998). The number of practices with network-connected PC's has doubled. Mainframe and mini computers, which were used in 30.7% of practices in 1994, were used in only 12% of practices in 2003. Thus the role of computers and the type of computer facilities employed in group medical practices has appreciably changed over the past decade.

One of the major problems of moving to IT systems is cost. A recent article in *USA Today* (Schmit, 2004) points out that wider use of computer software and hardware costs $10,000 to $20,000 per doctor and most of the benefits go to the insurers and hospital records. Doctor productivity drops 20% during the first three to six months after computer installation. Some possibilities for improvement are suggested by Bridges to Excellence, an employer coalition including GE and Ford Motor formed last year which pays eligible doctors $50 per patient, per year, to use technology to improve healthcare.

While this chapter provides a benchmark for the past decade's use of IT by physicians, its best use is as a foundation for further research. First of all, the consequences of the new HIPPA legislation may lead to more informational uses of IT in the physician's offices (Jonietz, 2003). Secondly, while the overall use of IT in key clinical functions remains low (Networks, 2000; 2001), new technologies are being developed on an almost daily basis. Electronic patient records are being utilized more frequently (Hassey, Gerrett & Wilson, 2001; Mondl, Szolonits & Kohane, 2001). There is a need to determine the use of computerized physician order entry (CPOE) systems, disease registries, and pharmaceutical surveillance systems. Patient-centered Internet applications are expanding. An example is PatientSite which allows access to patients' medical records (except for clinical notes). It also allows patients to schedule appointments online. Other systems tie in hospital-based IT with private practitioners. An example would be eICUs where hospital specialists can remotely track as many as 105 patients in intensive care. If problems arise, direct intervention can be signaled to the patient's on-site medical staff while the personal physician is being called (Turner, 2004). Another example is hospitals that provide online prescription renewal. These examples compose just a partial list. The key issue is that physicians are just beginning to utilize IT. In a recent study by BCG reported in the *Wall Street Journal* (Landro, 2002), only 42% of U.S. physicians are using electronic records or plan to do so in the near future. However, others have argued that "At the end of the day, a physician's value will depend on whether he or she can still connect to patients in this cyberspace odyssey" (Healy, 2004).

So will the majority of physicians end up going the same route as the early movers or will they demand new IT capabilities? Will these new applications of IT come from the U.S. or overseas? Given that IT is interconnecting the world, and governments worldwide strive to provide excellent medical services while containing costs, there is a need to glean information from world-wide practices. As of now, we do not know, but we have used an expanded form of this study in Taiwan in 2005-2006 and will do additional studies for both countries. The benchmarking done in this study, combined with periodic research assessing changes will provide the tools that researchers and practitioners need to best anticipate and manage the changes in medical practices that the future holds.

References

Burt, C. (2005). Use of computerized clinical support systems in medical settings: United States, 2001-2003. *Medical Benefits, 22*(9), 9-11.

Cordes, D., Rea, D., Rea, J., & Vuturo, A. (1995). Training the future physician manager: Assessing the results. *Safety Science, 20,* 349-352.

Dorenfest, S. I. A., Ltd. (2002). *Clinical systems fuel IT spending.* Retrieved August 15, 2002 from www.healthdatamanagement.com/html//ExpertStory. cfmDID=8959

Dutta, A., & Heda, S. (2000). Information systems architecture to support managed care business practices. *Decision Support Systems, 30,* 217-225.

Economist. (2005). The no-computer virus-IT in the healthcare industry. *Economist, 375*(8424), 65-68.

Florien, E. (2003). IT takes on the ER. *Fortune, November.*

Flower, J. (2003). Beyond the digital divide: Nothing about wiring physicians and hospitals is trivial. *Health Forum Journal, Winter,* 8-15.

Glasser, J. (1997). Return on investment. *Healthcare Informatics, June,* 134-138.

Griffith, T., & Sobol, M. (2000). Negotiating medical technology implementation: Overcoming power and stakeholder diversity. *International Journal of Healthcare Technology and Management, 2*(1-4), 375-392.

Hassey, A., Gerrett, D., & Wilson, A. (2001). A survey of validity and utility of electronic patient records in a general practice. *British Medical Journal, 322*(7299), 1401-1405.

Healy, B. (2004). 2004: A medical odyssey. *US News and World Report,* 61.

Hospital & Health Networks. (2000). *Healthcare's 100 Most Wired: Hospitals & Health Networks.*

Hospital & Health Networks. (2001). *Healthcare's 100 Most Wired: Hospitals & Health Networks.*

Jonietz, E. (2003). Paperless medicine. *Technology Review, April,* 59-66.

Landro, L. (2002). Unhealthy communication. *Wall Street Journal,* p. R12.

Lazarus, A. (1999). Down to business: A growing number of physicians recognize the value of an MBA. *Modern Physician, March,* 48-49.

Leroy, G., Chen, H., & Martinez, J. (2003). A shallow parser based on closed-class words to capture relations in biomedical text. *Journal of Biomedical Informatics, 36,* 145-158.

Liaw, M.-T., Chang, F.-W., Chang, H.-Y., & Lee, W. (2006). *The effect that gross revenue has on daily operations.* Unpublished paper, University of Texas at DFW, EMBA Taiwan.

Lipson, R. (1997). Back to school. *Health Systems Review, November/December,* 49-51.

Lowes, R. (2005). Expert help: Hire or outsource?. *Medical Economics, 82*(9), 23-25.

Magruder, C., Burke, M., Hann, N., & Ludovic, J. (2005). Using information technology to improve the public health system. *Journal of Public Health Management & Practice, 11*(2), 123-131.

McCauley, N., & Ala, M. (1992). The use of expert systems in the healthcare industry. *Information and Management, 22,* 227-235.

Miller, R., & Sim, I. (2004). Physicians' use of electronic medical records: Barriers and solutions. *Health Affairs, 23*(2), 116-127.

Mondl, K., Szolonits, P., & Kohane, I. (2001). Public standards and patients' control: How to keep electronic medical records accessible but private. *British Medical Journal, 322*(7281), 283-287.

MRI. (2002). *MRI fourth annual survey of EHR trends and usage.* Newton, MA: Medical Records Institute.

Palattao, K. (2004). Essential EMR functions: A perspective from the front lines. *Health Management Technology, 25*(11), 22-25.

Prater, E., & Roth, W. (2002). Medicine and the Internet: Opportunities in cyberspace. *MGMA Connexion, 2*(7), 24-27.

Prater, E., & Roth, W. (2003). Telemedicine: What's happening now?. *MGMA Connexion, 3*(1), 24-27.

Rodger, J., Pendharkar, P., & Paper, D. (1996). End-user perceptions of quality and information technology in healthcare. *The Journal of High Technology Management Research, 7*(2), 133-147.

Schmit, J. (2004). Healthcare's paper trail is costly route. *USA Today,* p. B1, 2.

Shine, K. (1996). Impact of information technology on medicine. *Technology in Society, 18*(2), 117-126.

Sobol, M., Alverson, M., & Lei, D. (1999). Barriers to the adoption of computerized technology in healthcare systems. *Topics in Health Information Management, 19*(4), 1-19.

Sobol, M. , Humphrey, J., & Jones, T. (1992). Hospital size and adoption of computer-based hospital information technologies. *Journal of Hospital Marketing, 7,* 173-195.

Sobol, M., & Woods, J. (2000). A ten-year update on the marketing life cycle of hospital information technologies. *Health Marketing Quarterly, 15*(1-2), 71-85.

Sobol, M., & Smith, G. (2001). The impact of IT adoption on hospital staffing and payroll. *International Journal of Healthcare Technology and Management, 3*(1).

Sobol, M., & Prater, E. (2006). Differences in computer usage for U.S. group medical practices: 1994 vs. 2003. *International Journal of Healthcare Information Systems and Informatics, 1*(1), 64-77.

Sukel, K. (2007). Looking abroad. *Healthcare Informatics, 24*(2), 60-61.

Tolle, K., Chen, H., & Chow, H.-H. (2000). Estimating drug/plasma concentration levels by applying neural networks to pharmacokinetic data sets. *Decision Support Systems, 30,* 139-151.

Turner, R. (2004). A high dose of tech. *US News and World Report, August 2,* p. 46-60.

Weill, P., & Broadbent, M. (1998). *Leveraging the new infrastructure: How market leaders capitalize on information technology.* Boston, MA: Harvard Business School.

Section III

HISI Implementation, Evaluation, and Practices

Chapter XIII

Decentralization of the Greek National Telemedicine System

Ioannis Apostolakis, National School of Public Health, Greece

Periklis Valsamos, Greek Ministry of Health and Social Solidarity, Greece

Iraklis Varlamis, Athens University of Economics and Business, Greece

Abstract

The demographic and geographic dispersion of Greece necessitates the adoption of telemedicine solutions in order to reduce patient transportation and waiting time. A centralized Telemedicine model proves insufficient to support the multitude of islands and other isolated areas of Greek mainland. This chapter records and analyzes the shortcomings and difficulties of the existing Greek Telemedicine system and suggests a more flexible, decentralized model, which upgrades the regional telemedicine centers into mid-range providers of telemedicine services. This reduces the burden of the central telemedicine unit, reduces reaction time in the offering of primary care without loosing in efficiency in more serious incidents. In this context, we list the necessary actions at the technical, operational and organizational levels for the smooth transition to a new system, as well as the advantages of this new structure.

The binding of the new regional telemedicine centers with the existing telemedicine system must be performed with the minimum cost. This presumes recording and reuse of the existing infrastructure, training of personnel and smooth transition to the new telemedicine structure. Based on the existing experiences, the specialized needs of the Greek National Healthcare System as well as the modern scientific developments, we present an action plan that covers technical and organizational aspects for the development and successful incorporation and management of the regional telemedicine centers in the Greek National Telemedicine System.

Introduction

The combined utilization of the information and telecommunication technologies for the provision of distant health and education services, in the context of telemedicine, offers important advantages in health systems and respectively in patients (Linkous, 2002). The most important are: (a) immediate access to scarce human and material resources (specialized doctors and expensive biomedical equipment) from remote primary care units, which lack of such resources; (b) reduction of medical errors; (c) improvement of provided health services at the local level; (d) reduction of costs and unnecessary patient transports; (e) offer of primary medical support to transport units; (f) facilitation of distant education and training programs (Apostolakis & Kastania, 2000); (g) large-scale review and analysis of medical data (i.e,. by geographical region); and (h) support of health advising briefings and so forth (Wootton, 1996; 2001).

Telemedicine is ideal for offering distant healthcare and medical consulting, but it proves insufficient when advanced healthcare issues must be solved. Primary diagnosis of common incidents can be easily performed from distance, while other more complex incidents demand detailed examination, medical tests and specialized doctors. Common incidents are more frequent than complex ones. As a result, a specialized practitioner is usually less busy than a general practitioner and intervenes less frequently to provide medical advices or diagnosis. A centralized telemedicine system usually has to deal with lack of general doctors or wrong utilization of specialized doctors for trivial incidents. In addition to this, such architectures result in increased information traffic between the dispersed medical units and the single telemedicine central.

This work suggests a dispersed telemedicine architecture with more than one nucleus that hierarchically serves medical requests, starting from local medical units that handle common incidents and delegate complex issues to higher levels. We consider that this approach is more flexible and efficient than the centralized equivalent and use the Greek Telemedicine System as a test bed. The demographic and geographic dispersion of Greece (multitude of islands, isolated highland regions, and unbalanced distribution of population) and the shortage of specialized resources (human and material) turn the existence of a telemedicine system, to a high priority issue. The suggested procedure can be easily applied to all countries that combine isolated mainland and island regions, as well as to countries with more than one population centers. In all cases, the decentralized architecture is preferable, since it reduces reaction time for simple cases, fully exploits specialized practitioners and reduces network traffic to the minimum.

The following section defines the scope of telemedicine and presents the basic Telemedicine models. Telemedicine applications in Greece and world wide are en-listed and the shortcomings and inefficiencies observed in the delivery of services so far are mentioned. The following section details the factors which suggest the evolution of the existing system, the development and incorporation of the regional telemedicine centers to the new telemedicine system. More specific, we illustrate the steps towards the effective embedment of the regional telemedicine centers to the existing structure, in an attempt to minimize the cost for equipment and training and guarantee the smooth transition to an integrated telemedicine system. Based on the existing experiences, the specialized needs of the Greek National Healthcare System and the modern scientific developments, we evaluate the feasibilty of this attempt. We then present the technical and organizational aspects of a proposed action plan for the development, introduction and management of the regional telemedicine centers at the Greek National Healthcare System. Finally, the last section contains the conclusions of our work.

Telemedicine: Models and Practices

Telemedicine refers to the use of telecommunications and information technologies for the delivery of medical services to the point of need. There are several defini-tions of telemedicine (Bashshur, 1996). Some of them are "narrower" covering only clinical services, while others have broader scope using telemedicine as an umbrella term covering clinical and non-clinical services (medical education, information and administrative services) (Lipson & Henderson, 1995). After the examination of several definitions, the Institute of Medicine has defined telemedicine as "the use of electronic information and communications technologies to provide and support healthcare when distance separates the participants" (Field, 1996). In this chapter, we use the broader definition of telemedicine.

Telemedicine is mainly used for the support of populations living in remote regions. It has mainly a supporting role, meaning that a general practitioner consulting a medical specialist or a medical specialist consulting another specialist. Remote monitoring of patients from their homes using devices like blood pressure monitors is a fast emerging service. Remote monitoring solutions that focus on chronic diseases are a new way of practicing telemedicine, usually referred by the term *tele-homecare*.

Telemedicine Models

According to the factor of time, telemedicine can be separated to real-time (synchronous) or asynchronous (store-and-forward) telemedicine (Table 1). Real-time (synchronous) telemedicine can be as simple as a telephone call or as complex as a robotic surgery. In order to take place, it requires the physical presence of both parties at the same time and a communication medium between them.

Store-and-forward telemedicine involves acquiring medical data (medical images, biosignals, etc.) and then transmitting them to a doctor/medical specialist for off-line assessment. It does not require the physical presence of both parties at the same time.

Furthermore, telemedicine can follow a centralized or distributed model (Vargas, 2002). In a centralized model, all regional telemedicine centers are connected to a secondary healthcare provider. Thus, it is not possible for them to communicate. On the contrary, in a distributed model, regional telemedicine centers have the ability to communicate between them as well. Obviously in both models (centralized and distributed), telemedicine can be conducted in a synchronous as well as an asynchronous manner.

Telemedicine Applications for Regional Medical Care

Telemedicine applications cover medical consultation, patient monitoring and counseling, treatment and therapy such as radiology, surgery, cardiology, and so forth (Roine et al., 2001) and the merits for doctors are numerous (cost cut, better treatment, faster response, etc.).

The concept of regionalization of medical care has been implemented in many countries since the 1940s and has re-appeared together with telemedicine in the

Table 1. The basic telemedicine models

	CENTRALIZED	DISTRIBUTED
Communication of regional telemedicine centers	Only, indirectly, through a central server	Directly
Ways of conducting telemedicine	Both synchronous and asynchronous	Both synchronous and asynchronous

Figure 1. A distributed telemedicine network for Greece

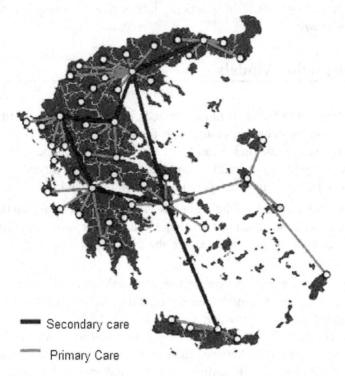

1990s. One ideology of regionalization appears to focus on the rationalization of service distribution and costs saving. Networks underlie virtual regions of telemedicine which must be integrated with real geographical regions. The choice between a centralized medical care unit and a distributed (hierarchical or not) network of telemedicine centers is affected by economical, political and strategic decisions (Cutchin, 2002).

Independently of the selected model, we must evaluate results based on the following three factors, according to the bibliography (Coughlan et al. 2006): a) Diagnostic accuracy, b) Cost (and its associated variables, e.g., benefit, utility, and so on), c) Patient satisfaction and use of services.

International Telemedicine Efforts

Although the implementation of telemedicine is still in progress, its role in the Healthcare Delivery System has been upgraded recently. In the USA, a great number of private health centers provide telemedicine services to their patients and most of the hospitals provide telemedicine services at home (*tele homecare*). In an attempt to standardize the delivery of care, the American Telemedicine Association (http://www.atmeda.org/) has defined specific requirements for the provision of telemedicine services. The general goal is the provision of nursing services at home and the development of self-care technology, in order to minimize the patient-doctor direct contact. Currently, services are designed for the chronic diseases, the urgent health incidents and the supervision and consultation of elderly people (ATA, 2006).

In Canada, emphasis is given mainly in the following areas of tele-health: (a) in telemedicine, (b) in distant continuous medical education, and (c) in *tele-homecare,* the utilization of telephone centers for the provision of remote medical consultation (Picot & Cradduck, 2000).

Telemedicine has been advanced in European countries as well. For example, Finland has an extended telemedicine network interconnecting health centers and hospitals over an ATM backbone. Arctic countries capitalize on the coverage of all regions and the equality in accessibility opportunities for urban and rural medical units (Arctic, 2003). Emphasis is given to the education of medical staff in distant regions, to the cooperation with adjacent networks and the distributed processing of medical incidents. Swedish project SJUNET provides an infrastructure for tele-healthcare by connecting all Swedish hospitals and primary care centers as well as some national authorities and vendors (Larson, 2003). Similar opportunities are developed in Central and South European countries, as part of a long-term plan for healthcare, for example, in the national telemedicine centers of Portugal and England.

In most European countries, there is a tendency to increase the telemedicine services offered at home. Primary health units offer services to the citizen, while, secondary health services (general hospitals) offer telemedicine services to the primary health units or directly to the citizens. In a broader planning of telemedicine services, specialized or university hospitals offer medical advices and exercise *tele-consulting.*

The developments in telecommunications are expected to boost telemedicine. The increase in network capacity and the ability to transfer huge data volumes in short time combined with the progress made in telemetry equipment, allowed the delivery of new telemedicine services (e.g., services that require real-time image, audio, video or data transmission, tele-homecare services, etc.). The evolution of wireless technologies removes space and time barriers and makes the direct contact and communication between patient and doctor feasible (Laxminarayan & Istepanian, 2000).

Finally, the evolution of information systems is expected to significantly improve the architecture of telemedicine services, increase re-usability and promote interoperability (Valsamos & Apostolakis, 2005). The recent trend in this era is the transition from "closed architecture" systems to open protocols-based systems, which use the Web for information exchange and services provision (Web-based information systems) (Bellazzi et Al., 2001; Varlamis, 2007).

Table 2. Summary of Telemedicine approaches world wide

Country	Action - Services	Model
USA	Tele-homecare, self-care	Centralized
Canada	Medical education, home care	Centralized
Finland (arctic countries)	Medical education, healthcare	Distributed
Sweden	Integrated healthcare services	Distributed

It is undeniable that technological evolution creates better conditions for the development of telemedicine. However, the critical factor for the success of such programs is the coordination, support and continuity of all efforts.

Telemedicine Projects in Greece

Several telemedicine applications have been developed in Greece since 1950, when Professor Skevos Zervos examined his first patient from a distance (Sotiriou, 1998). Efforts (Apostolakis, 2007) have been made from both public and private organizations in projects such as MERMAID (Anogianakis et al., 1998) and AMBULANCE (Kyriacou et al., 2003) even with a European scope (i.e., NIVEMES 1998). In a Greek telemedicine program, a joint work of "Sismanogleio" hospital and the medical physics laboratory, an extended telemedicine network has been developed, comprising about 40 interconnected health centers and community clinics with *tele-consulting* rooms for pneumonic, cardiac, urological, pathological and consular diseases. Educational programs for healthcare prevention and continuing medical education are also conducted. During VSAT and TALOS projects, Onassion Cardiac Surgery Center provided tele-cardiology services in North Aegean region. The HYGEIANET network allows the interconnection of the health centers with the University hospital of Crete and offers integrated health services to the region of Crete. The NIKA project connects Kimi hospital and Istiaia health center to the hospital of Halkida and delivers tele-dermatology and tele-cardiology services. The Regional Healthcare Network of Central Macedonia participates in the RESHEN (www.biomed.ntua.gr/reshen) project, which improves secure communication and information exchange between all levels of healthcare service providers—within the regional networks and between different regional networks in Europe (pilot implementation in Germany, Greece and Finland).

Table 3. Summary of telemedicine approaches in Greece

Name	Service	Area
MERMAID	medical emergencies	Maritime in general
NIVEMES	health provision, telemedicine, tele-consultation, videoconferencing	Ship vessels in Europe
AMBULANCE	telemedicine, home monitoring, vital signs and images transmission	Athens Greece, Nicosia Cyprus, Pisa Italy and Malmo Sweeden
Sismanogleio	pneumonic, cardiac, urological, pathological and consular diseases	Northern Greece and North Aegean
VSAT, TALOS	tele-cardiology	North Aegean
HYGEIANET	general	Crete
NIKA	tele-dermatology and tele-cardiology	Chalkis

Current State of Telemedicine in Greece

Despite the encouraging results of the previous efforts, the progress of telemedicine in Greece was not comparable to the initial expectations. The delay is due to many reasons:

- The lack of proper education in information and telecommunication technologies of medical and non-medical staff of the telemedicine centers and hospitals imposed tremendous difficulties in the effective operation of the system.

- The shortage of hospitals and telemedicine centers in expert staff significantly constrained the system's working hours.

- The inability to allocate permanent staff for the operation of the system in a 24/7 basis, hindered its real-time usage. The system failed to support urgent health incidents (synchronous operation mode) and was limited to asynchronous mode only (store-and-forward telemedicine) which is suitable for confronting chronic problems or offering distant education programs.

- The shortage in telecommunication and other facilities resulted in slow-operating systems. Telecommunications breakdown incidents were also increased.

- The lack of information technology protocols and standards resulted in "closed architecture" systems, with serious data exchange limitations (Valsamos & Apostolakis, 2005).

- The absence of a distributed, virtual electronic health record, which would permit the remote access to patient health data and history from any telemedicine system, also hindered the delivery of effective telemedicine services.

Additionally, several legal issues have arisen that need be solved for effectively delivering healthcare services. As far as it concerns the electronic health record, security and privacy issues relate to the visibility of health data and their secure transfer over telecommunication networks. As far as it concerns the medical diagnosis and the doctor's intervention in a distant incident, the problem of legal responsibility should be defined as prior to the practice of telemedicine (i.e., who is responsible for a therapy and how is this proven). Last, but not least, is the issue of decentralization of the existing telemedicine system, which is operated, controlled and supported by the university hospitals and specialized hospitals only. In order to distribute the load, we should exploit the medical equipment and staff of primary healthcare units and offer medical care on demand to isolated and distant areas. We should make use of general or specialized hospitals only when primary care is insufficient. The redistribution of tasks and responsibilities is expected to increase the efficiency of the National Telemedicine System.

The most important issue that must be considered for the successful operation of a Telemedicine System is the coordination of services and staff over a long-term action plan.

Technical, Organizational, and Functional Features of the Decentralized Model

The Suggested Model

The backbone of the suggested model is the hierarchical structure of the existing telemedicine system with the primary, secondary and tertiary healthcare providers operating harmonically for the efficient patient service. The suggested modifications are expected to reduce the workload of the secondary and tertiary health providers in urban areas and to enforce the role of the primary health providers in rural and isolated areas. The decentralized regional telemedicine centers will be the connecting node between primary healthcare and specialized care. Equipped with the necessary telemedicine equipment, they will be able to monitor, coordinate and support all regional healthcare units, provide diagnoses, advices and education where this is needed, and lighten the workload of general hospitals and specialized clinics. In this way, the provision of immediate medical care to the citizen is succeeded and the quality of diagnosis and consulting services is improved.

At the same time, the process of diagnosis and consulting provision is accelerated. In common medical incidents, assistance is delivered from the regional centers, using telemedicine services. As a result, general hospitals have less workload and more time to focus on the most difficult/demanding cases.

Figure 2. The suggested model's structure

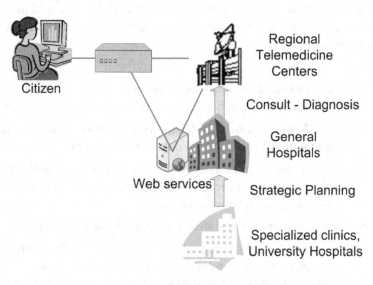

Another advantage of the suggested system is that tertiary healthcare providers (university and general hospitals) have more time to invest in the planning of a tele-health strategy and the provision of new prevention and briefing acts.

A crucial factor for the smooth transition to the suggested structure is the detailed listing of all technical, organizational and functional reformations that should be implemented. The examination of all factors and the estimation of costs and benefits from this reformation will show if the suggestion is eligible for the Greek telemedicine system.

Technical Characteristics

A critical factor for the effective operation of the new structure is the distribution of the workload between all involved parties. A first step is to define the responsibilities and authorizations of each involved party and to enumerate the required technical equipment for the diagnosis and examination processes. The first pre-requisite for a flexible and distributed telemedicine system is the existence of well-equipped regional centers. The second requirement is those centers to be interconnected effectively to the central coordinator and to consulting units. The last requirement is the digitization of medical information in accordance to broadly accepted standards.

A high-speed network connection paired with cable and satellite links (Clarke et al., 2001) will allow the immediate and uninterruptible transfer of medical data and diagnoses even in the most far-away/unreachable regions. The technical characteristics are synopsized to:

- Basic equipment of the local and home-based health units and connection of them with the fully equipped regional telemedicine centers. Analytically:
    o   Based on the needs, home telemetry devices for the supervision of patients and the transfer of medical data to the regional telemedicine centers.
    o   Primary health units in faraway regions with the essential medical equipment for conducting routine medical examinations and sending the results to the regional telemedicine centers.
    o   Fully equipped and staffed regional telemedicine centers.
    o   Connection of the home telemetry devices and the health units with the regional telemedicine centers. The connection will be made in local scale (prefecture, group of island) and must have above average data transfer rates due to the fact that it will carry the measures of the medical devices (picture, sound video) to the regional telemedicine centers where supervision and diagnosis will be conducted. In order to have continuous patient supervision, communication must be incessant. Therefore, we suggested the combined use of satellite and cable data telecommunications.
- Setup of the appropriate hardware and software at the regional health units allowing conducting diagnosis from a distance. In order to support such services, high-speed and high-availability network connection between regional telemedicine centers and hospital is demanded. In this way, the experience of secondary and tertiary staff will be utilized without the need for patient transfer.
- Usage of high-end equipment and high-skilled staff in secondary and tertiary health units in order to be capable to face complex incidents.
- Tertiary health units must be equipped with information systems which will collect, store, index and process medical data transferred form the regional telemedicine centers. These data can be used for the diagnosis and prevention of epidemic effects. Moreover, the concentration and process of statistical data allows the tertiary health units to check the new system's effective operation and schedule new tele-health acts.

The most important factors that should be considered in the process of medical information transfer are security and privacy. Patient data transferred over cable and wireless networks must be properly encrypted, in order to avoid unauthorized

Figure 3. Technical characteristics and functions per level

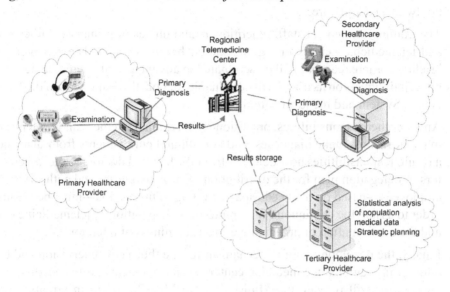

disclosure. Since primary diagnosis and examination results are collected in a central repository for further statistical analysis, extra care should be taken to remove any identification information.

Organizational Characteristics

The successful introduction of the regional telemedicine centers to the National Health System is an extremely complex process. The success of the whole project depends mainly on the effective organization and management of the distributed system in local and central level.

Regional telemedicine centers stand between primary healthcare units and hospitals. They serve local requests and act as a mediator to the central hospitals when it is needed. Telemedicine centers should have the appropriate coverage and responsiveness to telemedicine requests. An analysis of the medical profile of each region's population is required, in order to decide the appropriate location for each center.

Reformation in organizational level will indirectly affect the technical and human dimensions of the system. A strategic plan that defines the staff to be recruited, the equipments to be purchased and the redistribution in large scale is necessary. It is critical to develop a plan for continuous upgrade of existing equipment, continuous supervision and support of all regional centers (*online monitoring and support*) and also an action plan for the periodic maintenance and support of the system's hardware and software.

The training of medical staff, practitioners and nurses of primary healthcare units and telemedicine centers in regions should be provisioned. The arrangement of briefing conferences that will disseminate the advantages of telemedicine and will guide individuals on its usage will be valuable for both the employees of the National Health System and the local communities.

Among other responsibilities, practitioners in regional telemedicine centers should make decisions, make diagnoses, and consult and cure patients from distance. As a result, responsibilities now delegate from the hospital doctors to the general doctors. A delegation plan for the distribution of responsibilities and authorizations of employees—based on the needs and according to their skills—must be created, in order to assure the continuous and uninterrupted operation of telemedicine centers and the confrontation of urgent situations (i.e., illness of operators).

Finally, the development of a mechanism for the thorough supervision and evaluation of the regional telemedicine centers in management level is necessary. This mechanism will provide the Ministry of Health with useful information on the performance of each system node resulting in the improvement of the National Telemedicine System.

Operational Features: Telemedicine and Tele-Health Services

Telemedicine services are directly involved with medical applications and procedures of nursing, prevention and health education. Tele-health services have a broader application context, refer to health and nursing plans and are defined form doctors and medical experts. Both categories of services are based in great level to the usage of distance education and learning technologies

Telemedicine applications process and transfer sound, text, image and video through computers, faxes, scanners, e-mail and teleconference systems. Digitization and exchange of medical data aims to supply the medical experts—irrelevant to their position—with the highest possible level of information. Ulterior aim is the provision of same quality services at both central and far-away regions.

The medical and supporting services which can be offered to remote patients through the usage of computers and telecommunication networks are focus on three main categories:

- **Supervision-diagnosis-consultation:** transmission and interpretation of tomographies, radiograms, cardiograms, encephalogram, tele-dermatology, tele-radiology, virtual patient examination, tele-surgery, and so forth

- **Data/information processing:** Transfer of patent medical files, transmission of doctor's transcriptions and medical guidelines, access to medical databases centralization and organization of medical data
- **Education:** Connection with research centers, retrieval of medical bibliography, continuing education of doctors, nurses and other staff

Tele-Health is complementary to telemedicine and aims to a holistic confrontation of health subjects. It faces health and medical care problems in a broader context. Applications supported from computer science and telecommunication technologies:

- **Prevention planning:** Education in subjects like water clearness and basic hygiene, face of common health problems, promotion of prevention and check-ups, planned parenthood, care for pregnant women and newborns, safekeeping of personal hygiene and suitable nutrition
- **Education and training of healthcare service providers, medical staff and patients:** Prevention of diseases, infections and accidents, education on the provision of first aids
- The general management of the tele-health system

Use Cases

We will try to give a snapshot of the way the new model works with the help of two use cases.

a. For a **routine examination** to a remote village, the citizen goes to the local health unit where the first examinations are performed (temperature, pressure, cardiogram) and symptoms are written down. All information is forwarded to the regional telemedicine center. The doctor retrieves the patient's medical history (using the electronic medical record), examines the recorded symptoms and issues a diagnosis. The latter, paired with any notes and advices, are sent back to the remote health unit. Finally, examination results and notes are recorded to the patient's electronic health record for future use, and anonymously collected in a central repository for statistical reasons.

b. In a more **complex incident**, in which the initial exams do not lead to a straight diagnosis, the patient must be transferred to the closest regional center. Additional examinations and the consultation from a general doctor are incorporated to the second diagnosis. The doctor can have a teleconference with a specialized doctor in a general hospital, if needed. In the case of emergency, the incident is treated inside the regional center with the distant support of the hospital. Furthermore, the patient is transferred to the general hospital. All medical exams and diagnosis are transferred electronically to the hospital so that the specialized doctor has a clear view on the case before the patient's arrival.

c.   In the case of continuous **tele-homecare**, the patient uses the appropriate telemetry equipment and sends the results directly to the regional telemedicine center. Decision-support software, processes input data and patient's history and generates alerts to doctors who are responsible for the case. Doctors are able to monitor the patient status at any moment.

d.   In the case of **continuous medical training**, the tutor presents a medical case and the respective history and symptoms. The doctors who are trained from a distance must issue a diagnosis on this medical incident. The decisions and results are discussed in the teleconference that follows the course.

Feasibility Study

The eligibility and feasibility of the suggested solution should be measured in terms of *cost* and *gain* across all aforementioned axes: technical, organizational and functional.

Reformations in technical level include the re-distribution of existing medical staff and devices and possibly the de-centralization of general doctors towards the regional telemedicine centers and the primary healthcare units. The cost for this re-distribution is reasonable and permits the purchase of additional medical devices or the upgrade of existing ones. The transition to the new system does not require the engagement of more specialized doctors or the release from duty for other practitioners or nurses. So the personnel costs should remain stable. The adoption of cryptography techniques for the protection of personal medical data is of low cost, since these techniques have been extensively applied in other cases of sensitive data.

Reformations in organizational level can be summarized: in the definition of roles and responsibilities of nurses, general doctors and specialized doctors, the definition of data flow among the different healthcare providers. The most critical point in these reformations is the agreement on the legal responsibility regarding medical mistakes. Every one who is behind a medical mistake should undertake his/her responsibilities against the physical, financial or moral damage to the patient. This legal issue (Squifflet, 2003) is a matter of agreement between hospitals, doctors, nurses and patients and is outside the scope of this chapter.

As far as it concerns the functional dimension of the suggested system, it is expected that the new structure will bring many gains for patients and healthcare professionals. The delegation of responsibilities, the transfer of workload towards the regions and the reformation of the telemedicine services delivery will give more space and time to healthcare experts to design the strategic plan for tele-health. The money and time spent for the restructuring of the existing system and the re-distribution of its sources will be returned to the government and the citizens in the form of a national telemedicine system with fast response and a long-term national tele-health provision.

Action Plan

Based on the analysis above, it is obvious that the development and successful operation of regional telemedicine centers is a multi-faceted effort. The complexity of this effort and the weaknesses of the existing structures make necessary the creation of a transition plan. The plan should comprise:

- The recording of existing situation (structures, personnel, equipment, etc.)
- The reformation and re-distribution of existing infrastructure and the extension of the current system where it is absolutely necessary
- The pilot operation of a small number of regional telemedicine centers that will comply to the aforementioned specifications (technical, organizational and functional)
- Gradient extension of the network based on the pilot results
- Continuous monitoring of the telemedicine network operation and results feedback

The establishment of a coordinating group is necessary for the efficient transition to the new system. The group will comprise healthcare and technology experts, will be responsible for the monitoring of the transition and for the corroboration of all transformations. The group should be supervised by the Ministry of Health.

Conclusion

This chapter presented some of the approaches on the national and international level in the field of telemedicine. The analysis of the existing system uncovered its shortcomings and indicated the transition to a new national telemedicine system. The feasibility study proved that the creation of a new system from zero should be avoided, whereas a recording and redistribution of the existing infrastructure is advisable. The new model is expected to help us overcome existing problems and improve the quality of telemedicine services.

The coordinated effort in terms of an action plan and under the close supervision of the Ministry and a group of specialists will help us cover all organizational, functional and technical aspects of this multi-faceted problem. Telemedicine as a whole offers a great possibility for distant and low-cost services in high quality, given that several security, privacy and legal issues are solved.

References

Anogianakis, G., Maglavera, S., & Pomportsis, A. (1998). Relief for maritime medical emergencies through telematics. Information technology in biomedicine. *IEEE Transactions, 2,*(4), 254-260.

Apostolakis, I. (2007). *Health information systems,* (Papazisis eds.). Athens.

Apostolakis, I., & Kastania, A. (2000). Distant teaching in telemedicine: Why and how we do it. *Journal of Management and Health, 1*(1), 66-73.

Arctic. (2003). *Arctic telemedicine priorities, recommendations and proposed actions.* Report from the Arctic workshop in Tromso Norway.

ATA. (2006). *ATA's Federal policy recommendations for home telehealth and remote monitoring.* Retrieved September 7, 2006 fromhttp://www.american-telemed.org/news/policy_issues/FINA_%20DRAFTHome_Telehealth_Policy_ver3.5.pdf

Bashshur, R. (1995). On the definition and evaluation of telemedicine. *Telemedicine Journal, 1,* 19-30.

Bellazzi, R., Montani, S., Riva, A., & Stefanelli, M. (2001). Web-based telemedicine systems for home-care: Technical issues and experiences. *Computer Methods and Programs in Biomedicine, 64*(3), 175-187.

Clarke, M., Fragos, A., Jones, R., & Lioupis, D. (2001). Optimum delivery of telemedicine over low bandwidth satellite links, Engineering in medicine and biology society. *Proceedings of the 23rd Annual International Conference of the IEEE, 4,* 3606-3609.

Coughlan, J., Eatock, J., & Eldabi, T. (2006). Evaluating telemedicine: A focus on patient pathways. *International Journal of Technology Assessment in Healthcare, 22,* 136-142.

Cutchin, M. (2002). Virtual medical geographies: Conceptualizing telemedicine and regionalization. *Progress in Human Geography, 26*(1), 19-39.

Field, M. (1996). *Telemedicine: A guide to assessing telecommunications in healthcare.* Washington, D.C.: National Academy.

Grigsby, J., Kaehny, M., Schlenker, R., Shaughnessy, P., & Beale, S. (1993). *Telemedicine: Literature review and analytic framework.* Denver, CO: Center for Health Policy Research.

Koch, S. (2006). Home telehealth-current state and future trends. *International Journal of Medical Informatics, 75*(8), 565-576.

Kyriacou, E., Pavlopoulos, S., Berler, A., Neophytou, M., Bourka, A., Georgoulas, A., et al., (2003). *Multi-purpose healthcare telemedicine systems with mobile communication link support.* BioMedical Engineering (online), 2, 7.

Larson, M. (2003). *Sjunet–The national IT infrastructure for healthcare in Sweden.* Information and Communication Technology in the Arctic, an international conference of the Arctic Council. Retrieved May 23, 2007 from http://vefir. unak.is/ICTConference/Larson.pdf

Laxminarayan, S., & Istepanian, R. (2000). Unwired e-Med: The next generation of wireless and Internet telemedicine systems. *IEEE Transactions on Information Technology in Biomedicine, 4*(3), 189-193.

Linkous, J. (2002). Telemedicine: An overview. *Journal of Medical Practice Management, 18*(1), 24-27.

Lipson, L., & Henderson, T. (1995). *State initiatives to promote telemedicine.* Washington, D.C.: Intergovernmental Health Policy Project, George Washington University.

NIVEMES. (1998). *Network of integrated vertical medical services—targeting ship vessels and remote population.* Retrieved May 21, 2007 from http://ehto. org/ht_projects/html/dynamic/91.html

Picot, J., & Cradduck, T. (2000). *The tele-health industry in Canada: Industry profile and capability analysis executive summary & recommendations.* Prepared for the Life Sciences Branch, Canada.

Roine, R., Ohinmaa, A., & Hailey, D. (2001). Assessing telemedicine: A systematic review of the literature. *CMAJ, 165*(6), 777-779.

SJUNET. (2003). *Sjunet—the Swedish healthcare network.* Retrieved May 23, 2007 from www.itsweden.com/docfile/31930_Sjunet_the_swedish_healthcare_network.pdf

Sotiriou, D. (1998). *The history of Telemedicine in Greece.* In: O. Ferrer-Roca & M. Sosa-Iudicissa (Eds.), *Handbook of telemedicine.* IOS Press.

Squifflet, J. (2003). The medical responsibility: Current view from the council of physicians side. *Acta Chirurgicae Belgica, 103*(2), 120-123.

Valsamos, P., & Apostolakis, I. (2005). Interoperability and quality in information systems of healthcare units. *Second Hellenic Conference for the Quality in Healthcare,* NCSR. Demokritos.

Varlamis, I. (2007). A flexible model for the delivery of multi-facet information in patient–centric healthcare information systems. *The Electronic Journal for E-Commerce Tools & Applications,* Special Issue in Interoperability & Security in Medical Information Systems. http://minbar.cs.dartmouth.edu/greecom/ejeta/

Vargas, L. (2002). Organizational models of telemedicine and regional telemedicine networks. *Telemedicine Journal and e-Health, 8,* 71-79.

Wootton, R. (2001). Recent advances: Telemedicine. *BMJ, 323,* 557-560. Retrieved September 7, 2006 from: http://bmj.bmjjournals.com/cgi/content/full/323/7312/557

Wootton, R. (1996). Telemedicine: A cautious welcome. *BMJ, 313,* 1375-1377. Retrieved September 7, 2006 from http://bmj.bmjjournals.com/cgi/content/full/313/7069/1375

Chapter XIV

Perceived Level of Benefits and Risk Core Functionalities of an EHR System

Diane C. Davis, Southern Illinois University–Carbondale, USA

Minal Thakkar, Southern Illinois University–Carbondale, USA

Abstract

*The need to adopt an electronic health record (EHR) system in United States (U.S.) hospitals seems to be more and more obvious when evaluating the benefits of improved patient safety, quality of care, and efficiency. The purpose of the study was to identify the status of EHR systems in U.S. hospitals in regard to the core functionalities implemented (as identified by the Institute of Medicine) and to determine if there was a significant relationship between perceived level of benefit and risk with the use of each core functionality, as well as if there was a significant relationship between the status of the EHR system and size of hospital. A national survey of U.S. hospitals was conducted to answer the research questions. The results showed that 37% had some components in **all** of the core functionalities of an EHR system, while 27% were using at least **some** functionalities. Health information and data,*

*administrative processes, and results management were the three core functionalities
that a majority of hospitals had as a part of their EHR system. A significant positive
correlation between perceived benefits and risks was found in all of the eight core
functionalities. There was no significant relationship found between status of EHR
system and size of hospitals.*

Introduction

With the growing need to provide the right information to the right person anywhere
at anytime in today's global interconnected world, the U.S. healthcare industry has
been moving toward an electronic health record (EHR) system. The need to adopt
an EHR system in U.S. hospitals comes primarily from concerns regarding the
quality of healthcare. Results of two studies of large samples using 1984 and 1992
data "imply that at least 44,000 and perhaps as many as 98,000 Americans die in
hospitals each year as a result of medical errors" (Kohn, Corrigan, & Donaldson,
2000, p. 26). According to Aspden (as cited in Rippen & Yasnoff, 2004), universal
availability of healthcare information and decision support through the national health
information infrastructure can bring substantial improvements in patient safety and
quality of care. The EHR, which is defined as "a secure, real-time, point-of-care,
patient-centric information resource for clinicians" (HIMSS, 2003) is designed
to provide this point of access to patient health information where and when it is
needed by medical professionals.

EHR systems could save up to $81 billion in healthcare costs annually and improve
health care quality (Hillestad et al., 2005). Financially sound hospitals and physician offices are leaping into adopting EHR systems (Goldschmidt, 2005). At the
same time, some small hospitals and small physician offices are lagging behind in
the use of EHR systems creating a digital divide (Goldschmidt, 2005). This may be
due to lack of significant return on investment (ROI) in the short term, considering
the high costs associated with the adoption of EHR systems.

Currently there are various initiatives carried out by governing agencies and healthcare
associations in the area of promoting EHRs. David Brailer, national coordinator for
health information technology, emphasized the important role EHR systems play in
improving quality, increasing patient safety, increasing operational efficiency, and
reducing costs. In his report on "The Decade of Health Information Technology:
Delivering Consumer-centric and Information-rich Health Care: Framework for
Strategic Action," Brailer said that reimbursing physicians for using EHR systems
and reducing their risk of investing in them should accelerate the adoption of EHR
systems in physicians offices (as cited in Mon, 2004).

At a conference in Baltimore on April 27, 2004, President Bush announced that most Americans will have EHRs within the next 10 years to allow doctors and hospitals to share patient records nationwide. To build upon the progress already made in the area of health information technology standards over the last several years, he proposed the FY2005 budget to include $100 million for demonstration projects (Cassidy, 2004). This will help test the effectiveness of health information technology and establish best practices for more widespread adoption in the healthcare industry (Administration Unveils 10 Year Health Information ...., 2004).

Many organizations are working to develop initiatives and goals to help meet the needs of the healthcare industry. One initiative is electronic health information management (e-HIM) by the American Health Information Management Association (AHIMA). E-HIM goals are to: (1) promote the migration from paper to an electronic health information infrastructure, (2) reinvent how institutional and personal health information and records are managed, and (3) deliver measurable cost and quality results from improved information management ("AHIMA Mobilizes to Meet the e-HIM Call," 2003).

The Department of Health and Human Services (DHHS) charged a committee established by the IOM in May 2003 to:

• Provide guidance to DHHS on a set of "basic functionalities" that an electronic health record system should possess to promote patient safety.

The IOM committee considered functions, such as the types of data that should be available to providers when making clinical decisions (e.g., diagnoses, allergies, laboratory results); and the types of decision-support capabilities that should be present (e.g., the capability to alert providers to potential drug-drug interactions) (Institute of Medicine, 2003, p. 4).

Core functionalities of an EHR system and its components at that time as identified by the Institute of Medicine (IOM) committee were health information and data; results management; order entry/management; decision support; electronic communication and connectivity; patient support; administrative processes; and reporting and population health management. See the Appendix for a description of each of these functionalities.

Purpose and Goal of the Study

The overall goal of this study was to identify the core functionalities (as defined by IOM) being used by hospitals throughout the U.S. and the perceived level of benefits, costs, and risks associated with each of the functionalities. In order to meet this goal, a national survey was conducted to answer the following research questions:

- **RQ1:** What are the EHR core functionalities (such as health information and data, results management, order entry/management, decision support, electronic communication, patient support, administrative processes, reporting and population health management) utilized by healthcare systems?

- **RQ2:** Is there a significant difference between the status of the EHR system utilized and the size of the hospital (as measured by number of beds in the hospital)?

- **RQ3:** Is there a relationship between the perceived level of benefit and risk with the use of each of the core functionalities of an EHR system?

Related Work

The status and the effects of using an EHR system are topics of growing interest to researchers. The most comprehensive study on the trends and usage of EHR has been conducted on a yearly basis by the Medical Records Institute (2005). The major role of the largest number of the 280 provider respondents of the 2005 study was information technology (IT) managers and professionals (42%) of which 11% were health information managers or MIS/CIS managers (p. 3). The motivating factors or driving forces for implementing EHR systems that were marked by 75% or more of these respondents were the need to (1) improve clinical processes or workflow efficiency, (2) improve quality of care, (3) share patient record information with healthcare practitioners and professionals, and (4) reduce medical errors (p. 6). The only major barrier to implementation marked by a majority of respondents (57%) was lack of adequate funding or resources (p. 22).

In regard to specific applications or functions, the ones used by a majority of respondents were in the Administrative and Financial Application; the Data Capture, Review, and Update Capabilities; and E-mail categories. Those used by 50% or more in the Administrative and Financial category were in billing and accounts receivable (66%), claims processing (63%), scheduling (61%), patient appointments, (59%), registration/admissions (59%), and charge capture and/or coding (53%) (MRI, 2005, p. 11). In Data Capture, Review, and Update Capabilities, demographics (67%), laboratory results (52%), medications being taken (50%), and allergies (50%) were the ones used by the majority of respondents (p. 13). In the e-mail category, only e-mail between practitioners was used by a majority of respondents (57%).

A study conducted in 2004 by AHIMA showed the industry is continuing to see more movement toward the EHR. The study (as cited in Zender, 2005) was conducted by

Healthcare Informatics in collaboration with AHIMA at their 2004 national convention. It included 284 responses from respondents who primarily (80%) worked in clinical settings. Of these, 55% worked in hospitals while smaller groups worked in ambulatory care, long-term care, behavioral health, and others. A total of 83% of the respondents indicated they were HIM professionals (most having titles of director or manager). The study found that when organizations were asked to describe progress toward an EHR, 17% of respondents indicated extensively implemented; 26% indicated partially implemented; 27% said they were selecting, planning, or minimally implemented, and 21% indicated they were considering implementation and gathering information about it (Zender, 2005).

Medical personnel at the Adult Primary Care Clinic at the Medical University of South Carolina in Charleston, South Carolina, conducted a study to identify if the direct entry into the EHR system in the examination room by physicians had an effect on the physician-patient relationship as perceived by the patients themselves. They found the "use of the EHR had no negative impact on patients' perceived level of satisfaction with their physicians' interpersonal skills, the quality of the visit, or the perceived outcome of the care received" (Wagner et al., 2005, p. 38-39).

In a study conducted during the summer of 2004 by the American Academy of Family Physicians (AAFP), nearly 40% of respondents indicated they either completely converted to EHRs or were in the process of doing so and 24% with EHRs had purchased the system within the first half of the year (Carol, 2005). Cost seemed to be the primary barrier to EHR systems for physicians in small and medium-sized practices. According to Barbara Drury, an independent consultant of Pricare, a national consulting firm in Larkspur, CO (as cited in Carol, 2005), the median cost of implementing an EHR system was in the range of $30,000 per physician and could easily increase to $50,000 when including hardware, training, network upgrades, and IT services.

Previous research on EHR systems identified reducing medical errors, improving quality of care, conserving physician time, sharing patient information among healthcare practitioners, and workflow efficiency as the main benefits (Berman, 2004; Hier, Rothschild, LeMaistre, & Keeler, 2005; Valdes, Kibbie, Tolleson, Kunik, & Petersen, 2004). In regard to risks, privacy, security, and ROI were identified as major concerns (Bates, 2005; Hersh, 2004; Swartz, 2005). Few other studies conducted in the area of EHR reported the status of EHR systems in U.S. hospitals and physician offices (Gans, Kralewski, Hammons, & Dowd, 2005; "Small practices report success with EHRs," 2005; Valdes et al., 2004). These studies and other previous research conducted in the area of EHR systems studied the benefits, risks, and the extent of the usage of EHR applications and functions in U.S. hospitals and physician offices. They did not study the perceived level of benefits, risks, and costs associated with each of the core functionalities of an EHR system.

Methodology

In order to gain a better understanding of electronic record systems used in health-care systems and terminology related to electronic health systems, the researchers conducted interviews at three hospitals within a 65-mile radius. Seven healthcare and information systems professionals from the three hospitals were interviewed. After these interviews and a thorough review of the literature, a draft of a survey instrument was developed. It was designed to gather answers to the research questions stated above. The survey instrument was reviewed by a panel of experts, which included an additional group of medical personnel and information systems personnel in local hospitals. Revisions were made to the survey instrument based on the comments of the reviewers. The survey was then approved by the Human Subjects Committee at the university employing the researchers prior to pilot testing. Next, the survey was sent to eight randomly selected hospitals from a national list of hospitals for pilot testing. Comments from these experts were reviewed and used as feedback for final revision of the instrument.

A database of randomly selected 1000 member hospitals of the American Hospital Association was purchased from Third Wave Research. A mailing including a cover letter, survey instrument, and drawing describing the core functionalities as identified by the IOM, and self-addressed return envelope was mailed in February 2005 to the Director of Health Information of these 1000 randomly selected hospitals. A follow-up mailing was sent in March. The response rate was slightly less than 10% and the findings described on the following pages are based on the 90 usable surveys that were returned. Responses to this study were coded onto Scantron sheets and analyzed using SPSS, version 14.

Findings

Demographics of Respondents and Hospitals Surveyed

Fifty-eight percent of the respondents had 20 years or more of experience in the field; only 16% had less than 10 years. The mean for experience was 20 years. The majority of the respondents (61%) indicated their job title was health information manager or director of health information as seen in Table 1.

The specific titles in the miscellaneous "medical titles" category were Executive Director Physician Practice Network, Sr. VP Quality and Medical Staff Affairs, Transcription Coordinator, Coder in HIM, Patient Health Education Coordinator, and RN/DON. The titles in the miscellaneous "information systems" category were

Table 1. Job titles of respondents

Title	Number	Percent
Director (or Manager) of Health Information	54	61.36
Director (or Manager) of Medical Records	13	14.77
HIM Manager/Director and Privacy Officer	3	3.41
Chief Information Officer/VP of Information Systems	3	3.41
Miscellaneous Medical Titles	6	6.82
Miscellaneous Information Systems' Titles	4	4.55
Other	5	5.68
Total	88	100.00

Table 2. Number of beds in facility

Beds	Number	Percent	Percent from AHA Statistics*
Less than 100	30	34.88	47.46
100 – 199	24	27.91	23.86
200 - 299	12	13.95	12.75
300 - 399	7	8.14	7.13
400 - 499	7	8.14	3.51
500 or more	6	6.98	5.29
Total	86	100.00	100.00

*Based on AHA 2003 statistics of 4,895 U.S. community hospitals.

Systems Coordinator, Accounts Receivable /IT, Manager Patient Accounts/MIS, and Network Administrator. The "other" category contained respondents that indicated they had a title such as Chief Financial Officer, Operations Manager, Team Leader, or Resource Manager.

The average (mean) for the number of beds in the facility was 209. The smallest hospital had 12 beds and the largest had 1460 beds. Table 2 shows the number of beds per facility as grouped according to the groupings used by the American Hospital Association (AHA). The average for the number of beds in the entire healthcare system was 546, with the smallest containing 20 beds and the largest containing 6000 beds.

The average number of hospitals in the healthcare system was 14 with a range from 1 to 172; 48% of the systems had only one hospital; 43% had 2 to 28 hospitals. The remaining 9% had more than 50 hospitals in their entire healthcare system.

Table 3. Status of facility in regard to use of EHR system

Status of Facility	Number	Percent
Currently using some components in all the core functionalities of an EHR system	33	37.08
Currently using some functionalities of an EHR system	24	26.97
Currently using some electronic records systems and plan to interface these into an EHR system within the next two years	9	10.11
Currently using some electronic records systems and plan to interface these into an EHR system sometime between 2 and 5 years from now	13	14.61
Not currently using any electronic records systems, but plan to use an EHR system sometime in the future	10	11.24
Total	89	100.01

Table 4. Status of the core functionality within facility

Core Functionality	Already a part of the EHR system or it is interfaced with the EHR system	Plan to interface within the next 5 years	Do not plan to interface or Not sure
Health Information and Data	64%	32%	4%
Results Management	56%	35%	9%
Order Entry/Management	46%	46%	7%
Decision Support	35%	39%	26%
Electronic Communication and Connectivity	48%	36%	16%
Patient Support	21%	36%	42%
Administrative Processes	57%	25%	17%
Reporting and Population Health Management	39%	27%	34%

Research Question #1

During the literature review and the interviews with healthcare and IT professionals, it was found that an EHR system could be purchased with some or all of the core functionalities depending on the funds available to purchase the software system. In an attempt to determine where hospitals were in regard to the use of EHR systems, the respondents were asked two questions. First, they were asked to mark the status of their facility in regard to the use of an EHR system from a list of options as shown in Table 3. The largest number of the respondents (37%) indicated they currently used some components in all of the eight core functionalities and 27% used only some of the eight core functionalities of an EHR system. Table 3 shows the number of responses and their corresponding percentages.

Second, they were asked to mark the core functionalities of the EHR system that their facility had or planned to have within the next five years (Research Question #1). Health Information and Data, Results Management, and Administrative Processes were the only core functionalities that were currently part of or interfaced with the EHR system in more than 50% of the respondents' facilities. The responses are shown in Table 4.

Research Question # 2

To answer the second research question, which was to determine if there was a relationship between the status of the EHR system and the size of the hospital as measured by the number of beds in the hospital, a one-way ANOVA was conducted. The overall F did not reveal any significant differences among the groups as seen in Table 5 (the groups are the levels of EHR status as listed in Table 3). In other words,

Table 5. Status of EHR system compared to size of the hospital

Status of EHR	Sum of Squares	df	Mean Square	F	p-value
Between Groups	364250.21	4	91062.553	2.011	.101
Within Groups	3622448.1	80	45280.601		
Total	3986698.3	84			

Table 6. Mean of benefits, risks, and costs associated with each of the core functionalities

Functionality	Benefits	Risk Factors	Cost Justification
Health Information and Data	8.83	6.71	7.84
Results Management	8.64	6.96	7.74
Order Entry/Management	8.49	6.77	7.59
Decision Support	7.71	5.95	6.45
Electronic Communication and Connectivity	8.69	7.03	7.21
Patient Support	7.71	6.67	6.83
Administrative Processes	8.25	6.59	7.46
Reporting and Population Health Management	7.58	6.23	6.83

there was no relationship between the status of the EHR system and the size of the hospital. The significance of the results was assessed at the 0.05 alpha level.

General Benefits and Risks

The respondents were asked to evaluate the benefits, risk factors, and cost justification of the core functionalities for which they currently had interfaced or planned to interface into their EHR system within the next five years. They were to evaluate the core functionalities in regard to (1) the degree each one had benefits related to the delivery and quality of healthcare, (2) the degree each had risk factors in relation to cost, cultural change, security of information, dependency upon information, computer downtime, etc., and (3) the degree to whether or not each one was cost justifiable in regard to general terms such as whether the benefits in the long run outweighed the problems, risks, etc., and the anticipation that there would be some ROI in the future. The core functionality the respondents indicated as the most beneficial (one with the highest mean) was "health information and data," closely followed by "electronic communication and connectivity." The functionality with the greatest risk (highest mean for risk factors) was "electronic communication and connectivity," closely followed by "results management." The two functionalities that the respondents found to be the most cost justifiable were "health information and data" and "results management." The means for all three factors for each of the functionalities can be seen in Table 6.

Research Question #3

To answer the third research question, to determine if there was a relationship between perceived level of benefit and risk, a Pearson correlation was conducted. First, it was determined if an overall correlation existed between benefits and risks for each core functionality. Then the correlation was calculated again for each of the groups separately to test where the significance occurred and which group had a higher correlation between benefits and risks (those who had the functionality or with those who did not currently have it, but planned to within the next five years). Those who indicated they did not plan to have the core functionality or were not sure, were not included.

There was a significant positive correlation between benefits and risks for all eight core functionalities. The correlation was significant at the 0.01 alpha level. This positive correlation indicated that the respondents associated high benefits with high risks. For three of the eight core functionalities--Health Information and Data, Administrative Processes, and Reporting and Population Health Management--there was a significant positive correlation for both groups (those who already had it and those who planned to have it). For the other five functionalities, the significance existed only in the group that planned to have it. Therefore, for the group of hospitals who already had the core functionalities of an EHR system, the respondents did not seem to associate as high a risk with the benefits as those who were just in the planning stages.

In the area of Health Information and Data, the correlation was 0.544 between perceived benefits and risks. When looking at each group individually (those who had this functionality in their EHR system and those who planned to have it within the next five years), the correlation was twice as much for the group who planned to have this functionality (0.742) compared to those who already had it (0.361).

In the area of Results Management, there was again an overall high positive correlation between benefits and risks (0.578). However, this time when looking at the groups individually, a significant positive correlation (0.681) existed only in the group who planned to have this functionality (and not those who already had it). These results and those for the other core functionalities can be seen in Table 7.

Table 7. Correlation between perceived benefit and risk for each functionality (overall and individual correlation for groups respectively)

Core Functionality	Overall Correlation for Both Groups	Calculated p value	Correlation for Group that Already Had Functionality	Calculated p value	Correlation for Group that Planned to Have Functionality	Calculated p value
Health Information and Data	.544*	.000	.361*	.011	.742*	.000
Results Management	.578*	.000	.247	.120	.681*	.000
Order Entry/ Management	.597*	.000	.134	.444	.738*	.000
Decision Support	.694*	.000	.205	.337	.816*	.000
Electronic Communication and Connectivity	.533*	.000	.087	.626	.723*	.000
Patient Support	.664*	.000	.414	.125	.722*	.000
Administrative Processes	.619*	.000	.364*	.021	.936*	.000
Reporting and Population Health Management	.666*	.000	.396*	.033	.908*	.000

*p = 0.01

Discussion

The majority of the respondents (61%) indicated their job title was health information manager or director of health information. This is a much larger percent than the 11% of respondents to the 2005 Medical Records Institute's Survey of EHR trends and usage (which included physicians as well as those in other roles), but slightly less than the 83% from the AHIMA study which indicated they were HIM professionals. The average (mean) for the number of beds in the facility's surveyed was 209; 35% of the hospitals had less than 100 beds. The most recent American Hospital Association statistics for bed size of hospitals in the U.S. was consulted to determine if the study sample provided a qualitative representation of U.S. hospitals. Thirty-five percent of the hospitals responding to the survey reported 1 to 99 beds while the 2003 AHA statistics reported approximately 47% hospitals in the category of less than 100 beds. Therefore, this study had responses from fewer small hospitals than there were in the actual population of hospitals. However, for all the other categories of hospitals by bed size, it was pretty comparable, varying only 2 to 5% within each bed size category (AHA, 2003). See comparisons in Table 2.

The largest number of the respondents (37%) indicated they currently used some components in all of the eight core functionalities and 27% used only some of the eight core functionalities of an EHR system. The study conducted by AHIMA, although worded slightly differently, found that 17% of organizations indicated they had extensively implemented EHR systems and 26% indicated partially implemented (Zender, 2005). These two studies had a slightly different focus and way of analyzing the status of the EHR system. The AHIMA statement asked respondents to describe their organization's progress toward implementation of an EHR, and this study sought to discover the status of their facility in regard to the use of the EHR system by looking at how many of the core functionalities were used or interfaced into the EHR system.

The overall F in this study did not reveal any significant differences among the status of the facilities' use of an EHR system in relation to the size of hospital. However, other research indicated that some small hospitals and small physician offices were lagging behind in the use of EHR systems creating a digital divide (Goldschmidt, 2005). In order for EHR systems to be seamlessly used and offer the intended benefits, they must become more affordable and see some return on investment (ROI).

Health Information and Data, Results Management (lab test results, radiology procedures, and other results reporting), and Administrative Processes were the only core functionalities that were currently part of or interfaced with the EHR system in more than 50% of the respondents' facilities. This seems to correspond fairly closely to the MRI Survey which found that specific applications or functions used by at least a majority of respondents were in the Administrative and Financial Application; the Data Capture, Review, and Update Capabilities; and E-mail categories. Laboratory results, which fell under the category of Data Capture, Review, and Update Capabilities, of the MRI survey were used by over 50% of respondents.

There was a significant positive correlation between perceived level of benefits and risks for all core eight functionalities. For the majority of the core functionalities, the positive associations were stronger for those in the group that planned to have it (than the group that already had it). Since all the overall correlations between risk and benefits were positive, we can conclude that the respondents associated high benefits with high risks. For the group of hospitals who already had the core functionalities of an EHR system, the respondents did not seem to associate as high a risk with the benefits as those who were just in the planning stages. This may imply that once the functionality is implemented the perceived level of risk decreases.

Limitations

The study may have some limitations. First, the low response rate may make it difficult to generalize the findings to the total population. Second, although the study identified that a correlation existed between the risks and benefits for each of the core functionalities among the groups, it did not identify any specific risks or benefits for each of the functionalities.

Conclusion and Future Work

Each of the eight core functionalities can be adopted by hospitals individually or as an entire EHR system. This study identified the majority of the core functionalities used in the hospitals, as well as the correlation between the benefits and risks associated with these core functionalities. Other hospitals that are in the planning and information gathering stages can use this information to prioritize the core functionalities that they plan to adopt.

Based on the findings of this study, it is suggested that some of the high risks associated with EHR systems may be misconceptions by professionals in the field who have not yet adopted an EHR system. The benefits have been stated over and over again. However, little research has been done on the risks associated in using these systems. Future work in the area of EHRs should identify risks associated with the use of each of the core functionalities of an EHR system and ways to avoid these risks or come to the realization that they may not be as problematic as once thought.

This study identified a perceived level of cost associated with the benefits and risks in adopting each of the core functionalities. Since ROI is a barrier to adoption of EHR systems, future study of cost-benefit factors related to each of the core functionalities is recommended. An implication of this would be that hospitals and physicians will gain a better understanding of the cost factors related to each of the functionalities and be able to prioritize and procure the functionalities of an EHR system as needed.

References

Administration unveils 10 year health information technology strategic framework. (2004). *E-health initiative*. Retrieved August 28, 2004, from http://www.ehealthinitiative.org/initiatives/policy/administration.mspx

AHIMA mobilizes to meet the e-HIM call. (2003). *AHIMA Advantage, 7*(1), *1-3*.

American Hospital Association. (2005). *AHA hospital statistics: The comprehensive reference source for analysis and comparison of hospital trends*. Chicago: AHA, p. 10.

Bates, D. (2005). Physicians and ambulatory electronic health records. *Health Affairs, 24*(5), 1180-1189.

Berman, J. (2004). Safety centers and EMRs. *Health-IT world*. Retrieved August 11, 2004, from http://www.health-itworld.com/emag/050104/183.html

Carol, R. (2005). EHRs, the doctor will see you now. *Journal of American Health Information Management Association, 76*(4), 24-28.

Cassidy, B. S. (2004). Skills for success in managing an EHR environment. *Advance Online Editions for Health Information Professionals*. Retrieved June 18, 2004, from http://www.advanceforhim.com/common/Editorial/PrintFriendly.aspx?CC=34975

Gans, D., Kralewski, J., Hammons, T., & Dowd, B. (2005). Medical groups' adoption of electronic health records and information systems. *Health Affairs, 24*(5), 1323-1333.

Goldschmidt, P. G. (2005). HIT and MIS: Implications of health information technology and medical information systems. *Communications of the ACM, 48*(10), 69-74.

Hersh, W. (2004). Health care information technology: Progress and barriers. *Journal of the American Medical Association, 292*(18), 2273-2274.

Hier, D., Rothschild, A., LeMaistre, A., & Keeler, J. (2005). Differing faculty and house staff acceptance of an electronic health record. *International Journal of Medical Informatics, 74*(7/8), 657-662.

Hillestad, R., Bigelow, J., Bower, A., Girosi, F., Meili, R. et al. (2005). Can electronic medical record systems transform health care? Potential health benefits, savings, and costs. *Health Affairs, 24*(5), 1103-1117.

HIMSS. (2003). *Electronic health record definitional model version 1.0.* Retrieved July 26, 2004, from http://www.himss.org/content/mindmaps/EHR/multimaps/resources/resources.htm

Institute of Medicine. (2003). Key capabilities of an electronic health record system. Retrieved July 26, 2004, from http://books.nap.edu/html/ehr/NI000427.pdf

Kohn, L. T., Corrigan J. M., & Donaldson, M. S. (2000). *To err is human: Building a safer health system.* Washington, DC: National Academy Press.

Medical Records Institute. (2005). *Medical records institute's seventh annual survey of electronic health record trends and usage for 2005.* Retrieved October 5, 2005, from http://www.medrecinst.com/files/ehrsurvey05.pdf

Mon, D. T. (2004). Next steps for the EHR draft standard: Core functionality and conformance criteria key for accreditation. *Journal of American Health Information Management Association, 75*(10), 50-51.

Rippen, H. E., & Yasnoff, W. A. (2004). Building the national health information infrastructure. *Journal of American Health Information Management Association, 75*(5), 20-26.

Small practices report success with EHRs. (2005). *Family Practice Management, 12*(4), 40.

Swartz, N. (2005). Electronic medical records' risks feared. *Information Management Journal, 39*(3), 9.

Valdes, I., Kibbe, D., Tolleson, G., Kunik, M., & Petersen, L. (2004). Barriers to proliferation of electronic medical records. *Informatics in Primary Care, 12*(1), 3-9.

Wagner, K. A., Ward, D. M., Lee, F. W., White, A. W., Davis, K. S., & Clancy, D. E. (2005). Physicians, patients, and EHRs. *Journal of American Health Information Management Association, 76*(4), 38-41.

Zender, A. (2005). Ready for the EHR? A new survey measures EHR implementation and individual readiness. *Journal of American Health Information Management Association, 76*(3), 54-55.

Appendix A

1. **Health information and data:** A defined dataset that includes medical and nursing diagnoses, a medication list, allergies, demographics, clinical narratives, and laboratory test results for access by care providers when needed.

2. **Results management:** A feature to manage the lab test results, radiology procedures results, do results reporting, results notification, and multimedia support—images, waveforms, pictures, sounds.

3. **Order entry/management:** Computerized provider order entry (CPOE) for such areas as electronic prescribing, laboratory, microbiology, pathology, XR, ancillary, nursing, supplies, consults. Even with little or no decision support, they can still improve workflow processes by eliminating lost orders and ambiguities caused by illegible handwriting, generating related orders automatically.

4. **Decision support:** A computerized decision support system, which enhances clinical performance by providing drug alerts, other rule-based alerts, reminders, clinical guidelines, and pathways. It also helps in improving drug dosing, and drug selection. It can be used for chronic disease management, clinician work lists, diagnostic decision support, and automated real-time surveillance.

5. **Electronic communication and connectivity:** Electronic communication can be between provider-provider, patient-provider, trading partners such as pharmacies, insurers, laboratory, radiology, and among team members for coordination. Electronic connectivity includes integrated medical record within facility, within different facilities of the same healthcare system, and among different healthcare systems.

6. **Patient support:** Patient support includes patient education, family and informal caregiver education, data entered by patient, family, and/or information caregiver such as home monitoring

7. **Administrative processes:** Administrative processes include electronic scheduling systems for hospital admissions, inpatient and outpatient procedures, and identifying eligible or potential eligible patients for clinical trials.

8. **Reporting and population health management:** This feature would report patient safety and quality data, public health data, and disease registries. It makes the reporting process less labor-intensive and time-consuming (Institute of Medicine, 2003).

Chapter XV

Using Pocket PCs for Nurses' Shift Reports and Patient Care

Karen Chang, Purdue University, USA

Kyle D. Lutes, Purdue University, USA

Melanie L. Braswell, Purdue University, USA

Jacqueline K. Nielsen, Purdue University, USA

Abstract

Nurses working in hospitals with paper-based systems often face the challenge of inefficiency in providing quality nursing care. Two areas of inefficiency are shift-to-shift communication among nurses, and access to information related to patient care. An integrated IT system, consisting of Pocket PCs and a desktop PC interfaced to a hospital's mainframe system, was developed. The goal was to use mobile IT to give nurses easier access to patient information. This chapter describes the development of this system and reports the results of a pilot study: a comparison of time spent in taking and giving shift reports before and after the study and nurses' perceptions of the mobile IT system. Results showed a significant difference in taking shift reports and no significant difference in giving shift reports. Nurses stated that quick and easy access to updated patient information in the Pocket PC was very helpful, especially during mainframe downtime.

Introduction

The quality of the American healthcare delivery system has been problematic. The Institute of Medicine (IOM, 2001) identified six dimensions of quality: safe, effective, patient-centered, timely, efficient, and equitable. However, in hospitals with paper-based delivery systems, nurses often face challenges in meeting these expectations. Two areas of inefficiency are communication among nurses, and accessing information relevant to patient care.

Nurses use shift reports (also called handoffs or handovers) to communicate pertinent patient information to maintain the continuity of safe and effective care. However, the quality of shift reports has been criticized in several areas: missed information, irrelevant information, inaccurate information, inefficiencies, and lack of standardization (Currie, 2002; Sexton, Chan, Elliott, Stuart, Jayasuriya & Crookes, 2004). A better means to improve the quality of shift reports is urgently needed.

Three types of shift reports are commonly used: audiotape reports, face-to-face reports, or walking rounds. Audiotape reports do not require the presence of outgoing nurses and incoming nurses simultaneously. Outgoing nurses give reports by speaking into an audiotape recorder about one hour before the end of the shift. Incoming nurses listen to the audiotape reports at the beginning of the shift. Face-to-face reports occur in a designated room, such as an office or a conference room. Walking rounds occurs at the patient bedside. Face-to-face reports and walking rounds require all outgoing and incoming nurses be present at the same time. Face-to-face reports and walking rounds require more time than audiotape reports.

Audiotape reports have become prevalent since the 1990s. Audiotape reports may save about 15 minutes in each shift because outgoing nurses do not need to wait for incoming nurses to give reports (Mason, 2004). However, incoming nurses may spend about 30 to 60 minutes taking shift reports from the audiotape reports before starting to take care of their assigned patients. The majority of the time is spent on transcribing key information from audiotape reports to their self-designed paper worksheets. Nurses use self-designed paper worksheets to write key patient information (e.g., diagnosis, physical or psychosocial status, treatments, tests, etc.) and to organize patient care activities. Incoming nurses listen to the audiotape reports at the beginning of the shift and take notes on their self-designed worksheets or on any piece of paper (also called scraps) to organize patient care information (Hardey, Payne & Coleman, 2000). Nurses carry their worksheets in their pocket or on a clipboard, take notes about their patient care activities, and record updated information for later documentation and outgoing shift reports. Audiotape reports continue to limit nurses in providing care in a timely and efficient manner.

Nurses need to efficiently and effectively communicate information to provide safe, effective, and patient-centered care. When comprehensive patient information is transferred efficiently, nurses can identify patient needs, monitor patient conditions, prevent or detect complications, and implement physician orders safely and accurately. However, accessing all relevant information for patient care in the paper-based delivery system can be difficult and time-consuming. For example, when nurses need to know patient health history and health status, they need to find the patient's paper medical records, which could be misplaced or in use by other healthcare providers. When nurses need to know the results of a patient's most recent laboratory or diagnostic tests that are stored in the hospital's mainframe system, they need to go to a nursing station to log in to the mainframe to obtain the information. When nurses need to give unfamiliar medications, they need to look up the information in a drug reference, which could be misplaced or in use by other nurses, or outdated. If nurses give medications without accurate knowledge of drug information, such as safe dosage, rate of administration, drug interactions, and side effects, medication errors may occur. Thus, paper-based information systems are fraught with inefficiencies that can compromise patient care. Specifically, if nurses do not have pertinent patient information, they are ill-prepared to make appropriate clinical decisions. They may not detect or prevent complications due to medications, procedures or treatments, or may not provide adequate patient education to help patients care for themselves.

The Institute of Medicine (2001) asserted that information technology (IT) must be used in the 21st century to improve the quality of healthcare. The American Academy of Nursing Technology and Workforce urged the use of IT to support nurses' work and to eliminate waste and redundancy (Sensimeier, Raiford, Taylor & Weaver, 2002). President Bush (April 27, 2004) announced that electronic medical records (EMR) would be available for residents in the United States in 10 years. However, there are many barriers to integrating IT in the hospital, such as high cost, lack of support from physicians and administration, and lack of applications that are easy to use (Gillespie, 2002; Sensimeier et al., 2002). Thus, many hospitals are still using paper-based medical records and mainframe computer systems to store patient information.

Using "computers, handheld" as the key word in combination with other key words, such as "database nanagement systems, hospital information systems, hospital nursing staff, or nursing information systems" in MEDLINE and CINAHL, current clinical use of personal digital assistants (PDAs) was identified. There is an increasing trend in using PDAs in the healthcare field. For examples, orthopedic surgeons used programs loaded in the PDAs to access patient data in the office and the operating room (Laskin & Davis, 2004); a wireless PDA was developed for patient transport to monitor patient's vital signs (heart rate, three-lead electrocardiography, and SpO2) remotely (Lin et al., 2004); nurses used PDAs to collect utilization review data that were sent to hospital's mainframe system for quality evaluation; and physicians at Cedars-Sinai hospital in California used wireless PDAs to access patient EMRs wirelessly and used them during ward rounds or at shift changes (Shabot, 2002). The healthcare providers of Shock Trauma Intensive Care Unit at Intermountain Healthcare, Salt Lake City, used EMR and reported that they spent ten minutes for shift reports (Nelson et al., 2003). PDA users, including nurses, pharmacists, and physicians, report that PDAs are useful and effective tools for their patient care (Dee, Teolis, & Tod 2005; Honeybourne, Sutton & Ward, 2006). However, no studies were found regarding nurses' use of PDAs interfaced with the hospital mainframe system for shift reports.

A collaborative effort among Purdue's School of Nursing, Purdue's Department of Computer Technology, and a local hospital's nursing staff resulted in the development of the iCare system to improve the efficiency and effectiveness of shift reports in the paper-based medical records environment. This chapter reports the development of the iCare system and nurses' perceptions of the iCare system for shift reports and patient care. The iCare system consists of handheld computers (Pocket PCs, or PDAs), a desktop personal computer (PC), and a hospital's mainframe system (Figure 1). The goal of the iCare system is to use mobile IT, in the form of Pocket PCs, to give nurses easier access to patient information so that nurses have more time to provide quality patient care. Additionally, an electronic version of a worksheet similar to nurses' paper worksheets and audiotape reports was developed to improve the efficiency of communicating patient information between shifts.

Method

Design and Security Considerations

By design, Pocket PCs are small, mobile computing devices and can easily be lost or stolen. Privacy of patient information on the Pocket PCs was a serious concern. To protect this information, several layers of security were used. First, password protection was built into the Pocket PCs, which requires a password each time a Pocket PC was powered on. Second, the custom applications required nurses to log in using a unique user ID and password. And finally, all patient information used

Figure 1. The iCare system architecture

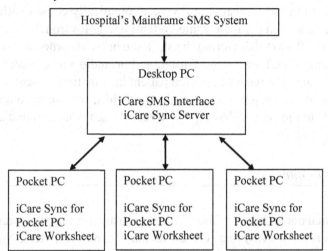

by the system was stored in encrypted and obfuscated files on the Pocket PCs and desktop PC.

Other considerations were technology-related. Because the hospital did not have a wireless network infrastructure in place, nor would they allow wireless networks to be installed, the iCare system was not developed to use wireless network access of any kind. Instead, the system required the nurses to send and receive patient information to and from a Pocket PC by periodically synchronizing it with the desktop PC through a sync cable.

In designing the study, a decision was made to limit the impact this research would have on the work load of the hospital IT staff. The project was designed so that no new custom mainframe programs or changes to the existing systems were required. Retrieving patient information from the hospital's mainframe computer system was done using custom software, designed by the second author.

After an analysis period and meeting with several of the nursing staff to understand the process of shift reports and the process of accessing the hospital's mainframe system for patient information, four custom software applications were developed. These were named "iCare SMS Interface," "iCare Worksheet for Pocket PCs," "iCare Sync for Pocket PCs," and "iCare Sync Server." An iterative process was used to simulate paper-based worksheets and audiotape shift reports during the development of the iCare Worksheet.

A desktop PC was centrally located in a unit of the hospital in which the study was carried out. A program on the central PC periodically accessed patient information from the hospital's mainframe computer systems for all patients in that unit. At the beginning of a shift, each nurse synchronized the Pocket PC by placing it in a cradle connected to the PC. Custom software automatically copied patient information, including data from the mainframe systems and notes from the nurses on previous shifts, to the Pocket PC. During the shift, the nurse recorded new notes about each patient using typed text, handwriting, and/or audio voice recordings. Whenever the nurse wanted to retrieve updated patient information, to send the notes to other nurses, or to give reports at the end of the shift, the nurse connected his or her Pocket PC to the central desktop PC where the software automatically copied any new patient notes.

iCare SMS Interface

The hospital tracked patient information using an information system from Siemens Health Services (SMS) that runs on its mainframe computers. Nurses access this system using dumb terminal hardware, or terminal emulation software running on PCs. To avoid changes to programs running on the mainframe system, the iCare Interface program was written to use a technique called "screen scraping" to gather patient information.

The iCare SMS Interface program functions by communicating with a terminal emulation component running on the same PC. The iCare SMS interface program sends keystrokes to the terminal emulation component that mimics the keystrokes a nurse might use when using the SMS system. When patient information is returned as text to the terminal emulator, the iCare SMS Interface program copies the text from the emulator screen buffer, reformats it, and saves it to encrypted files stored on the PC. Although not efficient by modern IT standards, screen scraping does provide an interface to legacy systems that cannot otherwise be modified to interface with a new system.

The iCare SMS Interface program was developed using Microsoft Visual Basic 6 and a terminal emulation component from Attachmate. These technologies were chosen for this application because it was developed by the authors primarily onsite at the hospital's IT department, and these technologies were already being used by the hospital's IT staff for other projects.

iCare Worksheet for Pocket PCs

The iCare Worksheet application is the primary program for nurses to use for shift reports and patient care management. It simulates nurses' self-designed paper worksheets to organize patient information and patient care activities. Nurses can view patient information either gathered from the mainframe system via iCare SMS Interface or recorded notes. They can also record new notes. The user interface allows

Figure 2. Categories of the iCare worksheet

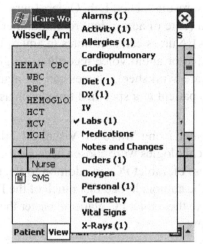

Note: Fictitious patient information shown. A number inside of parenthesis indicate the number of notes in that category.

Figure 3. An example of text, audio, and handwriting notes in the iCare Worksheet

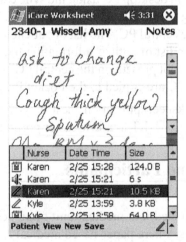

Note: Fictitious patient information shown. Red, blue, green, and black pen colors can be used when taking handwritten notes.

nurses to see a list of all patients in the unit. After selecting a patient, nurses can see information about the patient. Because of the limited screen space on a Pocket PC, information is grouped into various categories to make finding the information quicker (Figure 2). The patient information obtained from the mainframe system by the SMS Interface program is automatically sent to the categories of Allergies, Cardiopulmonary (test results), Diet, Lab, Orders (current medications and laboratory orders), Personal (date of admission, room number, physicians), and X-Rays (radiology test results). Nurses can take notes in any of the categories using either typed text, hand-written or audio voice recordings (Figure 3). Alarm features are also built into the iCare Worksheet. Nurses can set alarms to remind them to do certain tasks for each patient at a specified time, such as time to give medications or treatments.

This program was written using Microsoft Visual C# .NET and the .NET Compact Framework. These technologies were chosen because the study also included plans to test the effectiveness of Tablet PCs in addition to Pocket PCs for use by nurses. By using Visual C#, the authors hoped that much of the Pocket PC program source code could be ported to the Tablet PC platform easier than other software development tools would allow.

iCare Sync for Pocket PCs and iCare Sync Server

The iCare Sync for Pocket PCs and iCare Sync Server work in tandem to automatically copy patient information to and from the Pocket PCs. When a Pocket PC is connected to the central desktop PC using the sync cable, the iCare Sync for Pocket PCs program running on the Pocket PC establishes a connection to the iCare Sync Server running on the central PC. The list of patient information files on the Pocket PC is compared to the list of patient information files on the central PC. Any note files on the Pocket PC not present on the central PC are copied to the PC. Likewise, any note files on the PC are copied to the Pocket PC.

As with the iCare Worksheet application, the iCare Sync programs were developed using Microsoft Visual C# .NET to allow easier porting to the Tablet PC platform.

Study Setting and Participants

This study was conducted in a medical unit of an acute care hospital in the Midwestern United States, where paper-based medical records were used. In addition, key patient information was available using dumb terminals in the nurses' stations. There was no computer access at the bedside. A prospective pre- and post-test design was used to examine the efficiency and effectiveness of the iCare System for shift reports and patient care. Nurses of all shifts who worked during the study period participated in the study.

Procedure

Ten Dell Axim X5 Pocket PCs were used in the study because the maximum number of nurses working at one time on the unit was eight. All Pocket PCs were kept on the unit and maintained by unit staff. After the approval from the Institutional Review Board, this study was implemented over four weeks (two weeks of learning and two weeks of actual use). In the first week, six one-hour orientation sessions were provided. Nurses were encouraged to practice using the iCare Worksheet for shift reports. The purpose and the procedure of the study, confidentiality of collected data, and voluntary nature of participation were explained to participants. After consent was obtained, nurses learned to use Pocket PCs and the iCare Worksheet to find patient information, and take notes (text, handwritten, or voice format) in the iCare Worksheet. During the second week, nurses continued to practice using the iCare system for shift reports and patient care. In the third week, nurses used both the iCare Worksheet and audiotape for all shift reports. In the fourth week, the iCare Worksheet was the only means for shift reports and audiotape recorders were removed. Three nursing faculty members provided orientation and support for the iCare system. They visited the unit periodically during each shift and talked to every nurse to inquire about concerns or difficulties. They also helped each nurse to use the iCare Worksheet.

Questionnaires

To examine efficiency and effectiveness of using the iCare Worksheet, baseline information and perceptions of the iCare Worksheet questionnaires were used. Nurses were asked to indicate their comfort level using Pocket PC (very uncomfortable, somewhat uncomfortable, somewhat comfortable, and very comfortable) and the number of years working in the hospital and in the unit in the baseline information. Nurses were also asked to provide the average time spent in giving and taking shift reports before starting the study.

Perceptions of the iCare Worksheet were given to nurses at the end of the study in a self-addressed stamped envelope. Information obtained included: average time spent in giving reports and taking reports using the iCare Worksheet, positive and negative experiences in using the iCare Worksheet, and suggestions for improvement. In addition, nursing faculty who provided support during study period took anecdotal notes about nurses' comments and experiences in using the iCare system.

Table 1. Descriptive statistics of time spent (in minutes) for giving and taking shift reports using audiotape and iCare Worksheet methods

		Audiotape		iCare Worksheet	
		Giving Reports	Taking Reports	Giving Reports	Taking Reports
N	Valid	22	22	23	24
	Missing	4	4	3	2
Mean (S.D.)		23.05 (14.25)	24.95 (11.04)	20.21 (14.90)	16.41 (11.52)
Median		20	20	16.25	13
Minimum		7	10	0	3
Maximum		60	55	60	55

Table 2. Paired samples statistics—time spent (in minutes) in giving and taking shift reports—audiotape vs. iCare Worksheet

		Mean	N	SD
Pair 1	Time spent in giving reports per audiotape	23.05	22	14.25
	Time spent in giving reports per iCare worksheet	20.09	22	15.36
Pair 2	Time spent in taking reports per audiotape	25.20	20	11.32
	Time spent in taking reports per iCare Worksheet	16.38	20	11.77

		Paired Differences				
		Mean	SD	t	df	Sig. (2-tailed)
Pair 1	Time spent in giving reports per audiotape—time spent in giving reports per iCare worksheet	2.96	13.45	1.03	21	.314
Pair 2	Time spent in taking reports per audiotape—time spent in taking reports per iCare Worksheet	8.83	12.01	3.29	19	.004

* Paired samples statistics (exclude cases analysis by analysis) was performed.

Results

Baseline Information

Response rate was 74.3% (35 received iCare training, 26 responded to questionnaires; 4 of 26 contained incomplete data). The average years of working in the hospital was 12.62 (range = 1.5 – 36; S.D. = 10.61). The average years of working in this unit was 7.28 (range = 1 – 32, S.D. = 7.57). Most nurses reported that they were comfortable in using Pocket PC to find information (44% somewhat comfortable; 44% very comfortable).

Efficiency

Results of descriptive statistics showed that on average, nurses using the iCare Worksheet method spent 8.54 minutes less in taking reports (24.95 – 16.41 = 8.54) and 2.84 minutes less in giving reports (23.05 – 20.21 = 2.84) than the audiotape method (Table 1). The average total time spent in giving and taking shift reports using the iCare Worksheet method was 11.38 minutes less than the audiotape method.

Paired sample T-Test procedure showed significant differences in taking reports (t = 3.29, p = .004), but no significant differences in giving reports between these two methods (Table 2).

Perceived Benefits

Nurses wrote many positive comments about the accessibility of the iCare Worksheet. All respondents (n = 26) stated that quick access to patient information was very helpful. They were glad to see laboratory results, radiology reports, diagnoses, and medications at the beginning of the shift and while providing patient care. Several nurses gave examples to describe how the iCare Worksheet helped them provide patient care. For example, one patient had an emergency situation. A nurse responded and did not know this patient. She accessed information in the iCare Worksheet (code status and treatment) quickly so that she could provide proper care until support staff arrived. In another example, a nurse answered the call lights of other nurses' patients. She used information in the iCare Worksheet to answer patients' requests. A nurse answered physicians' and patients' questions about laboratory and diagnostic tests results promptly by accessing information in the iCare Worksheet. Three nurses reported that they were glad to have comprehensive patient information in the Pocket PC when the hospital's mainframe systems were unavailable.

Eight nurses wrote positive experiences about entering nurses' notes in the iCare Worksheet. They also reported that using the iCare Worksheet was faster than using audiotape to give reports to the next shift. In addition, being able to see nurses' notes of previous shift helped them know patients' condition quickly without duplicating work. One nurse liked to use the alarms feature. She set alarms to remind her when to give medications and treatments, to check laboratory results, and to call physicians.

Key Findings from Anecdotal Notes

Anecdotal notes provided further perceived benefits of the iCare system. Initially, nurses stated that they spent more time entering data into the iCare Worksheet than they did on their paper-based worksheets. Gradually, they began to voice the benefits of using the iCare Worksheet. They could readily access specific patient information in the iCare Worksheet without having to leave the patient's room to look up information in dumb terminals during physician rounds.

Taking notes in the iCare Worksheet involved a learning curve. Nurses who took notes in the iCare Worksheet stated that they became more proficient with repeated use. Some nurses voiced that the time required taking notes and synchronization was far less than the time required to manually abstract updated patient information from patient's medical records.

One nurse reported that an unexpected incident convinced more nurses to use the iCare system. One day, the hospital mainframe systems went down. No new orders or new diagnostic results could be retrieved on the dumb terminals. The only way to find this information was to call various departments. Physician rounding became quite challenging. On this particular day, nurses discovered that they could still access updated patient information in the iCare Worksheet if their Pocket PCs were synchronized. Subsequently, whenever there was an indication that hospital's mainframe systems would go down, there was a flurry of activity at the sync station.

Being able to access all patients' data was another significant nurse satisfier. Nurses covered for other nurses during meal breaks or time off the unit. With the iCare Worksheet, any nurse could access the most updated information on all patients. Nurses reported that this benefit did not exist with the paper-based worksheet. Some verbalized that they spent less time abstracting information from medical records and the mainframe system and had more time available for patient care.

A train-the-trainer strategy was used to have nurses helping nurses for orientation, training, and support. Many times, computer-based training was performed by computer personnel. Nurses with limited computer background tended to become apprehensive because they could not comprehend the information. When nursing faculty provided the training and were available to help them, they reported feeling less threatened in learning the new technology. Some nurses who began with apprehension due to limited computer skills became enthusiastic participants later.

Areas for Improvement and Suggestions

There was no consistent system to take notes in the iCare Worksheet. Some nurses entered useful notes and some nurses who were slow to use the technology did not enter notes. Some nurses worked only once or twice during the study period and were uncomfortable with the technology. To them, talking to the audiotape recorder was faster than entering notes on the Pocket PC. Scribbled handwriting was hard to read sometime. Voice notes could be hard to hear. Nurses would like to have had all information in one screen instead of going to each category to view. They would like to have had more information from the mainframe systems, such as physicians' dictated notes. They would like to print out patient reports and to use the iCare Worksheet along with computerized charting and physician-order entry system in the future.

The size of the Pocket PC was identified both as a positive and a negative. The portable size was beneficial for carrying and immediate access. The disadvantage was in reading reports with large amounts of data on a small screen, which necessitated a significant amount of side-to-side and up-and-down scrolling. They would like to have had a larger screen to view reports.

Several suggestions were related to hardware improvement. They would like to hear louder sounds for recorded notes, a lighter weight Pocket PC, a keyboard, and a longer battery life. They would like to have more sync stations, voice translation, faster handwriting recognition program, and a faster sync process. They also voiced a desire to see if the patient call lights system could be integrated with the Pocket PC in the future.

Discussion

The goal of the iCare system is to use an integrated IT system using Pocket PCs to give nurses working in hospitals with paper medical records and mainframe systems quick access to patient information and to improve quality patient care. Most of the nurses in this study were using this mobile technology for the first time. Initially, they were skeptical about using mobile technology. Results indicated that nurses enjoyed the quick access to pertinent patient information at any time and any place without patients' paper medical records or dumb terminals. Their comments and anecdotal notes indicated that the iCare system enabled them to have more time to provide quality patient care.

The iCare system shortens incoming nurses' time taking reports at the beginning of the shift. When the Pocket PC is synchronized with the central PC, pertinent and updated patient information can be viewed in the iCare Worksheet. There is less information that nurses need to write down. However, the iCare system does not save nurses' time when giving reports. The discrepancy reflects variations of how each nurse uses the iCare Worksheet. One nurse indicated that she spent zero minutes in giving reports while another nurse identified that she spent 60 minutes in giving reports. The first nurse wrote notes throughout the shift while caring for patients. This nurse used iCare Worksheet the same way as using the paper-based worksheet, in an ongoing fashion throughout the shift. The second nurse tried to enter notes in the iCare Worksheet at the end of the shift to give the report. The second nurse did not use this technology the way it was intended and thus took 60 minutes to give her report. IT can be a tough sell to nursing staffs (Gillespie, 2002). Strategies are needed to help nurses embrace the technology to use it in a consistent manner.

The iCare Worksheet provides a standard format to record and retrieve patient information. This format decreases variability in transferring and communicating patient information among nurses. In the paper-based worksheet system, there is no consistency. Each nurse uses his or her own system to transfer and communicate patient information for patient care and shift reports. Variability increases risks for errors. The iCare Worksheet has the potential to improve the quality of nursing care by standardizing nurses' information transfer and communication in the hospital with paper-based medical records and the mainframe system. The situation-background-assessment-recommendation model (SBAR) developed by Leonard and colleagues (2004) was designed to improve the quality of communication between healthcare professionals. This model can be integrated into the iCare Worksheet to enhance communication between shifts in the future development.

In this study, nurses expressed the benefits of accessing information in the PDA. They hoped to access more information relevant to patient care (physician's dictated notes, physicians' and healthcare facilities' phone numbers) and to use the PDA to document patient care. These findings converge with a study of nurses' preferences and needs of assistive computing devices (Mihailidis, Krones & Boger, 2006).

At the end of this study, it was also identified that nursing students could benefit from using the iCare Worksheet to access key patient information instead of look- ing for paper medical records, which are often used by other healthcare providers. Thus, the hospital allowed the iCare system to be placed in two additional units for students to use during the school year. The iCare Worksheet was loaded in both Pocket PCs and Tablet PCs for students to use. Preliminary students' feedback showed the preference of using Tablet PC rather than Pocket PC. This could be explained in part because students not only needed to access pertinent patient data to provide appropriate care but also had to record and analyze specific data as part of their course requirements. The Tablet PC was preferred because they could both access patient data and complete their synthesis evaluations during clinical.

This project was limited to four weeks, but the impact of this study continues to be experienced. Prior to this study, the hospital's nursing administrators had not considered using Pocket PCs for nurses. After the study, the hospital's nursing administrators saw the benefits of using Pocket PCs to access patient information in the mainframe, but chose not to expand the iCare system hospital wide because the hospital was going to change the mainframe system to another vendor. An effort to refine iCare Worksheet to interface with the new mainframe system has been sought to continue this technology for nurses as long as the hospital is using the paper-based medical records and the mainframe system.

Conclusion

This study demonstrated that the use of mobile technology, integrated with a hospital's mainframe system, improved the efficiency of communication in shift reports and in accessing information relevant to patient care. Nurses in the study perceived that with quick access to pertinent information in the Pocket PC, they could provide better patient care. This technology provided a standardized means to communicate patient information from shift to shift. However, whether or not the patients perceived an improvement in their care as a result of nurses using this technology was not examined in this study. The future goal of this project is to revise the iCare Worksheet to better meet nurses' needs to communicate patient information from shift to shift. A larger and longer study will be conducted in the future.

At the beginning of the study, it was unclear if nurses would be receptive because they had become accustomed to the paper-based system and audiotape reports. However, as they identified the benefits of having quick access to patient information with the mobile technology, they gradually responded positively to the iCare system. At the conclusion of the study, they eagerly offered suggestions for improvement. They even requested to continue using the Pocket PCs after the study ended.

The iCare system has great potential for use in hospitals that use paper-based medical records and mainframe systems. Hospitals face many constraints to fully implement IT for nurses, such as costs, human factors, regulation and standards, technology, and information systems (Schneider, 1997; Androwich et al., 2003; Blair, 2003; Thakkar & Davis, 2006). As hospitals decide to move away from mainframe systems to EMR systems, the iCare system could be a valuable tool to help nurses during the interim.

In the future, the iCare Worksheet could be further improved by engaging nurses in the process of refinement. The iCare system could incorporate advanced technology, such as wireless network infrastructure, to expedite communication, information access, and synchronization. Tablet PC could be the solution for small screen issues. Further studies using Tablet PC in the integrated IT system are warranted and underway by the authors.

References

Androwich, I., Bickford, C., Button, P., Hunter, K., Murphy, J., & Sensmeier, J. (2003). *Clinical information systems: A framework for reaching the vision.* Washington, D.C.: American Medical Informatics Association and American Nurses Association.

Blair, J. (2003). The electronic health record today: The Medical Records Institute's annual survey shows the trends and challenges ahead. *Healthcare Informatics, 20*(1), 45-46.

Bush, G. (2004). *Executive order: 13335: Incentives for the use of health information technology and establishing the position of the national health information technology coordinator.* Retrieved July 15, 2007 from http://www.whitehouse. gov/news/releases/2004/04/20040427-4.html

Currie, J. (2002). Improving the efficiency of patient handover. *Emergency Nurse, 10*(3), 24-27.

Dee, C., Teolis, M., & Todd, A. (2005). Physicians' use of the personal digital assistant (PDA) in clinical decision making. *Journal of the Medical Library Association, 93*(4), 480-486.

Gillespie, G. (2002). IT: Often a tough sell to nursing staffs. *Health Data Management, 10*(4), 56.

Hardey, M., Payne, S., & Coleman, P. (2000). 'Scraps': Hidden nursing information and its influence on the delivery of care. *Journal of Advanced Nursing, 32*(1), 208-214.

Honeybourne, C., Sutton, S., & Ward, L. (2006). Knowledge in the palm of your hands: PDAs in the clinical setting. *Health Information and Libraries Journal, 23*(1), 51-59.

Institute of Medicine. (2001). *Crossing the quality chasm—a new health system for the 21st century.* National Academy Press, Institute of Medicine.

Laskin, R., & Davis, J. (2004). The use of a personal digital assistant in orthopaedic surgical practice. *Clinical Orthopaedics & Related Research, 421,* 91-98.

Lanway, C., & Graham, P. (2003). Mobile documentation. Wireless PDAs boost job satisfaction for utilization review nurses. *Healthcare Informatics, 20*(10), 80.

Leonard, M., Graham, S., & Bonacum, D. (2004). The human factor: The critical importance of effective teamwork and communication in providing safe care. *Quality & Safety in Healthcare, 13*(Supplement 1), 85-90.

Lin, Y., Jan, I., Ko, P., Chen, Y., Wong, J., & Jan, G. (2004). A wireless PDA-based physiological monitoring system for patient transport. *IEEE Transactions on Information Technology in Biomedicine, 8*(4), 439-447.

Mihailidis, A., Krones, L., & Boger, J. (2006). Assistive computing devices: A pilot study to explore nurses' preferences and needs. *CIN: Computers, Informatics, Nursing, 24*(6), 328-336.

Nelson, E., Batalden, P., Homa, K., Godfrey, M., Campbell, C., Headrick, L., et al. (2003). Microsystems in healthcare: Part 2. Creating a rich information environment. *Joint Commission Journal on Quality & Safety, 29*(1), 5-15.

Schneider, P. (1997). Married to the mainframe. *Healthcare Informatics, 14*(9), 37-38, 40-42, 44-46.

Sensimeier, J., Raiford, R., Taylor, S., & Weaver, C. (2002). Using innovative technology to enhance patient care delivery. *American Academy of Nursing Technology and Workforce Conference.* Washington, D.C. Retrieved May 16, 2005 from http://www.himss.org/content/files/AANNsgSummitHIMS-SFINAL_18770.pdf

Sexton, A., Chan, C., Elliott, M., Stuart, J., Jayasuriya, R., & Crookes, P. (2004). Nursing handovers: Do we really need them?. *Journal of Nursing Management, 12*(1), 37-42.

Shabot, M. (2002). Wireless technologies in medicine. *Cedars-Sinai NET Journal.* Retrieved June 14, 2005 from http://www.csmc.edu/pdf/Wireless.pdf.

Thakkar, M., & Davis, D. (2006). Risks, barriers, and benefits of EHR systems: A comparative study based on size of hospital. *Perspectives in Health Information Management, 3,* 19.

Chapter XVI

Evaluation of a Tool to Enhance Searching for Useful Medical Information on the Internet

David Parry, Auckland University of Technology, New Zealand

Abstract

Evidence-based medicine (EBM) requires appropriate information to be available to clinicians at the point of care. Electronic sources of information may fulfill this need but require a high level of skill to use successfully. This chapter describes the rationale and initial testing of a system to allow collaborative searching and ontology construction for professional groups in the health sector. The approach is based around the use of a browser using a fuzzy ontology based on the National library of medicine (NLM) unified medical language system (UMLS). The results suggest that a tool that can assist users in finding information by recording their preferences and preferred meaning of text words can be usable by healthcare professionals. This approach may provide high-quality information for professionals in the future.

Introduction

Evidence-based medicine (Sackett, Richardson, Rosenberg & Haynes, 1997) has become increasingly important in the modern healthcare industry. Indeed the concept of basing practice on evidence is even extending to the software engineering industry (Kitchenham, Dyba & Jorgensen, 2004). Care that is not based on evidence has become increasingly indefensible from professional, safety and economic points of view. Electronic access to high-quality information can improve the professional knowledge of clinicians (Leung et al., 2003), and is very popular (Westbrook, Gosling & Coiera, 2004). However there are a number of difficulties associated with providing high-quality information to support EBM.

Assessing and finding appropriate information is difficult and can be time-consuming. This is partly due to the continuing difficulty users have in navigating the interfaces used by various systems and also because of the lack of training available. Indeed if the concept of just-in-time information retrieval, as an aid to clinical decision-making at the point of care is to be realized (Gardner, 1997), then complex time-consuming strategies performed by trained users are not possible. Recent work, looking at the usage of the Clinical Information access program (CIAP) in New South Wales (Gosling, Westbrook & Coiera, 2003), has emphasized cultural barriers to use of online sources of information in a clinical setting, and this includes a perceived lack of skill in information retrieval by clinicians. Consumer medical information is also now being provided by government agencies for example NHSdirect in the UK (UK National Health Service, 2007), and Medline Plus in the USA (U.S. National Library of Medicine, 2007). Privately funded consumer portals are also becoming more common such as WebMD (WebMD Inc., 2005).

In assessing the usefulness of information sources, a framework to identify the aspects that are important needs to be established. Existing well-known frameworks such as health on the net (HON) (Health on the Net Foundation, 2003), and Netscoring® (Centrale Sante, 2001), are more concerned with the sources and reliability of the information than its usefulness. Three dimensions of usefulness have been identified, based partly on the work of (Sackett et al., 1997), and some of the limits used in PUBMED, and other information sources. They are information quality, clinical relevance and clinical usefulness,. The aspects of each dimension are outlined in Tables 1-3.

Diversity

Both the users and sources of information are characterized by diversity, and current examples of information portals reflect this. The CIAP system, described by Moody & Shanks (1999), is particularly interesting as a "top-down" approach to

Table 1. Information quality

Aspect	Comments
Peer-review	World Wide Web (WWW) sites as well as journals may now have peer-review in place.
Randomized Controlled Trial (RCT)	This is the gold standard for clinical interventions although many interventions have not been subjected to this process. There are also issues of the quality and power of a trial. In some cases meta-analysis can cause smaller trials to loose credibility.
High citation number	This is more of a rule of thumb than an absolute factor. If the source is frequently cited then it indicates that large numbers of authors have found it relevant. It is perfectly possible that a particularly bad study may have a high citation index, or that the index may be inflated for other reasons such as age of the reference. It is possible to infer that references cited in 'good' documents are more likely to be good themselves but this is dangerous to extend too far.
Recent	This depends on the rate of change of the field. Documents in very active research areas are more likely to have a shorter useful life than those in slow-moving or moribund areas.
Significant result	A document containing information that a treatment or diagnostic method is effective, and that this effect is large, is likely to be more useful than one that does not. If there is a traditional treatment that is shown to be ineffective then this also is significant.
Authoritative source	For electronic sources of information, the Health on the Net Code of conduct can give some guidance—otherwise, inclusion by indexes or directories, for example, MEDLINE or Cochrane, can lend authority. The author affiliation can be an important issue here. An automated system for "authoritativeness" is described by Farahat, Nunberg, Chen, and Heylighen (2002).
Usability	Traditional Web usability, for example, Neilson's heuristics (Neilson, 2000), and also in terms of technical issues such as plug-ins media, and so forth

providing evidence at the point of care. Having multiple database systems, with many different interfaces and means of searching can only increase the obstacles to effective use of these tools. Even the CIAP system has over 40 different, searchable, databases available, each with its own quirks, not to mention the individual journals, and tools such as Google.

Aside from the differences in professional education—which will influence the use of preferred search terms—along with the clinical usefulness indicators, users may also have fundamental differences in their understanding of the meaning of terms. The need to share understanding of the meaning of search terms has been a driver in the use of ontologies (Noy & McGuinness, 2001), and indeed (Musen, 2001) assigned ontology use and creation the central role in medical informatics. A general view of a system to support reaching for useful medical information is illustrated in Figure 1. Key elements include the use of multiple information sources accessed through a single browser, an ontology-supported scheme for query expansion and refinement, and the identification of users as members of a professional group, with expertise in particular domains and five levels of expertise based on the Dreyfus, Dreyfus, & Athanasiou (1986) classification.

Table 2. Clinical relevance

Aspect	Notes
Human	Although animal studies, or theoretical ones may be of great use—for example, in the case of poisoning or electric shock, human studies are often essential.
Correct sex	Included in this is whether the interventions are safe for pregnant women, and the variation in body sizes and compositions between the sexes.
Age group relevance	Various age bands are used, or bands that reflect characteristics of the individual rather than his or her age.
Specialty is appropriate	Information designed for one medical specialty may not be appropriate for others, for example, between pathologists and other clinicians. Similarly the information requirements of different clinical groups, for example, physiotherapists and surgeons treating a patient with an artificial hip may have different needs.
Appropriate language	Is this information in a suitable language for use by clinicians, or is it designed for lay people? In this situation, the information may be too imprecise to be of use. In the opposite case, the information may be too technical.

Table 3. Clinical usefulness

Aspect	Comments
Appropriate to stage of encounter (e.g., therapy, diagnosis, etc.)	This also excludes information that is purely of a research nature, if better information for the clinical decision is available. However such information can be useful if it casts doubt on current clinical practice, or can help explain otherwise unexpected results.
Deals with available tools	This includes such aspects as whether the drugs or procedures involved are licensed or available in the location, and acceptable in terms of cultural factors and cost.
Suitable format	Are the documents or information sources able to be read by the user; correct language, is a machine reader available? Concrete examples of this include different varieties of microfiche, or PDF files that may require large bandwidths for download.
Available in a timely fashion	Broadly, the information may be available immediately (read off the screen—a time period of seconds), quickly (within the library or searching area—a time period of minutes), after a short pause (if documents need to be retrieved from a nearby site—a time period of hours) or after a long time (if the document needs to be specially ordered or generated—a time period of days).
Useful for exclusion	That is, the information source confirms that a potential diagnosis or treatment is not correct.

This approach sees members of a professional group as shared owners of the meaning of terms used within documents that are used by that group. Having shared ontologies emphasizes that not only individual terms, but the relationship between them and the underlying concepts they signify represent a key aspect of membership of the group. It is suggested that the appropriate scale of support for information retrieval for health information is not always the individual, or the entire population, but somewhere in between. The experience of walking through a music shop illustrates this point— people who enjoy classical music use very different classification schemes than those who listen to hip-hop—for example composer, orchestra,

Figure 1. The overall system

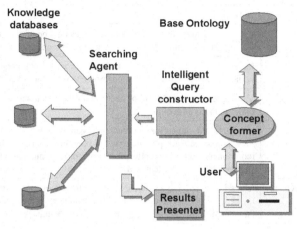

Figure 2. The fuzzy ontology

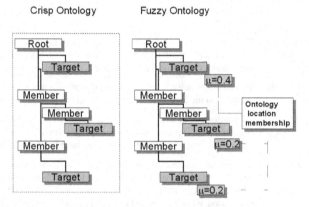

Figure 3. The results browser

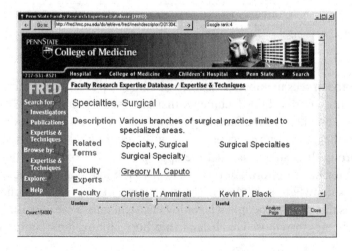

Figure 4. The system components

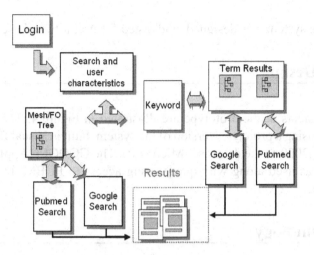

Table 4. Multiple occurrence examples: "Pain"

Term	Concept ID	Parent	Depth	Root term
Pain	G11.561.796.444	Sensation	4	Musculoskeletal, Neural, and Ocular Physiology
Pain	F02.830.816.444	Sensation	4	Psychological Phenomena and Processes
Pain	C23.888.646	Signs and Symptoms	3	Pathological Conditions, Signs and Symptoms
Pain	C23.888.592.612	Neurologic Manifestations	4	Pathological Conditions, Signs and Symptoms
Pain	C10.597.617	Neurologic Manifestations	3	Nervous System Diseases

conductor, rather than artist, genre and even region of origin. Nevertheless, such schemes do exist, and the music lovers involved do not appear to find the lack of consistency problematic.

The next section deals with the methods used to construct a system to see if such an approach is valuable, the section after that describes the case study and prototype usability testing. The Results section includes the results of the evaluation, followed by the Discussion section which discusses the significance of such an approach.

Methods

A prototype system was designed, and tested for usability and usefulness.

System Design

The components of the prototype are illustrated in Figure 4. The case study was performed using a prototype version of the system, built in Visual Basic.NET, using SQL server 2000 as the database (Microsoft). The GOOGLE Application program interface was used along with query string access to PUBMED, to provide two date sources.

Fuzzy Ontology

The concept of a "fuzzy ontology" was introduced in Parry (2004b). Effectively, this approach reuses a current ontology—in this case the MeSH hierarchy (U.S. National Library of Medicine, 2001), and assigns a particular membership value to each multiply occurring term in each location

Table 4 demonstrates how these issues arise in existing ontologies. "Pain" occurs in five locations in the MeSH ontology. Because the term is located in a number of different places, query expansion for this term is difficult, because there are wide numbers of "related" terms. For this reason, the MeSH hierarchy was adapted in order to allow users to assign membership values to term, location pairs, via a machine learning system, described in Parry (2004a). The case study was designed partly to investigate different methods of learning these relations, but all the searches were performed using the original MeSH hierarchy terms, without the use of fuzzy ontology support.

Case Study

The setting was an academic department of obstetrics and gynecology, and only elements of the MeSH tree relevant to this domain were included. Ethical approval was obtained, and eight users were allocated one hour each to use the system. During user number 8's study, the database was corrupted and she was unable to complete any testing; she was therefore not included in any analysis. This is a small number of users but Neilson (2000) points out that usability testing can often be successful with small groups. In fact, the whole department only comprised less than ten faculty members, and as with many systems designed for professional use, the pool of users is actually quite small.

The users were asked to perform the following tasks:

a.   Log into the system and select the appropriate demographic, and area of interest

b.   Perform a search using the "obstetric" keyword on the Google interface. This was done mostly to familiarize the users with the system, in particular the appropriate use of the mouse and the use of the + anchor in lists to expand them, as in windows explorer.

c.   They then performed another search using terms of their own choosing, again using the Google interface.

d.   With the open browser windows, they were asked to rate a number of the pages shown in terms of usefulness via the slider. They were also asked to perform an analysis on pages that they rated highly. In most cases, this amounted to around five pages.

e.   They were then asked to perform a similar task using the full MeSH tree.

Table 5. User group details

Number	Job description	Professional group	Computer experience	Gender	Age Range
1	Senior Academic	Doctor, interest in MFM	Moderate	Male	50+
2	Senior Academic	Doctor interest in MFM	Moderate	Female	50+
3	Junior Academic	Doctor, interest in REI	High	Female	30+
4	Research Midwife	Midwife background, clinical researcher	Moderate	Female	50+
5	New Consultant	Doctor, General Obstetrics and Gynaecology	Moderate	Female	30+
6	Senior Academic	Doctor, interest in Contraception	High	Female	40+
7	Junior Academic	Doctor, interest in Infertility	Moderate	Female	30+
8	New Consultant	Doctor, General Obstetrics and Gynaecology	Moderate	Female	30+

Results

The results of the study are based around the usability questionnaire responses and user comments. The questionnaire used in the study was adapted from one of those generated from the site provided by Perlman (2001). This questionnaire was originally reported in Davis (1989), and has subsequently been used in a number of studies. This questionnaire focuses on the use of a system for work-related tasks, and the scale runs from -2 to +2, to allow a 0 for neutrality. All the questions are phrased so that a positive result implies satisfaction with the system. One of the most interesting aspects of this questionnaire is that it specifically links ease of use and usefulness. The original work suggested that increased perceived ease of use has a causal influence on perceived usefulness. However, more recent work (Segars & Grover, 1993) appears to suggest that this analysis is not complete. It is suggested that in turn, an information system that is perceived as useful must be retrieving useful information.

Overall, the perceived usefulness was rated as X=1.16 (SD 1.21) and the perceived ease of use at X=1.53 (SD 0.29). This compares favorably with similar scores in the technology acceptance model, for example, in Henderson and Divett (2003), dealing with electronic shopping, where ease of use was 1.25 and usefulness was 0.96 when converted to the same scale as used in this work. Ease of use could be expected to be rated more highly as the situation for testing was somewhat artificial.

Comments about the system were recorded and general satisfaction seemed quite high. Of particular interest was the ease of use of the analysis system, despite the fact there were bugs in this version, which allowed duplicate words to occur in the pick list. There was certainly a preference towards identifying positive (very, somewhat relevant), rather than negative (irrelevant, unwanted) words. The users preferred to analyze those documents they found useful, and tended to ignore those they found useless.

One aspect of particular benefit was the presentation of the derived MeSH keywords, which allowed the user to reconsider her search before it began. General observations of users included the fact that they found dealing with large numbers of windows a little confusing. By attempting to improve visibility, the use of multiple windows tended to remove the obvious focus. Mouse movement became more uncertain when there were overlapping windows and the users were often uncertain as to the difference between closing and minimizing windows. In many cases, the users maximized the active window.

One of the recurring themes was the uncertainty of whether such a system was primarily for medical professionals or for patients. When browsing the documents recovered via Google, the users were sometimes surprised to find what they regarded as legitimate medical pages amongst the obviously patient-centered ones. This is an unexpected benefit of using multiple search engines—multiple search strategies

Table 6. Initial group satisfaction (Please refer to the appendix for the full questions)

Question	User 1	User 2	User 3	User 4	User 5	User 6	User 7	Mean
Perceived Usefulness								
1 (Quick)	0	2	1	1	1	2	2	1.26
2 (Performance)	0	1	0	0	1	2	2	0.86
3 (Productivity)	2	1	1	0	1	2	2	1.29
4 (Effectiveness)	1	1	0	0	1	2	2	1.00
5 (Easier)	1	1	0	1	1	2	2	1.14
6 (Useful)	1	1	2	1	1	2	2	1.43
Perceived Ease of Use								
7 (Easy to Learn)	2	1	2	2	2	2	2	1.86
8 (Easy to Control)	-1	2	1	2	2	1	2	1.29
9 (Clear Interact)	2	2	1	2	1	1	2	1.57
10 (Flexible)	-1	2	1	2	1	1	2	1.14
11 (Skill)	2	2	2	2	1	2	2	1.86
12 (Easy to Use)	0	2	1	2	1	2	2	1.43

are used simultaneously. Various meta-engines already use this approach, but they currently do not appear to use non-commercial data sources such as PubMed.

Discussion

Finding and applying appropriate information is one of the key tasks of the knowledge worker (Kidd, 1994). There exists a vast body of knowledge in electronic form for workers and patients in the health sector. However, finding appropriate knowledge is difficult and time consuming. Fears of inappropriate information being provided abound (Eysenbach, 2002). In order to fully realize the potential benefits of electronic knowledge sources, they must be appropriate for their use and usable by the potential beneficiaries. Understanding the knowledge requirements of users in this domain, and providing appropriate tools for such users remains a great challenge for informatics professionals. This chapter has attempted to set up a framework for future research in the area of appropriate knowledge sources, based around a user perspective. The importance of delimiting different user groups within the health sector has also been identified. In addition, a prototype system for combining knowledge from different sources in an integrated way has been tested for usability and potential usefulness. These results suggest that an integrated knowledge discovery system for medical professional is desirable, and that the prototype represents a useful start in this direction. It is hoped that further research in this area will continue, in particular in the following areas: the replacement of the executable form of the system with a browser based client server system that will allow much larger user groups to interact with it, and provide a substantial base for learning about group preferences. Mobile and wireless information retrieval may be more appropriately integrated into clinical workflow, especially by means of "information appliances" (Eustice et al., 1999). More research needs to be undertaken in the use and standardization of aspects of information reliability, usefulness and relevance to improve research and classification in this area, especially from the perspective of the clinical worker. The "Semantic Web" (Berners-Lee, Hendler, & Lassila, 2001) may be helpful in allowing seamless pulling-together of information from diverse sources. However, the interface between information sources designed for consumers and those designed for professionals remains fluid, and this requires continuing study. This is epitomized by the rise of user-generated content in the form of community tagging, blogging, Wikis, and so forth, the so called "Web 2.0" (O'Reilly, 2005). There are obvious difficulties in making effective use of less formal information sources, which may never conform to the appropriate standards (Miller, Hongsermeier, Neumann & Gilman, 2004), but nevertheless are still valuable. Fortunately, humans have proved resilient in their quest for useful information for many millennia and encoding this wisdom in computer systems should not be an impossible challenge.

References

Berners-Lee, T., Hendler, J., & Lassila, O. (2001). The Semantic Web. *Scientific American, May,* 29-37.

Centrale Sante. (2001). *Net Scoring ®: Criteria to assess the quality of health Internet information.* Retrieved July 1, 2007 from http://www.chu-rouen. fr/netscoring/netscoringeng.html.

Davis, F. (1989). Perceived usefulness, perceived ease of use, and user acceptance of information technology. *MIS Quarterly, 13*(3), 319-340.

Dreyfus, H., Dreyfus, S., & Athanasiou, T. (1986). *Mind over machine: The power of human intuition and expertise in the era of the computer.* Oxford: Blackwell.

Eustice, K., Lehman, T., Morales, A., Munson, M., Edlund, S., & Guillen, M. (1999). A universal information appliance. *IBM Systems Journal, 38*(4), 575-601.

Eysenbach, G. (2002). Infodemiology: The epidemiology of (mis)information. *The American Journal of Medicine, 113*(9), 763-765.

Farahat, A., Nunberg, G., Chen, F., & Heylighen, F. (2002). AuGEAS: Authoritativeness grading, estimation, and sorting: Collective Intelligence and its Implementation. *Computational & Mathematical Organization Theory, 5*(3), 194-202.

Gardner, M. (1997). Information retrieval at the point of care. *British Medical Journal, 314,* 950-953.

Gosling, A., Westbrook, J., & Coiera, E. (2003). Variation in the use of online clinical evidence: A qualitative analysis. *International Journal of Medical Informatics, 69*(1), 1-16.

Health on the Net Foundation. (2003). *HON code of conduct.* Retrieved December 31, 2003 from http://www.hon.ch/honcode/conduct.html

Henderson, R., & Divett, M. (2003). Perceived usefulness, ease of use and electronic supermarket use. *International Journal of Human-Computer Studies, 59*(3), 383-395.

Kidd, A. (1994). *The marks are on the knowledge worker.* Paper presented at the Human factors in computing systems: Celebrating interdependence. Boston.

Kitchenham, B., Dyba, T., & Jorgensen, M. (2004). *Evidence-based software engineering,* (pp. 273-281).

Leung, G., Johnston, J., Tin, K., Wong, I., Ho, L.-M., Lam, W., et al. (2003). Randomised controlled trial of clinical decision support tools to improve learning of evidence-based medicine in medical students. *British Medical Journal, 327*(7423), 1090-1090.

Miller, E., Hongsermeier, T., Neumann, E., & Gilman, B. (2004). *W3C Semantic Web healthcare and life sciences interest group.* Retrieved June 6, 2006 from http://www.w3.org/2001/sw/hcls/

Moody, D., & Shanks, G. (1999). *Using knowledge management and the Internet to support evidence-based practice: A medical case study.* Paper presented at the the 10th Australasian Conference on Information Systems. Victoria University, Wellington.

Musen, M. (2001). *Creating and using ontologies: What informatics is all about.* Paper presented at the Medinfo 2001. London.

Neilson, J. (2000). *Designing Web usability.* Indianapolis, IN: New Riders.

Noy, N., & McGuinness, D. (2001). *Ontology development 101: A guide to creating your first ontology.* Stanford, CA: Stanford University.

O'Reilly, T. (2005). *What Is Web 2.0? Design Patterns and Business Models for the Next Generation of Software.* Retrieved July 1, 2007 from http://www.oreillynet.com/pub/a/oreilly/tim/news/2005/09/30/what-is-web-20.html

Parry, D. (2004a). *Fuzzification of a standard ontology to encourage reuse.* Paper presented at the 2004 IEEE International Conference on Information Reuse and Integration (IEEE IRI-2004). Las Vegas, NV.

Parry, D. (2004b). A fuzzy ontology for medical document retrieval. In: M. Purvis (Ed.), *The Australasian workshop on data mining and Web intelligence* (Vol. 32, pp. 121-126). Dunedin: Australian Computer Society.

Perlman, G. (2001). *Web-based user interface evaluation with questionnaires.* Retrieved March 1, 2003 from http://www.acm.org/~perlman/

Sackett, D., Richardson, W., Rosenberg, W., & Haynes, B. (1997). *Evidence-based medicine—how to practice and teach EBM.* Churchill Livingstone.

Segars, A., & Grover, V. (1993). Re-examining perceived ease of use and usefulness: A confirmatory factor analysis. *MIS Quarterly, 17*(4), 517-526.

U.S. National Library of Medicine. (2001). *Medical subject headings.* Retrieved January 11, 2002 from http://www.nlm.nih.gov/mesh/

U.S. National Library of Medicine. (2007). *Medline plus.* Retrieved July 1, 2007 from http://www.nlm.nih.gov/medlineplus/

UK National Health Service. (2007). *NHS direct.* Retrieved June 1, 2007 from http://www.nhsdirect.nhs.uk/

WebMD Inc. (2005). *WebMD.* Retrieved July 1, 2007 from http://www.webmd.com

Westbrook, J., Gosling, A., & Coiera, E. (2004). Do clinicians use online evidence to support patient care? A study of 55,000 clinicians. *Journal of the American Medical Informatics Association, 11*(2), 113-121.

Section IV

HISI Policies and Knowledge Transfer Processes

Chapter XVII

Applying Personal Health Informatics to Create Effective Patient-Centered E-Health

E. Vance Wilson, The University of Toledo, USA

Abstract

E-health use is increasing worldwide, but no current e-health paradigm fulfills the complete range of users' needs for Web-enabled healthcare services. Moreover, a number of obstacles exist that could make it difficult for e-health to meet users' expectations, especially in the case where the users are patients. These dilemmas cloud the future of e-health, as promoters of e-commerce, personal health records, and consumer health informatics paradigms vie to create e-health applications while being hampered by the implicit constraints of each perspective. This chapter presents an alternative approach for designing and developing e-health titled personal health informatics (PHI). PHI was developed to overcome the limitations of preceding paradigms while incorporating their best features. The chapter goes on to describe how PHI can be applied to create effective patient-centered e-health for delivery by healthcare organizations to their own patients.

Introduction

E-health is broadly defined as "health services and information delivered or enhanced through the Internet" (Eysenbach, 2001). Overall use of e-health continues to expand worldwide. Harris Interactive reports the number of Americans who have searched for health information online has increased to 117 million, and 85% of these individuals searched within the month prior to being surveyed (Krane, 2005). Outside the U.S. and Europe, e-health use has grown more slowly (e.g., see Holliday & Tam, 2004). But even in these areas further expansion seems likely as the World Health Organization and similar groups ramp up efforts to increase availability of e-health in developing nations (Kwankam, 2004; WHO, 2005).

Although some aspects of successful e-health are well-established, such as the need to provide encyclopedic health content, other aspects are less obvious. For example:

- Which services should be deployed online and how should users interface with these services?

- If communication is offered, what is the best way to coordinate this to balance needs of the public with those of healthcare representatives, for example, physicians and clinic staff?

- How should personal health records (PHR) be incorporated into e-health, who "owns" the data in these records, and what (if any) data should PHR share with records of the healthcare provider, insurer, and payer, such as employer or government agency?

These are no idle questions to the health informatics and IT practitioners who must design and deploy e-health applications. Given the large number of healthcare providers who currently are investing in e-health as an important part of organizational strategy (Lazarus, 2001; Martin, Yen & Tan, 2002), learning how to create successful e-health applications is a key topic for both research and practice.

In developing effective approaches for designers and developers of e-health, I propose that it will be helpful to view e-health, as broadly defined above, from a user-centered perspective that can incorporate best practices of preceding e-health paradigms without being limited by their implicit constraints. This chapter presents the foundational concepts underlying this approach and then describes how the approach can provide guidance in the specific context of e-health applications that healthcare providers develop to serve their own patients.

Paradigms of E-Health

E-health is a broad domain that describes numerous aspects of the convergence of healthcare and Internet technology (Oh, Rizo, Enkin & Jadad, 2005). A frequently-cited definition by Eysenbach highlights e-health's interdisciplinary underpinnings.

E-health is an emerging field in the intersection of medical informatics, public health and business, referring to health services and information delivered or enhanced through the Internet and related technologies. In a broader sense, the term characterizes not only a technical development, but also a state-of-mind, a way of thinking, an attitude, and a commitment for networked, global thinking, to improve healthcare locally, regionally, and worldwide by using information and communication technology (Eysenbach, 2001).

Indeed, "state-of-mind" has been much more critical to e-health than is the case for most other major Internet applications, such as online banking. Historically, three major paradigms have played key roles in developing e-health to its current state. Although each paradigm has been important in promoting specific feature sets and in raising overall awareness of e-health, I will argue that all have essential constraints that make it impossible to fulfill the complete range of users' needs for online health services.

E-Commerce Paradigm

Prominent early developers of e-health services operated within an *e-commerce* paradigm, in which vendors expected to profit from users paying directly for products and services acquired through the site or from advertisers paying for exposure to users. Typically, vendors were not affiliated with healthcare providers, thus they are essentially constrained from providing services that link individuals with their own physician, clinic, or pharmacy. Although numerous vendors developed e-health within the e-commerce paradigm, few survived the ensuing shakeout due to failure to provide value to customers or adequately control costs, lack of effective revenue models, or simple inability to ensure sustainable competitive advantage (Itagaki, Berlin & Schatz, 2002; Rovenpor, 2003). Among the prominent e-health ventures representing the e-commerce paradigm, such as DrKoop.com, MediConsult.com, and PlanetRx.com, only a handful remain. The best-known of these is WebMD, which provides an exceptionally wide range of health services but continues to struggle toward profitability.

Personal Health Record Paradigm

A second approach to e-health that was based initially on profit motives is the *personal health record* (PHR) paradigm. The PHR is defined as

an electronic, universally available, lifelong resource of health information needed by individuals to make health decisions. Individuals own and manage the information in the PHR, which comes from healthcare providers and the individual. The PHR is maintained in a secure and private environment, with the individual determining rights of access. The PHR is separate from and does not replace the legal record of any provider (AHIMA, 2005).

The idea of computerized storage of personal health data is not new. A number of vendors introduced PHR products during the 1990s both as standalone software and online services. To date, demand for commercial PHR products has been low—only 2% of individuals who maintain health records use purchased PHR software (Taylor, 2004)—and none of these products has gained financial success (Holt, 2005). However, several factors may prompt increased use of PHRs in the near term. First, the U.S. public gained increased awareness of the value of *portable* health records as a result of the massive human displacement and damage to healthcare facilities sustained from hurricanes during 2005. This awareness is likely to affect public sentiment and governmental policies for some time to come (Kloss, 2005). Second, PHR software is continuing to improve. Current offerings have become easier to use and are more fully capable of integrating health resources beyond the individual's immediate data, such as linking to relevant medical journals and FDA drug information (Campbell, 2005). Finally, researchers are beginning to study how individuals go about maintaining health records in non-computerized settings, and this research is clarifying the opportunities and constraints that PHR developers face. For example, two recent studies in this area assess the importance of privacy and security in health records (Taylor, 2004) and shed light on the diverse strategies that individuals prefer to employ in storing health records (Moen & Brennan, 2005). Even if PHRs gain wider acceptance, however, this paradigm is essentially constrained by its data-centric focus. Less data-centric services, for example, relating to communication and peer-group support, are accorded little attention within the PHR paradigm.

Consumer Health Informatics Paradigm

Although healthcare providers did not participate strongly in early stages of e-health development (Lazarus, 2001), these organizations recently have been instrumental in developing e-health within a *consumer health informatics* (CHI) paradigm. CHI is "a branch of medical informatics that analyzes consumers' needs for information; studies and implements methods for making information accessible to consumers; and models and integrates consumers' preferences into medical information systems" (Eysenbach, 2000). Where e-commerce vendors hoped to achieve competitive advantage, healthcare provider organizations appear to be driven more by concerns of achieving *competitive equity,* both with competing providers as well as commercial e-health sites. Because CHI is produced by healthcare provider organizations, e-health produced within this paradigm has been oriented toward augmenting customer service, increasing healthcare delivery quality, and containing costs rather than selling products, services, or advertising access. Although the CHI paradigm is designed to address needs of the individual user, it inherently takes an organizational perspective that imposes a passive view of users as consumers of information. This represents an essential constraint, as provision of services in which the user is an active information *provider* has not typically been a priority for e-health applications created within the CHI paradigm.

Personal Health Informatics

Each of the three historical paradigms described above identifies an area of need in the overall population of e-health users. However, none addresses the total range of needs that users identify. In the case of patients, for example, these include communicating with physicians and clinic staff, arranging services (e.g., scheduling appointments and renewing prescriptions), checking bills and making payments, viewing lab results, accessing records of procedures, tests, and immunizations, receiving online alerts, monitoring chronic conditions, and interacting with online support communities (e.g., patient chat groups), in addition to accessing encyclopedic health information (Harris, 2000; Taylor & Leitman, 2002; Fox, 2005). Patients also want the ability to control their personal data, to ensure that record-keeping aspects of e-health are interoperable and portable, and to be assured of privacy and security (Taylor, 2004; Holt, 2005).

In order to capture the complete set of knowledge and skills necessary to create e-health applications that meet users' needs, I propose it is essential to consider a new paradigm that can transcend limitations while incorporating best practices of the three paradigms discussed previously. Because of its user-centered focus, in which e-health is viewed from the perspective of an individual in the role of information provider as well as information consumer, this paradigm is titled *personal health informatics* (PHI). PHI is defined as the knowledge, skills, practices, and research perspectives necessary to develop e-health that is effective, efficient, and user-centered (Wilson, 2006a).

A conceptual model of PHI is presented in Figure 1. Four structural components define the content of PHI within three focal areas. *Web e-service infrastructure* is the hardware, software, and networking capabilities that support all e-health functions. Because e-health is primarily service-oriented, the *informatics focus* in PHI centers on infrastructure that is specialized for e-service presentation and delivery. *Personal health management* and *user-centered development* comprise the *personal focus* that PHI presents to individual users. User-centered development methods provide tools for eliciting user needs, designing solutions, and evaluating the utility of these solutions in meeting user needs. Personal health management addresses individual practices as well as psychological, social, and cultural aspects of the management, storage, and retrieval of personal health information. Personal health management and the *health informatics domain* combine in the *healthcare focus* of PHI. Content within the health informatics domain addresses the skills, knowledge, and surrounding use of IT within the subject health area(s).

For practitioners to enter the health informatics and IT workforce with sufficient preparation to develop e-health that can fully support individual users' needs, training is needed in each of the structural areas of PHI that are presented in Figure 1. None of these areas is beyond the grasp of college students or working health-IT practitioners. However, the combination of content areas represents a set of specializations that are rarely combined in current academic programs. Thus, for the time being, PHI training will necessarily have to be "pieced together" to some extent from existing textbooks, research reports, and industry cases. In the following sections, I address content and training issues relating to each structural component of PHI.

Web E-Service Infrastructure

E-health is essentially a form of e-service, defined as a service provided over electronic networks such as the Internet (Rust & Lemon, 2001). Thus, texts that focus on development and administration of Web e-service infrastructure will be applicable to PHI. Texts that address the general topic of e-commerce are typically less applicable, as large portions of these dwell on factors that are not central to e-health, such as general business models, marketing and consumer behavior issues, and methods for increasing online sales. Web infrastructure changes rapidly, so texts in this area must not be allowed to become stale. New texts should be chosen based upon inclusion of emerging technologies, such as mobile devices, speech recognition, and natural language parsers, as well as effective coverage of more mature technologies, such as XHTML, database connectivity, and network communications.

Figure 1. Conceptual model of key PHI structural components

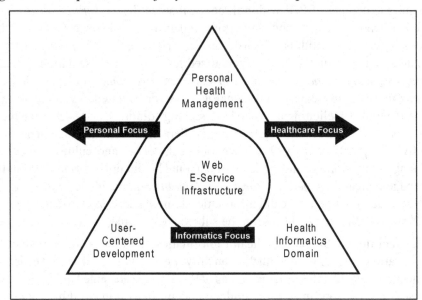

User-Centered Development

User-centered development refers to a software development process that incorporates the user viewpoint, assesses user needs, and validates that user needs are met. There are two complementary approaches to this process that will be valuable to students of PHI. The first of these is the *design guide* approach. Design guides emphasize generic or context-specific design principles, such as the following example for use of color on Web sites.

In the physical world, color has embedded meaning, usually culturally-based. In the American culture, at a simplistic level, red means stop and green means go, red means hot and blue means cold, black means death and white means birth, and green represents money and greed. These embedded meanings of color differ from culture to culture; for instance, the color white is symbolic not of birth, but of a funeral in Japan or India (Lazar, 2001).

Design guides are valuable in establishing general guidelines in conventional use of design features and in broadening students' appreciation of ways that others' perspectives may differ from their own.

The second approach emphasizes the *design process* by establishing an algorithmic approach or "how-to guidance" for developing functionality and user interface features. For example, the SALVO method (Wilson & Connolly, 2000) guides readers through five development stages. The first three of these are planning stages in which designers specify user needs, adopt a technology-specific design guide, and leverage appropriate matches between technology and user needs to enhance user abilities and support user disabilities. Once planning stages are initially completed, developers perform visualization techniques including mock-ups to elicit user feedback early in the development cycle. Visualization is followed by an observation stage in which designers observe and evaluate attempts by users to perform representative tasks using the mock-up or completed software. SALVO takes an iterative approach to development, and it is accepted throughout the development cycle that prior stages and sequences of stages can be repeated as necessary. The design process approach provides PHI students with a methodology and specific tools for customizing e-health to meet the needs of a specific user audience, which may differ substantially, for example, between a macular degeneration support group and the general public.

Personal Health Management

Personal health management is an emerging area of research, and new findings will likely emerge that add appreciably to current knowledge in this field. Although it may be too early to look for texts that focus on personal health management, good empirical studies and cases are available that would be highly applicable to PHI. One exemplar is a study by Moen and Brennan (2005) that investigates strategies for health information management (HIM) that are applied by individuals in their own homes. Their research identifies four HIM strategies:

- **Just-in-time:** Information is kept with the person at most times in anticipation of immediate need

- **Just-at-hand:** Information is stored in familiar, highly accessible locations, often serving as a reminder

- **Just-in-case:** Information is stored to be accessible in case of need, but out of view

- **Just-because:** Information is retained in interim storage pending a decision to file or discard it

This study presents several important implications for developers of HIM software that would be highly relevant for PHI students to consider and discuss. These include effects of trade-offs between information accessibility and visibility on the success of individuals' efforts to coordinate HIM, implications of the high degree of reliance individuals place on paper-based records, and design decisions that would be necessary to align electronic records to support the differentiated storage strategies that individuals are found to prefer.

Health Informatics Domain

The health informatics domain encompasses use of IT to support the delivery of healthcare services (including communication, coordination, logistics, and other business processes) as well as applicable practices and procedures that surround use of IT in the healthcare setting. It is important to recognize that, while the health informatics domain is a key component of PHI, it is not the central element of e-health from the *user's* perspective. In order to preserve a user-centered focus, it is essential that distinctive components of PHI should not be replaced by health informatics courses that focus on IT from a perspective that is internal to the organization (i.e., managerial or technical). Where PHI is taught within an existing health informatics program, a range of courses will already be in place to effectively cover topics in the domain. Where PHI is taught in technology programs, topics in the health informatics domain may be covered effectively by traditional health informatics or medical informatics texts.

Suggested Modes of Training Organization

PHI training does not necessarily require development of new academic programs. Specialized subject areas can be presented to health-IT audiences within professional seminars and continuing education programs and to student audiences by augmenting existing health informatics or technology programs, such as information systems, computer science, or information science (Wilson, 2006b). As a specialization in a health informatics program which already incorporates domain coverage, in-depth PHI training can be achieved by a curriculum that offers one course-equivalent each in user-centered development and personal health management, and up to two courses in Web e-service infrastructure. If two courses are offered, the first should focus on basic development methods including XHTML, XML, and simple database connectivity and the second on administration issues and advanced development methods including Web services, mobile applications, and emerging technologies.

As an augmentation to a technology program which already incorporates Web e-service infrastructure coverage, substantial depth of PHI training can be achieved by offering a specialization with one course-equivalent in each of user-centered development, personal health management, and health informatics. A final alternative for college students is to offer a basic introduction to each of these subjects within a single course-equivalent. Although not ideal for career preparation, this alternative could be an effective way to direct technology-area undergraduates toward careers and further educational opportunities in the field of health informatics and IT.

The Need for Patient-Centered E-Health

Patients comprise a large and growing constituency of e-health users (Krane, 2005), and surveys indicate there is very high interest among patients in increased access to provider e-health for a variety of specific interaction needs, for example, physician-patient communication (Taylor & Leitman, 2002). Leaders in the medical community are coming to recognize that patients *expect* to be empowered in making healthcare decisions (Institute of Medicine, 2001), and that the expectation of personal control is especially strong for e-health applications (Markle Foundation, 2004; Lafky, Tulu & Horan, 2006). However, healthcare provider organizations have only recently begun to provide their patients with online access to healthcare services, and numerous factors can obstruct development of effective e-health applications within this context. Examples of these factors include:

- Financial disincentives for participation by outside parties (i.e., participants in e-health other than the patient, including physicians and provider administration)
- Reduced work quality resulting from participation by outside parties
- Reluctance of outside parties to relinquish control to patients
- Restrictive interpretation of privacy and security regulations
- Discomfort of patients and other key parties with computing environments

A complete discussion of obstructions and means for overcoming them is beyond the scope of this chapter (for such a discussion, see Tan, Cheng, & Rogers, 2002). However, I argue that *patient-centered e-health* can help to meet patients' expectations and thereby avoid or mitigate obstructions to availability and use of e-health.

Guiding Principles for Creating Patient-Centered E-Health

In order to meet patients' expectations, it is essential for developers to focus on several guiding principles that are distinct from alternative approaches. Specifically, these are:

1. Focus on desired interactions in which the patient is an active participant
2. Incorporate only those services that meet the expressed needs of patients or that are validated against patient needs
3. Be understandable to patients
4. Provide easy access for patients to completely manage and control functionality
5. Provide support for interaction with outside parties (e.g., physicians and pharmacy) and with other healthcare information systems (e.g., hospital billing)

These principles correspond to a large extent with user-centered development principles that are known to be important to success of Web applications across numerous contexts outside the domain of healthcare (Lazar, 2001).

Principle 1 focuses on patient *involvement*, thereby distinguishing patient-centered e-health from other applications, such as telemedicine, where the patient is primarily an object of the interaction rather than an active participant. Principle 2 addresses patient *interest* and specifically cautions against relying on untested assumptions about patients as a basis for e-health design. By emphasizing patients' involvement and interest, the first two principles help to ensure that patients will have inherent motivation to use related e-health applications. They also guide the process of eliciting patients' interaction needs and mapping these to e-health services. The remaining principles center on accessibility and source of control.

Principle 3 proposes that e-health information and communication should be understandable to patients. Some researchers argue that it is patients' own health literacy that must increase in order for e-health to succeed (Norman & Skinner, 2006). However, this type of idealistic mindset ignores, first, that patients' *need* for healthcare services is not dependent upon their literacy level and, second, that patients can benefit greatly if e-health designers make the effort to incorporate simple explanations and illustrations where these are practical. Many individuals who are only marginally literate have proved to be highly capable of interacting with online applications, such as banking, when they are provided with effective interface support. Further, requiring patients to be highly literate in order to use e-health is no more defensible logically than requiring high literacy in order to schedule medical examinations or other healthcare services that the provider may offer. From the patient's perspective, e-health is simply an extension of the providers' other services, thus it is reasonable for patients to expect e-health to be generally understandable and for the provider to offer mechanisms by which better explanations can be obtained if these are needed.

Principle 4 presents a clear statement that ultimate control of patient-centered e-health must flow to the patient. Increasing patients' involvement in e-health has been promoted recently as part of the U.S. plan for "Delivering consumer-centric and information-rich healthcare" (Thompson & Brailler, 2004). However, achieving patient control faces two key obstacles. First, medical institutions are only slowly moving away from a firmly-embedded authoritarian or "paternalistic" model of physician-patient relationships (Emanuel & Emanuel, 1992) in which physicians expect to control virtually all aspects of their interaction with patients (Eysenbach & Jadad, 2001). Embedded cultural practices can take significant time to change, even in the face of substantial social pressures. Therefore, it is foreseeable in the near term that many physicians and other outside parties will resist allowing patients to exercise complete control over e-health or other aspects of healthcare. Second, healthcare provider organizations are reluctant to open up healthcare information systems (HIS) to access by patients. Reluctance is based on several factors, none of which is necessarily unreasonable. Providers have the responsibility to maintain privacy and security of patient and provider data, which could be compromised by increasing accessibility of the HIS. Significant labor expenditures are likely to be necessary in order to interconnect HIS with e-health, and it may be difficult for providers to identify ways that these expenses can be offset by increased income. Furthermore, access to HIS may be structurally blocked by disparate storage and communication formats among various proprietary systems. Lack of access to the provider's HIS or to specific parts, such as medical records and test results, leaves patients with relatively little to control, as the resulting e-health application will not offer direct interaction with key functions, such as billing and appointment scheduling. Thus, it is important to develop strategies that can economically enhance access to HIS without compromising security or that can establish alternatives to direct access, for example, by applying a data warehouse model where only a copy of the original data is accessible to patients. It also is key to promote among physicians and clinical staff the understanding that patients have the right to play a central role in their own healthcare decisions.

Principle 5 emphasizes that interaction with outside parties is essential for creating effective patient-centered e-health. Technical approaches can be important to achieve interoperability, as demonstrated by Wilson and Lankton (2003) in their proposal of a guided-mail system as an alternative to e-mail for patient-physician communication. However, social issues should not be overlooked in achieving interoperability, as these may be even more important than technical aspects in motivating outside parties to participate. For example, patients embrace the idea of having access to their own medical records, yet physicians are skeptical that patients would benefit from access and worry that their workload would increase if records became available (Ross, Todd, Moore, Beaty, Wittevrongel & Lin, 2005).

By addressing these five principles, developers can work to create e-health that is centered on patients' needs and meaningful in its capabilities. It may be anticipated that other design principles will also apply, for example, requirements arising from privacy and security regulations. However, care should be taken to ensure that these do not unnecessarily obstruct any of the five principles of patient-centered e-health that are enumerated above.

Personal Health Informatics and Patient-Centered E-Health

Through a joint focus on patients (personal focus), healthcare, and informatics, the PHI approach provides valuable tools for satisfying the guiding principles of patient-centered e-health.

- Background knowledge that includes user-centered development methods and personal health management (PHI personal focus) is key in understanding how to elicit patients' perceptions regarding which interactions and e-health services they desire (Principles 1 and 2) and assess comprehensibility and usability of e-health application prototypes (Principles 3 and 4).

- Training in Web e-service infrastructure (PHI informatics focus) provides technical skills necessary to develop accessible controls for patients to use in managing e-health functions (Principle 4) and to enable connections to disparate healthcare IS (Principle 5).

- Knowledge of the health informatics domain (PHI healthcare focus) enables effective interfacing with specialized healthcare IS, which frequently implements specialized protocols and nomenclatures (Principle 5).

Patient surveys consistently show a groundswell of desire for e-health applications that meet patients' specific needs, including needs for electronic support for managing personal health information (Taylor, 2004), patient-physician communication (Taylor & Leitman, 2002), and high-quality online health information (Krane, 2005). The PHI approach can effectively integrate the skills, knowledge, and patient-centered perspective that are necessary to meet these growing patient demands.

Conclusion

Although not always profitable for commercial vendors, e-health has been very beneficial to users, who already conduct many types of transactions and information searches on the Internet and strongly desire to be able to access healthcare services and information in the same manner. Patients comprise a large and growing constituency of e-health users, and I have argued in this chapter that the interests of this population would be served best by creating e-health from the patient's perspective. The guiding principles outlined above take important steps toward the goal of patient-centered e-health. Yet this goal faces numerous obstacles, including fears of financial disincentives and reduced work quality for outside parties who are called upon to participate. In order to be effective, patient-centered e-health initiatives will require champions who will be aided by establishment of training programs, identification of best practices, and development of a shared identity. I propose that PHI offers a practical approach to undertake these actions.

References

AHIMA. (2005). The role of the personal health record in the EHR. *Journal of AHIMA, 76*(7), 64A-64D.

Campbell, R. (2005). Getting to the good information: PHRs and consumer health informatics. *Journal of AHIMA, 76*(10), 46-49.

Emanuel, E., & Emanuel, L. (1992). Four models of the physician-patient relationship. *JAMA, 267*(16), 2221-2226.

Eysenbach, G. (2000). Consumer health informatics. *British Medical Journal, 320*(7251), 1713-1716.

Eysenbach, G. (2001). What is e-health? *Journal of Medical Internet Research, 3*(2), article e20.

Eysenbach, G., & Jadad, A. (2001). Evidence-based patient choice and consumer health informatics in the Internet age. *Journal of Medical Internet Research, 3*(2), article e19.

Fox, S. (2005). *Health information online.* Pew Internet & American Life Project. Retrieved December 13, 2005 from www.pewinternet.org

Harris. (2000). *Healthcare satisfaction study.* Harris Interactive/ARiA Marketing Final Report. Retrieved December 13, 2005 from http://www.harrisinteractive.com/news/downloads/HarrisAriaHCSatRpt.PDF

Holt, M. (2005). *An archaeology of the commercial PHR movement.* Presentation to QTC-CGU Symposium. The many faces of person-centric electronic health systems: A national symposium to examine use-cases for healthy, chronically ill and disabled user communities. Claremont, CA.

Institute of Medicine. (2001). *Crossing the quality chasm.* Washington, D.C.: Institute of Medicine, National Academies Press.

Itagaki, M., Berlin, R., & Schatz, B. (2002). The rise and fall of e-health: Lessons from the first generation of Internet healthcare. *Medscape General Medicine, 4*(2). Retrieved December 13, 2005 from http://www.medscape.com/viewarticle/431144_Print

Kloss, L. (2005). Greater urgency, sharper focus for PHRs. *Journal of AHIMA, 76*(10), 27.

Krane, D. (2005). Number of "cyberchondriacs" —U.S. adults who go online for health information—increases to estimated 117 million. *Healthcare News, 8*(5). Retrieved December 13, 2005 from http://www.harrisinteractive.com/news/newsletters_healthcare.asp

Kwankam, S. (2004). What e-health can offer?. *Bulletin of the World Health Organization, 82*(10), 800-802.

Lafky, D., Tulu, B., & Horan, T. (2006). A user-driven approach to personal health records. *Communications of the Association for Information Systems, 17,* 1028-1041.

Lazar, J. (2001). *User-centered Web development.* Sudbury, MA: Jones and Bartlett.

Lazarus, I. (2001). Separating myth from reality in e-health initiatives. *Managed Healthcare Executive, June,* 33-36.

Markle Foundation. (2004). *Achieving electronic connectivity in healthcare.* Markle Foundation.

Martin, S., Yen, D., & Tan, J. (2002). E-health: Impacts of Internet technologies on various healthcare and services sectors. *International Journal of Healthcare Technology and Management, 4*(1-2), 71-86.

Moen, A., & Brennan, P. (2005). Health@Home: The work of health information management in the household (HIMH): Implications for consumer health informatics (CHI) innovations. *Journal of the American Medical Informatics Association, 12*(6), 648-656.

Norman, C., & Skinner, H. E-Health literacy: Essential skills for consumer health in a networked world. *Journal of Medical Internet Research, 8*(2), article e9.

Oh, H., Rizo, C., Enkin, M., & Jadad, A. (2005). What is e-health?: A systematic review of published definitions. *Journal of Medical Internet Research, 7*(1), article e1.

Rovenpor, J. (2003). Explaining the e-commerce shakeout. *E-Service Journal, 3*(1), 53-76.

Rust, R., & Lemon, K. (2001). E-service and the consumer. *International Journal of E-Commerce, 5*(3), 85-102.

Tan, J., Cheng, W., & Rogers, W. (2002). From telemedicine to e-health: Uncovering new frontiers of biomedical research, clinical applications & public health services delivery. *Journal of Computer Information Systems, 42*(5), 7-18.

Taylor, H. (2004). Two in five adults keep personal or family health records and almost everybody thinks this is a good idea: Electronic health records likely to grow rapidly. *Healthcare News, 4*(10). Retrieved December 13, 2005 from http://www.harrisinteractive.com/news/newsletters_healthcare.asp

Taylor, H., & Leitman, R. (2002). Patient/physician online communication: Many patients want it, would pay for it, and it would influence their choice of doctors and health plans. *Healthcare News, 2*(8). Retrieved December 13, 2005 from http://www.harrisinteractive.com/news/newsletters_healthcare.asp

Thompson, T., & Brailler, D. (2004). *The decade of health information technology: Delivering consumer-centric and information-rich healthcare.* Washington, D.C.: Department of Health and Human Services.

WHO. (2005). E-health: Report by the Secretariat. *World Health Organization, 58th World Health Assembly.*

Wilson, E. (2006a). The case for e-health in the information systems curriculum. *Issues in Information Systems, 7*(1), 299-304.

Wilson, E. (2006b). Building better e-health through a personal health informatics pedagogy. *International Journal of Healthcare Information Systems and Informatics, 1*(3), 69-76.

Wilson, E., & Connolly, J. (2000). SALVO: A basic method for user interface development. *Journal of Informatics Education & Research, 1*(2), 29-39.

Wilson, E., & Lankton, N. (2003). Strategic implications of asynchronous healthcare communication. *International Journal of Healthcare Technology and Management, 5*(3-5), 213-231.

Wilson, E., & Lankton, N. (2004). Modeling patients' acceptance of provider-delivered e-health. *Journal of the American Medical Informatics Association, 11*(4), 241-248.

Chapter XVIII

The Impact of Certification on Healthcare Information Technology Use

Neset Hikmet, University of South Florida, USA

Anol Bhattacherjee, University of South Florida, USA

Abstract

This study examines the effects of certifications such as JCAHO on healthcare information technology (HIT) usage in healthcare organizations and user satisfaction with such usage. Using survey data collected from healthcare administrators in a nation-wide sample of 347 hospitals and long-term care facilities, we provide evidence that certifications do indeed enhance HIT usage and user satisfaction, at least within specialized user groups such as healthcare administrators. We further demonstrate that this increase in HIT usage due to certifications increases with facility size and is more prominent for larger hospitals than for smaller long-term care facilities, though the same cannot be said of user satisfaction. Our study suggests that certifications can be used as a valuable tool for motivating HIT usage, while also drawing attention to an under-examined area of HIT research.

Introduction

As the cost of healthcare has soared in the United States, rising to $2 trillion or 16% of GDP in 2005 (CMS, 2007), the role and use of healthcare information technology (HIT) has come into increased focus. HIT, in this context, refers to a wide range of clinical systems such as electronic medical records (EMR), computerized physician order entry (CPOE), and pharmacy information systems, and administrative systems such as patient billing systems, budgeting systems, and scheduling systems, that are expected to streamline healthcare delivery to patients, improve healthcare quality, and reduce delivery costs. In the report presented to the U.S. Congress by the Medicare Payment Advisory Commission (2004), HIT was identified as having the potential to significantly improve the quality, safety, and efficiency of healthcare. A similar report by the National Health Leadership Council (2005) identified HIT as the critical foundation for promoting health system reform, generating productivity and performance improvement, and producing significant cost reduction in healthcare expenditures.

As healthcare organizations face increasing pressure to invest in HIT, many healthcare managers are struggling to find ways to motivate physicians, nurses, and administrators to use the implemented HIT. Clearly, technology deployment is futile if users do not use the technology, use it inappropriately, or find ways to circumvent its usage. For instance, in 2003, doctors at the prestigious Cedars-Sinai Medical Center at Los Angeles rebelled against their newly installed CPOE system, complaining that the system was too great a distraction from their medical duties, forcing the withdrawal of a system that was already online in two-thirds of the 870-bed hospital (Freudenheim, 2004). The Leapfrog Group (an advisory group associated with the National Academy of Sciences) estimated that, of the nation's 300 non-governmental hospitals (6% of all hospitals in the U.S.) that have implemented comprehensive HIT systems, only 40 of these systems (less than 1%) are routinely used by of doctors for ordering prescriptions and laboratory tests (Freudenheim, 2004).

One practice that is expected to motivate HIT use among hospital administrators similar to professional certification (Chow, 2001) is agency certification (Pawlson & O'Kane, 2002; Dodd, 2004; Watcher, 2004). Professional certification of an individual is an implication that s/he is qualified in that profession attained by specific training, experience and knowledge and maintains such status periodical evaluation. Similarly, an institution certified by an accrediting agency would focus on its internal activities and enhance its processes in order to be in compliance with the standards that have been established by that agency. Thus, many hospitals nationwide seek certification from the Joint Commission of Accreditation of Healthcare Organizations (JCAHO) to demonstrate their commitment to quality in healthcare delivery which requires receiving a passing score on standards that is set forth. Receiving JCAHO accreditation also meets eligibility requirements for participation in the government's Medicare and Medicaid programs (Associated Press, 2004). A significant requirement of JCAHO certification is continuous monitoring and tracking of a variety of operational statistics such as design of new services, implementation of safety plans, and infection control, which requires intensive record keeping and information processing. Furthermore, information management, potentially using HIT, is a key concern in the JCAHO certification process, including management of patient-related information, use of comparative information, and patient-related information (www.jcaho.org). Such laborious and tedious tasks can be alleviated and streamlined by the use of HIT. Furthermore, most recently, JCAHO is field-testing a provision that would move hospitals toward more rapid adoption of electronic health records and other high-tech systems as a way to improve the accuracy of patient identification (*DoBias, 2006*). Hence, it is incumbent upon healthcare administrators to use the available HIT appropriately in order to meet and maintain JCAHO certification status for their facility with more effective information gathering practices based on real-time measurements.

In this chapter, we examine whether certifications such as JCAHO are indeed effective in motivating HIT use among administrators in healthcare settings. Additionally, we are interested in knowing whether JCAHO-induced HIT usage patterns vary across different types of healthcare organizations such as hospitals and long-term care facilities. Given the size and revenue differences between hospitals and long-term care facilities and the consequent availability of slack financial and technological resources to devote to HIT-driven quality initiatives such as JCAHO certifications, one may expect the motivation for JCAHO and HIT usage to be different across these organizations. Furthermore, given the broader scale and scope of hospital operations relative to long-term care facilities, the benefits of JCAHO may be disproportionately larger for the former than the latter.

Examining these issues is important for both practical and research reasons. From a practical standpoint, though JCAHO certification is eagerly sought by healthcare facilities nationwide, there is no evidence yet that such certification indeed yields significant quality and performance gains through the use of HIT. Though certification may be one potential tool in a manager's arsenal to motivate organizational HIT use, at least within certain user groups such as healthcare administrators, to the best of our knowledge, no prior study has yet examined whether such certifications are effective in the first place. Our study addresses this gap by examining the effect of certifications on HIT use by using field survey data collected from a random national sample of healthcare executives working for JCAHO certified and non-certified hospitals and long-term care facilities. If certifications are indeed effective in enhancing HIT usage and improving healthcare delivery, as expected, then organizational investments in such certifications and/or similar quality initiatives will be cost-justified. Furthermore, our study may also provide some evidence as to which type of healthcare organization stands to benefit most from JCAHO certification and related HIT usage.

From a research perspective, understanding the role of certifications is interesting also because much of the prior research on HIT usage has focused almost exclusively on user perceptions of the usefulness and ease of use of a given HIT, users' personal attributes such as information-seeking preference and Internet dependence, and situational characteristics such as healthcare needs (e.g., Wilson & Lankton, 2004). However, currently we know little about what organizational and/or structural factors can motivate given HIT deployment and usage among healthcare organizations to improve healthcare delivery (Hikmet et al., 2007). For instance, one of the stated concerns of the U.S. government is to understand organizational factors that enable or hinder HIT use among healthcare organizations (AHCPR, 1998). The ultimate goal of our work is to provoke enough interest among academics to study the underlying structural factors, such as certifications that may help explain why HIT deployment is more successful in some organizations and less successful in others.

The rest of the chapter proceeds as follows. In the next section, we present our research hypotheses and theoretical rationale for the same. In the third section, we describe our empirical methods for data collection and analysis to test our hypotheses. Following this, we discuss our observed findings and their implications and limitations. The chapter concludes with a summary of our key findings and suggestions for future research.

Research Hypotheses

JCAHO is a non-profit organization whose mission is "to continuously improve the safety and quality of care provided to the public through the provision of healthcare accreditation and related services that support performance improvement in healthcare organizations" (www.jcaho.org). As part of their accreditation procedure, JCAHO has been independently auditing the operational and quality performances of healthcare facilities in the U.S., once every three years, since 1994. Even though JCAHO certification is not mandatory for hospitals or other healthcare facilities, it is a prestigious award that implies that the facility is in compliance with the standards set by the accrediting organization and routinely implements and evaluates required quality indicators in all functional areas of the organization, including management of information (Watcher, 2004). Further, JCAHO certification is required for a healthcare facility to participate in Medicare and Medicaid programs, which are often large revenue sources for many healthcare organizations.

The JCAHO accreditation or re-accreditation process is based on a site visit, during which the JCAHO team evaluates how well a hospital meets more than 500 standards specified in the Accreditation Manual for Hospitals. This data is then aggregated into 46 "grid elements," 16 "performance areas," an overall performance score (on a 0 to 100 scale), and an accreditation decision (e.g., accreditation with commendation, conditional accreditation, accreditation denied, unaccredited, etc.). One key performance area recently added to the certification process is the "management of information," which includes grid elements such as information management planning, availability of patient-specific information, data collection and analysis, literature to support decision making, and use of comparative information. JCAHO certification requires formal evaluations of each of the metrics just mentioned and an ongoing organizational commitment to meeting JCAHO standards, performance elements, and scoring requirements.

JCAHO accreditation and re-accreditation procedures require hospital administrators to continuously monitor and document a wide variety of healthcare and patient safety statistics, such as adverse drug events and infection occurrences. Though JCAHO does not regulate what kind of HIT should be deployed or how it should be used or managed, it does encourage HIT usage as a reliable and timely means for tracking patient and healthcare quality information. For example, Standard IM.1.10 in JCAHO manual relates to information planning: "The hospital plans and designs information management processes to meet internal and external information needs;" and Standard IM.4.10 addresses information-based decision making: "The information management system provides information for use in decision making." The heavy record keeping, information processing, and periodical reporting needs imposed by JCAHO are therefore expected to motivate healthcare executives to aggressively deploy and utilize HIT to conform to JCAHO needs. Furthermore, meeting the JCAHO objectives by virtue of their HIT usage can be expected to enhance healthcare administrators' satisfaction with HIT usage, in consonance with positive associations between technology usage and user satisfaction reported in the information technology implementation literature (DeLone & McLean, 1992). These expectations lead us to hypothesize:

H1: *Administrators in JCAHO certified facilities have (a) higher HIT use and (b) higher user satisfaction than those in non-JCAHO certified facilities.*

JCAHO accreditation and re-accreditation require substantial financial and technological resources on the part of the accredited facility. Sophisticated HIT systems and applications are required to continuously track and monitor a wide variety of JCAHO performance and quality metrics and take remedial actions if things go wrong. A high level of financial resources and technological expertise is required to not only achieve such capability, but also to maintain it over the long-term. Larger organizations such as hospitals are likely to have more slack resources to devote to HIT investments than smaller organizations such as long-term care facilities. Once the appropriate HIT system is implemented, the better fit between the technology and administrators' tasks (e.g., tracking JCAHO metrics, etc.) may be expected to enhance their actual usage of HIT. Further, larger organizations, by virtue of their greater scale and scope of operations, are often able to distribute the benefits of JCAHO certifications over a wider array of services and divisions, resulting in greater satisfaction among healthcare administrators. Hence, we propose:

H2: *The effect of JCAHO certification on (a) higher HIT use and (b) higher user satisfaction is greater for administrators of hospitals than for long-term care facilities.*

Research Methodology

Survey Approach

Empirical data for testing our hypotheses was collected via a mail survey of healthcare administrators in hospitals and long-term care facilities throughout the United States. We focused specifically on healthcare administrators as the key informant in our study because these individuals were responsible for meeting JCAHO tracking and reporting needs and were expected to use HIT systems to do so. Our sampling frame consisted of a list of healthcare organizations purchased from a list broker that specializes in healthcare mailing lists. This list included the name, address, and type of healthcare facilities (e.g., hospital, long-term care) throughout the U.S., along with the names, addresses, phone numbers, and titles of senior executives (e.g., chief executive officers, presidents, managers, supervisors) in those organizations. A stratified sampling scheme was utilized, in which we categorized organizations in the sampling frame into three strata based on facility type: hospitals, long-term care facilities (e.g., nursing homes or assisted living facilities), and community health centers. A sample of 6,713 respondents, divided proportionally (10% of each population stratum) among the three strata, was selected randomly as targets of our survey research.

Our survey followed the approach recommended by Dillman (1978), intended to maximize response rates and minimize non-response bias. Using this approach, we first sent out postcards to our target respondents informing them of the pending arrival of a survey questionnaire regarding the role and use of information technology in the healthcare sector and soliciting their participation in this survey. Twenty postcards were returned as "non-deliverable" due to invalid addresses or the addressee having moved to a different organization. Valid subjects were then mailed the questionnaire booklet, along with a personalized cover letter and a postage-paid envelope for mailing back responses. Five weeks later, the questionnaire was mailed to non-respondents again, followed five weeks later by a reminder card urging them for the third time to respond to the survey if they had not already done so.

Table 1. Population and sample distributions

		Sampling frame	Percent	Study Survey	Percent
Position	Upper Management	4642	69.4	398	72.2
	Administrative Staff	2051	30.6	152	27.6
Facility	Hospital	1666	24.9	144	26.1
	Long-Term Care	3671	54.8	316	57.4
	Community Health Centers and Others	1356	20.3	91	16.7

Following this multi-round survey, 550 surveys were returned, for an overall response rate of 8.2%. To test for non-response bias, we conducted two multinomial distribution tests comparing the distribution of facility type (hospitals and long-term care, vs. community health centers) and respondents' position (upper management vs. administrative staff) in our sample with that of the population (as aggregated from the facility data provided by our mailing list provider). Chi-square analyses for these differences were non-significant for both facility type ($\chi2=5.61$, p=0.16) and respondent's position ($\chi2=2.53$, p=0.11), suggesting that our sample was reasonably representative of the target population. The population and sample distribution for these two dimensions are shown in Table 1.

The community health centers stratum was dropped from further analysis because very few of the responding centers were JCAHO certified or were interested in JCAHO certification. Additionally, being local, non-profit, and community-owned, and serving low income and other underserved communities, the vision and operational structure of community health centers were significantly different than that of hospitals and long-term care facilities. This divergence in vision and goals likely resulted in different motivations for HIT use or non-use in these facilities, further justifying their omission from our data sample. However, the remaining two strata were retained in our study because of higher levels of JCAHO certifications in these strata. Furthermore, hospitals were much larger in size (in bed count and number of employees), scope of operations (e.g., procedures served), and availability of resources than long-term care facilities. Hence, these facilities can respectively be considered to be proxies of large and mid-sized organizations. A comparative examination of these two facility types therefore not only helped us assess the generalizability of the effect of certifications, but also helped us examine whether organizational size might have had some influence on the hypothesized effect.

Variable Operationalization

Our two independent variables of interest were certification (presence vs. absence of JCAHO accreditation) and facility type (hospitals vs. long-term care facilities), and our two dependent variables were HIT usage and user satisfaction. The independent variables were captured as single fill-in measures in our survey questionnaire (e.g., whether the facility was JCAHO certified or not, and whether it was a hospital or a long-term care facility).

HIT usage was measured as the number of hours respondents (healthcare administrators) used HIT per day. Specifically, our survey questionnaire asked respondents (healthcare executives) to enter the number of hours they spent per week at work using 10 common HIT applications, such as reporting systems, billing systems, and error tracking systems. Self-reported hours across these ten categories were added to create an overall HIT use score for that respondent. This detailed elaboration of usage statistics across different HIT was expected to elicit the respondents' true level of usage, which is often masked in self-reported usage measures employing Likert and similar scales.

User satisfaction with HIT use was computed by summing two seven-point Likert-scaled items (anchored between "strongly disagree" and "strongly agree") that asked respondents the extent to which they were satisfied with the HIT available at their workplace and the level of support they received from HIT staff at work. This satisfaction scale was based on a similar scale developed and validated by Tan and Lo (1990). The Likert scale was appropriate for this measure because satisfaction was a perceptual construct and is best measured as such.

Data Analysis and Findings

Sample Characteristics

Following two rounds of reminders, our field survey resulted in an effective sample size of 347. This sample consisted of 115 hospitals and 232 long-term care facilities. Overall, 156 of the 347 facilities in our sample were JCAHO certified, and 191 were not. Ninety-eight of the 115 hospitals in our sample (85.2%) were JCAHO-certified, but only 58 of the 232 long-term care facilities (25.1%) enjoyed this certification, demonstrating a divergent pattern of JCAHO certification between these groups. This pattern is indicative of the organizational makeup of these two facility groups. Many long-term care facilities have fewer employees and perform tasks of less complexity in comparison to hospitals, thus making their recording and reporting activities a less important task for administrative staff and consequently resulting in the reduced dependence on JCAHO certification. Sample breakdown by groups, along with HIT use and user satisfaction means within each group are reported in Table 2.

Table 2. Descriptive statistics

Facility Type		Certification		
		JCAHO Certified	Non-Certified	Total
Hospital	Number of observations (%) Mean HIT use Mean user satisfaction	98 (85.2%) 59.82 10.10	17 (14.8%) 25.24 8.35	115 (100%)
Long-term care	Number of observations (%) Mean HIT use Mean user satisfaction	58 (25.1%) 25.34 9.89	174 (74.9%) 22.20 8.98	232 (100%)

Legend:

HIT use scores were calculated as a sum of ten items that captured the number of hours spent by respondent on using ten common HIT applications in the healthcare sector, such as reporting, billing systems, forecasting, and so forth.

User satisfaction scores were calculated as a sum of two 1-7 Likert scales. Hence, overall satisfaction scores for each respondent ranged from 2 to 14.

Figure 1. Health information technology use

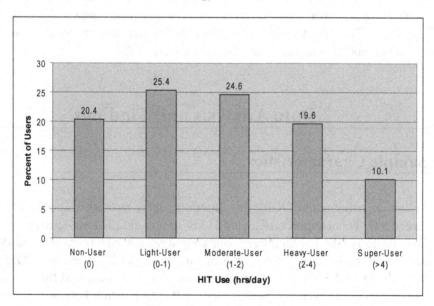

For descriptive analysis, we classified respondents into five categories based on their overall level of self-reported HIT use: (1) non-users: 0 hours per day, (2) light users: 1 hour or less per day, (3) moderate users: 1-2 hours per day, (4) heavy users: 2-4 hours per day, and (5) super users: more than 4 hours per day. This classification was based on an initial pilot study of healthcare executives (Hikmet & Burns, 2004). The frequency distribution of HIT use is shown graphically in Figure 1. It is interesting to note from this figure that more than 20% of the healthcare administrators in our sample did not use HIT at all, and more than 70% spend two hours or less per day on work-related HIT use. While this apparent low level of use may reflect respondents' time constraints at work, the required tracking and reporting by JCAHO and similar regulatory organizations are not bound by such constraints.

Hypotheses Testing

To test for the two hypotheses stated earlier, we first conducted a two-way multivariate analysis of variance (MANOVA) test to examine whether our two independent variables, certification (JCAHO vs. non-JCAHO) and facility type (hospitals vs. long-term care facilities), and their interaction had any significant effects on our two dependent variables of interest: HIT use and user satisfaction. MANOVA results, shown in Table 3, were significant for both certification ($F=8.34$, $p<0.001$) and facility type ($F=3.67$, $p=0.026$), while the interaction term between the two variables was weakly significant ($F=0.97$, $p=0.053$).

Next, we conducted follow-up analysis of variance (ANOVA) to examine which of the dependent variables experienced significant effects. As seen in Table 3, certification had a significant effect on both HIT use ($F=7.17$, $p=0.008$) and user satisfaction ($F=9.46$, $p=0.002$), when controlled for facility type. In contrast, facility type had a significant effect on HIT use ($F=7.10$, $p=0.008$), but not on user satisfaction ($F=0.250$, $p=0.618$), when certification was controlled. The interaction between certification and facility type also had a significant effect on HIT use ($F=4.98$, $p=0.026$), but not on satisfaction ($F=0.94$, $p=0.332$).

These analyses validate our first hypothesis that JCAHO certifications not only increases HIT use among healthcare administrators (Hypothesis H1a), but also increases user satisfaction with such use (Hypothesis H1b). HIT usage was more pronounced in larger facilities such as hospitals than in mid-sized facilities such as long-term care facilities, but user satisfaction experienced no such differential effect across facility types. Focusing on the interaction effect posited in the second hypothesis, we find that JCAHO certification had a stronger effect on motivating HIT use among hospital administrators than those in long-term care facilities (validating Hypothesis H2a), but did not increase user satisfaction among hospital administrators significantly more than those in long-term care facilities (failing to support Hypothesis H2b). Implications of these findings are discussed in the next section.

Discussion and Conclusion

Implications for Practice

The findings of our study confirm that healthcare managers can indeed motivate HIT usage within their organizations by proactively engaging in and obtaining certifications such as JCAHO. The incentive to maintain JCAHO accreditation works as an adequate incentive for healthcare administrators to use HIT systems appropriately to meet the monitoring and reporting requirements of JCAHO. Furthermore, administrators appear to be satisfied with their HIT usage, despite the demanding needs of JCAHO accreditation and re-accreditation. However, we do not have any evidence to examine whether this higher level of use among healthcare administrators translates into higher usage among other user groups such as physicians or nurses. Additional studies, with different subject populations, are required to examine those trends.

Hospitals in our study experienced a larger increase in HIT use from JCAHO certification than long-term care facilities. Extrapolating this size effect, we expect that smaller-sized organizations such as doctors' offices stand to benefit least from certifications and, hence, certification programs may not be a worthwhile investment for smaller organizations such as long-term care facilities and community health centers. Furthermore, user satisfaction is expected to remain relatively invariant across facility types between JCAHO certified and non-certified groups. Hence, managers should measure HIT usage and not user satisfaction to evaluate the outcome of JCAHO certification process, and more so for smaller facilities.

Implications for Research

Our study contributes to HIT research by providing preliminary empirical evidence regarding the role of certifications on HIT use and user satisfaction in healthcare organizations. Though such certifications undoubtedly enhance an organization's stature and prestige in its community and signal its commitment on quality processes, their effect on HIT use in particular was unclear and unexamined prior to this study.

Our study also draws attention to organizational factors such as certifications that managers can control to motivate HIT usage within their organizations. While much of the prior HIT usage research has focused on personal or cognitive factors, such as perceived usefulness and perceived ease of use as antecedents of HIT usage and user satisfaction (e.g., Wilson & Lankton, 2004), and has demonstrated good predictive abilities, it is worth noting that such factors cannot be controlled by managers and are therefore less relevant from a practitioner standpoint. In that sense, our study goes beyond predicting HIT usage to the more relevant question of examining how organizations can proactively manipulate HIT use through certifications.

Though our study was conducted in a healthcare setting, our findings can be expected to be generalizable to other industry sectors. For instance, many firms in other industries seek certification such as ISO 9001:2000 and ISO 13483:2003 from the International Standards Organization to signal their commitment to similar quality improvement and process management initiatives. Software firms often participate in Capability Maturity Model (CMM) certification initiatives from the Software Engineering Institute for similar reasons. However, additional studies are required to test for these effects.

Limitations of the Study

Finally, like most other empirical studies, our research was not without limitations. First, this study was conducted within the narrow context of healthcare organizations. Hence, our findings may not be readily generalizable to other industry sectors without conducting additional studies to test our reported effects in other industry contexts (e.g., manufacturing or service). Second, we viewed certification as an instance of a quality initiative, since such certification requires prior evaluation of organizational processes and procedures in accordance with the certification agency's norms and expectations. However, one may debate whether certification is an accurate or reasonable proxy of quality programs. Hence, the value and importance of our findings may be limited in instances where certification is not consistent with organizational quality initiatives. Third, the nature and substance of certifications vary widely across certification agencies, their scale and scope of certification, and certification metrics employed. Though JCAHO certification is viewed as being one of the most comprehensive and prestigious quality certifications in the healthcare industry, similar certifications from other agencies may be less valued. Such variance in certification quality may mitigate the nature of HIT use effects across certification agencies.

Future Research Directions

This study examined only two of several organizational factors, namely certifications and facility type (size), that can motivate HIT usage and user satisfaction among healthcare organizations. There may be more such organizational factors with comparable or greater predictive ability, and we encourage future research to uncover and investigate those factors. Second, we observed that the effects of some of these organizational factors are invariant for user satisfaction, while varying for HIT usage. Since HIT usage tends to be positively correlated with user satisfaction, this divergence of effects is theoretically perplexing. Additional research is required to examine potential reasons for such divergence. Third, future research can also examine the generalizability of our study's findings across other industry sectors (e.g., financial or technology), across other user groups (e.g., physicians or nurses), and across other forms of certification (e.g., ISO-9000 or CMM).

References

Agency for Healthcare Policy and Research (AHCPR). (1998). *Effective dissemination of health and clinical information and research findings*. Retrieved January 20, 1999 from http://www.ahrq.org.

Associated Press. (2004). *Alta Bates risks loss of accreditation over negative audit*. Retrieved from http://www.signonsandiego.com/news/state/ 20041114-0931-caltabatesproblems.html

Chow, W. (2001). Ethical belief and behavior of managers using information technology for decision making in Hong Kong. *Journal of Managerial Psychology, 16*(4), 258-267.

CMS. (2007). Center for Medicare and Medicaid services. Retrieved July 2, 2007 from http://www.cms.hhs.gov/NationalHealthExpendData/downloads/highlights.pdf

DoBias, M. (2006). JCAHO floats IT to propel safety. *Modern Healthcare, 36*(49), 14-15.

Dillman, D. (1978). *Mail and telephone surveys*. New York, NY: John Wiley & Sons.

Dodd, A. (2004). Accreditation as a catalyst for institutional effectiveness. *New Directions for Institutional Research, n123*, 13-25.

Freudenheim, M. (2004). Many hospitals resist computerized patient care. *New York Times*. Retrieved February 2, 2006 from http://www.nytimes.com/2004/04/06/technology/06errors.html

Hikmet, N., & Burns, M. (2004). Healthcare executives: The association between external factors, use, and their perceptions of health information technology. *Proceedings of the 10ᵗʰ Americas Conference on Information Systems*. New York.

Hikmet, N., Bhattacherjee, A., Menachemi, N., Kayhan, V., & Brooks, R. (2007). The role of organizational factors in the adoption of healthcare information technology in Florida hospitals. *Healthcare Management Science, 10*(4).

Medical Library Association librarian's guide to JCAHO survey. (2006). Retrieved March 1, 2006 from http://www.mlanet.org/resources/jcaho.html#Q1

Pawlson, L., & O'Kane, M. (2002). Professionalism, regulation, and the market: Impact on accountability for quality of care. *Health Affairs, 21*(3), 200-207.

Tan, B., & Lo, T. (1990). Validation of a user satisfaction instrument for office automation success. *Information & Management, 18*(4), 203-208.

Watcher, R. (2004). The end of the beginning: Patient safety five years after 'to err is human'. *Health Affairs,* hlthaff.w4.534

Wilson, E., & Lankton, N. (2004). Modeling patients' acceptance of provider de-livered e-health. *Journal of the American Medical Informatics Association, 11*(4), 241-248.

Chapter XIX

The Competitive Forces Facing E-Health

Nilmini Wickramasinghe, Stuart Graduate School of Business, USA

Santosh Misra, Cleveland State University, USA

Arnold Jenkins, John Hopkins Hospital, USA

Douglas R. Vogel, City University of Hong Kong, China

Abstract

Superior access, quality, and value of healthcare services has become a national priority for healthcare to combat the exponentially increasing costs of healthcare expenditure. E-Health in its many forms and possibilities appears to offer a panacea for facilitating the necessary transformation for healthcare. While a plethora of e-health initiatives keep mushrooming both nationally and globally, there exists to date no unified system to evaluate these respective initiatives and assess their relative strengths and deficiencies in realizing superior access, quality and value of healthcare services. Our research serves to address this void. This is done by focusing on the following three key components: (1) understanding the Web of players (regulators, payers, providers, healthcare organizations, suppliers, and last but not least patients) and how e-health can modify the interactions between these players as well as create added value healthcare services, (2) understand the competitive forces facing e-health organizations and the role of the Internet in modifying these forces, and 3) from analyzing the Web of players combined with the competitive forces for e-health organizations we develop a framework that serves to identify the key forces facing an e-health and suggestions of how such an organization can structure itself to be e-health prepared.

Introduction

E-health is a broad term that encompasses many different activities related to the use of the Internet for the delivery of healthcare service. Healthcare professionals are extending the use of the Internet to include a source of evidence-based consumer information as well as to facilitate the research of protocols for healthcare delivery, accessing laboratory and medical records, and performing second opinion consults (Sharma & Wickramasinghe, 2005; Sharma, Wickramasingeh, Xu, & Ahmed, 2006). Moreover, the Internet is being used by patients to become more knowledgeable about health practices as seen from their questions to their physicians (Gargeya & Sorrell, 2005).

Although, a relatively new term and unheard of prior to 1999, e-health has now become the latest "e-buzzword" used to characterize not only "Internet medicine," but also virtually everything related to computers and medicine (Sharma et al., 2006; Von Lubitz & Wickramasinghe, 2006). The scope and boundary of e-health, as well as e-heath organizations, is still evolving. However one can only imagine it will grow rapidly especially given that governments in both U.S. and Europe, and organizations such as WHO (World Healthcare Organization) are advocating that e-health be on the top of all healthcare agendas and an integral component of any healthcare delivery initiative (Von Lubitz et al., 2006).

Given the growth and variety of e-health initiatives, it becomes important to examine the forces affecting these initiatives and factors leading to the success of e-health. To date, little research examines metrics of measurement pertaining to e-health initiatives or their economic value. What are the forces of competition affecting e-heath? Are the competitive forces constrained by external considerations? Is the issue of competition an appropriate concern for e-health? If so, what are the strong and weak competitive forces? We argue that analysis of these forces would lead us to understand the long-term sustainability of any e-health initiative.

Traditional Competitive Forces

The starting point for understanding the competitive forces facing any e-health initiative lies in understanding the fundamentals of traditional competitive forces that impact all industries and then how the Internet as a disruptive technology has impacted these forces.

The strategy of an organization has two major components (Hendersen & Venkatraman, 1993). These are (1) formulation--making decisions regarding the mission, goals, and objectives of the organization and (2) implementation--making decisions regarding how the organization can structure itself to realize its goal and carryout specific activites. For today's healthcare organizations the goals, mission, and objectives all focus around access, quality, and value and realizing this value proposition for healthcare then becomes the key (Wickramasinghe, Fadlalla, Geisler, & Schaffer, 2005). Essentially, the goal of strategic management is to find a "fit" between the organization and its environment that maximizes its performance (Hofer, 1975). This then describes the market-based view of the firm and has been predominantly developed and pushed by the frameworks of Michael Porter. The first of Porter's famous frameworks is the generic strategies (Porter, 1980).

The use of technology must always enable or enhance the businesses objectives and strategies of the organization. This is particularly true for 21st Century organizations where many of their key operations and functions are so heavily reliant on technology and the demand for information and knowledge is so critical. A firms' relative competitive position (i.e., its ability to perform above or below the industry average is determined by its competitive advantage). Porter (1980) identified three generic strategies that impact a firm's competitive advantage. These include cost, focus, and differentiation. Furthermore, Porter himself notes that two and only two basic forms of competitive advantage typically exist:

1. Cost leadership.
2. Differentiation.

Firms can use these two forms of competitive advantage to either compete across a broad scope of an industry or to focus on competing in specific niches; thereby, leading to three generic strategies. Porter (ibid) notes that firms should be cautious about pursuing more than one generic strategy; namely cost, differentiation, and focus. For example, if a cost leadership strategy is adopted it is unlikely that a firm can also maintain and sustain differentiation since it would not be possible to simultaneously pursue the costly capital investment or maintain high operating costs required for differentiation and thus in the long run the firm has a confused strategy which leads to failure.

In order to design and develop ones strategy, an organization should first perform an industry analysis. Porters Five Forces or Competitive Forces model is most useful (Porter, 1980, 1985). Figure 1 depicts this model. Essentially, Porter has taken concepts from micro-economics and modeled them in terms of five key forces that together outline the rules of competition and attractiveness of the industry.

Figure 1. Porter's competitive (Five) forces model

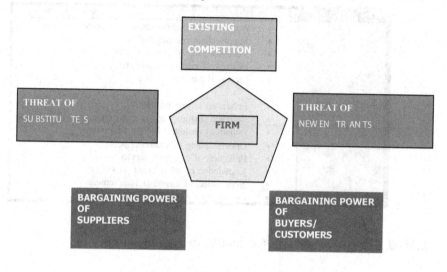

The forces are as follows:

1. **Threat of new entrant:** A company new to the industry that could take away market share from the incumbent firms.

2. **Threat of substitute:** An alternative means that could take market share from product/service offered by the firms in the industry.

3. **Bargaining power of buyers:** The strength of buyers or groups of buyers within the industry relative to the firms.

4. **Bargaining power of suppliers:** The strength of suppliers relative to the firms in the industry.

5. **Rivalry of existing competition:** Relative position and market share of major competitors.

The collective strength of these five forces determines the attractiveness of the industry and thus the potential for superior financial performance by influencing prices, costs, and the level of capital investment required (Porter, 1985). Once a thorough industry analysis has occurred, it is generally easier for a firm to determine which generic strategy makes most sense for it to pursue and enables the firm to exploit most of its core competencies in its existing environment.

Table 1. The three e-opportunity domains and their components

Components	
e-operations	• Automation of administrative processes • Supply-chain reconfiguration • Reengineering of primary infrastructure • Intensive competitive procurement • Increased parenting value
e-marketing	• Enhanced selling process • Enhance customer usage experience • Enhanced customer buying experience
e-services	• Understanding of customer needs • Provision of customer service • Knowledge of all relevant providers • Negotiation of customer requirements • Construction of customer options

Table 2. The e-opportunities for healthcare organizations

Components	
e-operations	• Internet-based supply purchasing • Prescription writing, formulary checking, and interaction checking using hand-held devices
e-marketing	• Delivery of consumer health content and wellness management tools over the Internet • Use of consumer health profiles to suggest disease management and wellness programs
e-services	• Patient-provider communication and transaction applications • Web-based applications to support the clinical conversation between referring and consulting physicians
Crossing multiple domains	• Increasing the level of information content in the product • Increasing the information intensity along the supply chain • Increase in the dispersion of information

Role of the Internet of the Competitive Forces

Feeny (2001) presents a framework that highlights the strategic opportunities afforded to organizations by using the Internet. In particular, he highlights three e-opportunity domains. Table 1 details these domain and their respective components.

E-Opportunities in Healthcare

Given the three areas of e-opportunities previously discussed, Glaser (2002) identifies several key e-opportunities for healthcare. Table 2 details these.

Web of Players in Healthcare

Figure 2 depicts the Web of healthcare players and the key elements of the any e-health architecture that serves to support the interactions between and within this Web of players. In order to fully capture the flows of information it is necessary to first identify the primary producers and consumers of data and information within the healthcare system. At the center of the information flows is the HCIS (healthcare information system, i.e., the e-health network) because not only does it connect the key players within the healthcare system in an efficient and effective manner, but also it forms the central repository for key information such as patient medical records, billing, and treatment details. Hence, the HCIS provides the foundation for supporting the information flows and decision making throughout the healthcare system. Figure 2 then represents a macro view of the inter-relationships between the key players within this system as well as the sources, destinations and flows of information between these players and the pivotal role of the HCIS.

Healthcare procedures such as medical diagnostics, treatment decisions, and consequent effecting of these decisions, prevention, communication, and equipment usage can be thought of as iatric in nature (Wickramasinghe & Fadlalla, 2004). Integral to these iatric procedures is the generating and processing of information (Wickramasinghe & Fadlalla, 2004). The patient naturally provides key information at the time of a clinical visit or other interaction with his/her provider. Such a visit also generates other information including insurance information, medical history, and treatment protocols (if applicable) which must satisfy regulatory requirements, payer directives and, obviously, the healthcare organization's informational needs. Thus, we see that from a single intervention many forms and types of information are captured, generated, and then disseminated throughout the healthcare system. All this information and its flows must satisfy some common integrity characteristics such as accuracy, consistency, reliability, completeness, usefulness, usability, and manipulability. Consequently, generating a level of trust and confidence in the information's content and processes. Since the information flows across various organizational boundaries, the challenge of ensuring information integrity is further compounded because any integrity problems will propagate with ripple effects following the same trajectory as the information itself. Given the high degree of inter-relatedness between the various players, the consequences of poor quality information (such as the cost of information integrity problems) are multiplied and far reaching. This highlights the need for robust, well designed, and well managed

Figure 2. Web of e-health players adapted from Wickramasinghe et al 2004

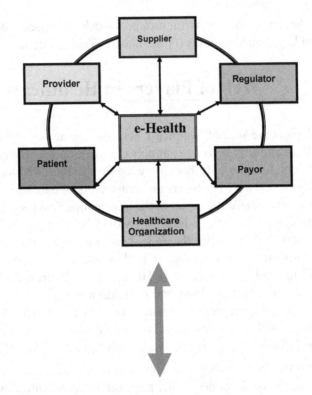

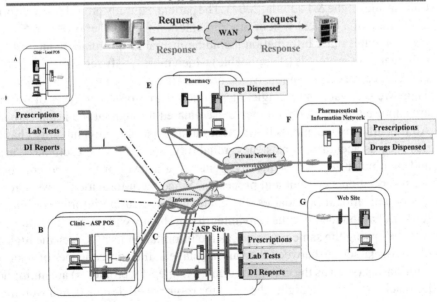

HCIS (Wickramasinghe & Fadlalla, 2004). Such a perspective should not be limited to new systems, but rather, equally and perhaps of even more importance should be applied to existing systems as well.

Modeling the Competitive Forces in E-Health

In order to model e-health, let us first construct a general model of the competitive forces pertaining to e-business. E-business is not simply offering traditional products and services on line. It requires broad-scale asset redeployment and process changes, which ultimately serve as the basis for a company's competitive advantage in today's Digital Economy. For this study, the e-business model could be broken into components such as; products and services, customer value, pricing component, revenue source, the cost component, and asset model as shown in Figure 3.

The prime objective of business model is to make money (La Monica, 2000). The various components of business model as shown in Figure 1 work together to create profit margins for the business. First of all, the electronic business model should offer products and services online. These products and services should be differentiated with competitors by low price or unique customer value. The products are differentiated if customers perceive some value in these that other products do not have. Differentiation can be done by offering different product features, timing, location, service, product mix, linkage between functions, etc. (Afuah & Tucci,

Figure 3. Generic e-business model components

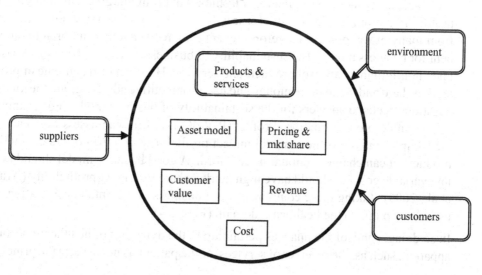

Figure 4. e-health business model components

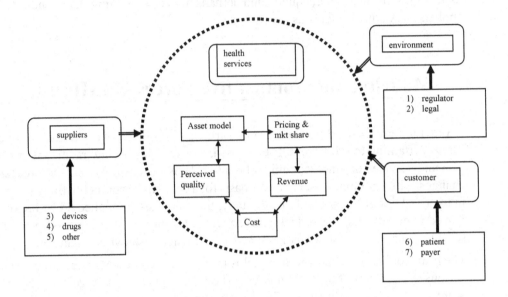

2000). Customer value can be judged whether firm offering its customers something distinctive or at a lower cost than its competitors. The success of business model depends upon how does the firm price the value? An important part of profiting from the value that firms offer customers is to price it properly. For pricing, market shares and margins would be most critical. The good business model should strive for high market share and thus firm should devise strategies accordingly. Pricing of products depends upon the cost and asset model of the firm. The cost (fixed cost + variable cost) should be spread in a fashion that profit margins remain high. The profits in electronic business model case will not only come from sales but may come from many other sources. Therefore, revenue source is another important component for business model. The sustainability of business model can be gauged based upon non-imitable nature of products and services. How can firm continue improve market share and make more money and have competitive advantage are the kind of questions needs to answers for the sustainability of business model. For example; using simple profits equation; Profits=(P-Vc)Q-Fc , firm can assess how each of the components of business model impact profitability. If a firm offers distinctive products, it can charge premium price P for it. A good business model should keep low variable cost but should have high market share for higher profitability (Afuah et al., 2000). Taking these components of a business model into consideration, let us now map this to the healthcare domain (Figure 4).

In so doing, some of the nuances pertaining to the dynamics of healthcare become apparent; such as, the receiver of services, or the patient, is not usually the principal payer. Moreover, the model serves to underscore that for e-health initiatives to truly add value and be sustainable the dynamics of a generic e-business model must be satisfied. Hence, some determination needs to be made regarding Vc, Fc, P, and Q in this context.

To understand these dynamics more easily let us consider a case study example of the implementation of an electronic patient record.

Case Study

The Johns Hopkins Medicine Center for Information Services Public LAN (JPL) is a computer network designed to provide patient care providers access to clinical applications. This computer network is utilized by all types of patient care providers in both inpatient and out patient services. These providers include, but not limited to, doctors, interns, fellows, nurses, unit clerks, pharmacists, nutritionists, and admission specialists. In this article, an examination of the history of the Public LAN, the current state of the LAN, and the future of the Public LAN will be examined. Since its inception the Public LAN as been the leader in efficiency and innovation for Desktop Computing Services (DCS), a division of Information Technology @ Johns Hopkins (IT@Hopkins).

Introduction of the Public LAN

During the spring of 1996, JHMCIS and a group of doctors developed an in-house application to provide patient care. This application is called Electronic Patient Record or EPR. The application was to be used in patient areas for tracking patient record. These records can then be viewed by other clinicians throughout the hospital. A second application was introduced at the same time to provide a graphical user interface to many of the hospital's mainframe and mid-range systems. This application is Host Interface Program or HIP. The challenge at this stage was to provide a computer system that could be used by the doctors that would allow EPR and HIP to be used to provide patient care and at the same time have a desktop system that was secure.

These desktops were to be deployed in medical exam rooms and the major problem was having a desktop that could provide these applications to the clinicians without allowing the clinicians or patients the ability to access the operating system and the computer configuration. This led to the development of the Public Desktop.

The Public desktop is a Microsoft Windows based desktop that has the clinical applications installed, as well as an Internet browser and the Microsoft Office suite. The challenge was managing these systems in areas with limited access during business hours as they were in use by clinicians providing patient care. The operating system was secured and limited access was given to the users. The users were not able to install any applications or download any programs.

The Public LAN started out with 70 desktops in three clinical areas. The Harriet Lane Clinic, which is an outpatient clinic for pediatrics, the neonatal intensive care unit, and the adolescent outpatient clinic. This pilot lasted approximately six months. During the next three years, the Public LAN grew to 1100 desktops.

The Growth of the Public LAN

Today the Public LAN supports over 1800 desktops and many clinical applications. During the first three years of the Public LAN, the number of systems reached over 1100 systems. Included in this growth, not only the number of devices supported, but the number of applications that were supported on these desktops. The driving forces of these changes were outdated clinical applications that were being replaced with client server applications and the millennium with applications that were not year 2000 compliant.

During this time, the application supported grew to include BDM, a new pharmacy application, Vision—a nutrition application and ClicTate, a pediatrics version of EPR. With the intention of more clinical applications moving from the mainframe and mid-range systems to client server applications, the desktops are going to need to be able to handle these additional applications.

The process of managing these systems became a challenge as well. Since the desktops were standardized, DCS was able to implement Microsoft's System Management Server (SMS). This allowed not only the ability to manage these desktops, but also distribute software, inventory the hardware, and software of a specific system, and provide remote control capabilities. SMS was included when the pilot of the Public LAN was deployed but its true value was not realized until the rapid growth of the LAN.

The Public LAN Today

The Public LAN today is well over 1800 desktops, supporting more than 30 clinical applications. Most of these applications are still accessed via HIP, however more client server applications are also supported. The additional client server applications have lead to different configurations of the desktop's application software or "flavors" of Public workstations. Currently there are currently many different configurations for the Public Workstations. These different configurations include:

- Standard configuration.
- Training configuration.
- Wilmer Eye Clinic configuration.
- Pharmacy configuration.
- Nutrition configuration.
- Provider Order Entry configuration.
- Operating room configuration.
- DCOM image viewing configuration.
- Eclypsis Point of Care configuration.
- Procedure Reporting System configuration.
- OB/GYN Configuration.

These different configurations can be on a few as 20 desktops to as many as 600, where the standard configuration is on all of the desktops. The standard configuration is:

- Windows XP Professional.
- EPR.
- HIP.
- Internet Explorer.
- Microsoft Office Suite.
- Adobe Reader.
- Calculator.

The additional configurations are based on adding additional clinical applications to the desktops. In addition, many of the systems have multiple clinical applications installed.

The Lessons Learned

During the growth of the Public LAN, many lessons have been learned. These lessons include best practices for desktops management, application management and deployment, and reduction in the total cost of ownership of a desktop.

The current network is supported by three desktop technicians, which is an average of 600 plus desktops per technician. Desktop Computing Services needed to have a way to manage these systems not only located at the East Baltimore campus, but at other campuses within the Baltimore metropolitan area. The use of Microsoft Systems Management Software (SMS) was deployed to allow desktop management. SMS allows a technician the ability to remote control in to a desktop and perform work as if they were at the desktop. This capability also allows the support staff to view the process of the user and see the error as it happened. SMS also is used to deploy application software to the desktop.

Due to the increased number of clinical applications, the number of different application software configurations increased. In order to manage this DCS used SMS for application deployment. DCS is able to determine the application software installed on the desktop and perform upgrades to the software. The upgrade to an application is preformed by using SMS to "push" and install the software on the desktop without any user intervention. Therefore, and application could be upgraded or installed without having to visit the desktop.

With the integration of SMS to manage the desktops, this has reduced the total cost of ownership of supporting the Public LAN. This decrease is realized by having a ratio of one desktop technician per 600 desktops. DCS is able to remote control the desktop; this prevents the technician from have in walk across campus to help a user. In addition, the installation of applications and upgrades to applications is completed on many systems at once without having to visit each individual desktop. Also, DCS has secured the desktop to prevent the users from accessing the operating system and the hard drive. If the users were able to access the operating system and download and install applications, including spyware, this would greatly increase the support costs of the desktop.

The Future of the Public LAN

The future of the Public LAN at Johns Hopkins Hospital is ever evolving. The needs of the clinicians for resources to provide patient care are continually changing. With patients bringing medical records in on CD-ROM to access to network resources the Public LAN must evolve to meet these needs. In order to meet these needs the Public LAN support staff is required to find clever and innovative ways to provide these resources. New hardware is being added to the Public desktops to allow viewing of clinical data on CD-ROM, the use of USB keys for file storage has been enabled and logging in with a personal account.

The ability for a clinician to login with their personal account allows them to access network resources. These resources include access to network file servers and departmental file servers. In order for a clinician to use a personal account they are required to have a timeout of their session. The timeout of the session will log the user off after a certain amount of idle time. The reason for this is to prevent others from accessing information and to prevent non Johns Hopkins employees to access data and network resources.

The future of the Public LAN is ever evolving. The Johns Hopkins Hospital is building two new clinical towers that will be state of the art. The devices that provide patient care will also need to be state of the art and provide clinicians the ability to provide patient care in a completely paperless, film-less, and wireless network. The Public LAN will be able to provide these solutions and will realize the benefits of these efforts, as patients are cared for more efficiently and effectively.

Mapping the Case to the Model

The implementation of the EPR at Johns' Hopkins represents a relatively common e-health initiative in the current healthcare environment. The EPR enables the seamless flow of patient data and thus facilitates the delivery of efficient and effective quality healthcare to the patient. This is certainly professed as a key benefit for the embracing of EPR in most instances.

The e-health sustainability model however, suggests that one must analyze the micro- and meso-dynamics more closely to actually determine the sustainability of such an initiative. Specifically, it is necessary to capture key factors including, perceived quality, fixed and variable costs, price and market share and quantity and then look at the interaction of these factors before sustainability of the initiative can be pronounced. However, this is beyond the scope of this article but will form the focus of future research.

What can be noted at this point and will be research in more detail in future work is the size or scale of the e-health initiative. Returning to the simple profit equation Profits=(P-Vc)Q-Fc, in the case scenario above, fixed costs will be constant and Vc for any EPR will be marginal given the generic nature of the program and the applications of it by various providers hence we hypothesis that the sustainability of the EPR would increase with Q the quantity or size. Thus, the larger the EPR initiative the more likely it is to be sustainable. Quantitative data to support the relationship between scope and quantity and impact of ICTs in general in healthcare settings can be found in previous studies (Wickramasinghe & Lamb, 2002; Wickramasinghe & Silvers, 2003).

Discussion

In mapping the John's Hopkins case to the model in Figure 4, we can see that the reality of an e-health initiative involves the interactions of various groups of stakeholders. Knowledge management provides an umbrella under which we may discuss a number of opportunities and raise issues relative to components of the business model. The vision of collaboration between components of the business model recognized as stakeholders is one of great opportunity. Stakeholders in this case include suppliers, the firm, the customer, and the government as a key representative of the environment. Each stakeholder brings to the table talent, resources, and differentiated perspectives that, together, create a robust whole in addressing problems and projects. For example, suppliers can be a source of knowledge that can assist the firm in delivering cost effective products and services. Customers are an additional source of knowledge in terms of personal history and preferences. The firm can manage knowledge in a form that maximizes the probability of value added products and services. The government can serve as a catalyst to create an environment conducive to knowledge exchange and management.

Unfortunately, great opportunities do not always turn into reality. Collaboration successes between suppliers, the firm, and its customers much less the government can, sadly, be few and far between. In addition to strengths and distinctions, each stakeholder also brings to the table residual weaknesses and biases that can scuttle the best of collaborative intentions. For example, internal firm bureaucracy can easily drive out the best of suppler intentions and customer good will. Problems can easily be left unaddressed and efforts can easily fail as reality drives out vision. This can be exacerbated by cultural norms and historical behaviors embedded in government policies.

A case in point is the handling of SARS. Levels of suffering and unnecessary deaths were, in part, a result of lack of collaboration between stakeholders. In this case, government agencies (specifically the hospital authorities) were negligent in sharing information and allocating resources amongst hospitals. The hospitals, however, were not guilt free and were accused of withholding information to customers including patients and their families. Further, the relationship between suppliers and hospitals was insufficient to respond to the need for supplies. Shortages were evident and supplies misapplied in circumstances that could have been adverted through collaboration. The situation was further strained as lack of information sharing across governments and excessive bureaucratic delay inhibited quick action to rapidly respond to changing circumstances. In summary, stakeholder collaboration could have, arguably, avoided hardship at individual and societal levels. Unfortunately, it didn't happen and the World Health Organization (WHO) was, rightly, exasperated.

Experiences with SARS have sensitized stakeholders at all levels with respect to effectively dealing with potential pandemics e.g., H5N1-based bird flu. Over the past months, we have already seen a much higher level of information exchange and collaboration than existed in the lead-up to SARS. Governments have more readily shared information and established channels for dealing with global adversity. Hospitals have begun preparations including emergency response practice. Suppliers have opened historically propriety processes and licenses to enable extended manufacturing capability (e.g., Roche with Tamiflu, as but one example). Customers have sought (and obtained) information relative to prevention and preparation for a variety of circumstances as well as acted as a source of information back to appropriate authorities regarding infectious incidences, e.g., bird flock deaths. Numerous conferences with multiple stakeholders present have provided forums for knowledge sharing, enhanced understanding leading towards the creation of action plans. In short, bird flu threats have galvanized stakeholders in a way that was unseen in the handling of SARS, in part, as a result of witnessing and experiencing hardship.

Knowledge management provides a focus that can enhance the probability of success in encouraging and sustaining broad-based stakeholder collaboration. Formalized knowledge management promotes the ultimate desire for the benefits of stakeholder collaboration to be sufficiently well developed and supported to offset inherent weaknesses. Knowledge management plays a key role in assuring that aspects of information creation, sharing, and dissemination compatible with multiple stakeholder objectives can be successfully achieved (Alavi & Leidner, 2001). Problems are often beyond the scope of any particular stakeholder, which encourages cooperation in order for success to be attained (Van de Ven, Angle, & Poole, 2000).

The concept of suppler, firm, customer, and government collaboration is sound but operationalization is difficult and fraught with problems. This doesn't suggest that the concept should be abandoned, just managed, and supported. Sadly, this situation is not unique (Lyytinen & Rose, 2003). The missing element is often cooperative knowledge creation and exchange. Each element of the collaboration needs a better understanding and focus on cooperation. Unfortunately, this doesn't naturally exist and easily turns antagonistic. Cooperation is difficult to achieve even when linkages are in place. It is far too easy to say that "details can be worked out." Unfortunately, the "devil" is in the detail. Towards that end, stakeholder collaboration in achieving knowledge management objectives is paramount.

Conclusion

The underlying goal for healthcare is to provide cost effective quality treatment (i.e., realize its value proposition in this challenging environment). In order to do this healthcare needs to maximize its information management techniques and make prudent use of ICTs (Information Communication Technologies). In such a context e-health initiatives will clearly play a dominant role in healthcare delivery. This has been underscored by leaders of US and the EU as well as leading bodies such as the World Healthcare Organization (WHO) that focus on global healthcare issues and policy. Moreover, Both European and US authorities define their initiatives primarily in terms of medical information technology centering on computerized patient record [CPR] or, in more acceptable parlance, the HER electronic health record as referred to by WHO. Hence, e-health is here to stay. What becomes critical then is the sustainability of these e-health initiatives and their ability to bring benefits to the key actor in healthcare, the patient.

This article has set out to delve into the abyss of e-health sustainability. A logical starting place to us seemed to identify the primary drivers in a generic e-business model and then map them into healthcare. Our e-health sustainability model then serves to identify the critical factors and important dynamics faced by any e-health initiative. In addition, we identified the importance of scale and scope economies in this process through the mapping of case study data. Finally, we noted that it is necessary to incorporate the techniques and strategies of knowledge management if superior collaboration between the multiple stakeholders is to ensue. Through the example of SARS we underscored how important this aspect is not only to the sustainability of e-health but in order to realize effective healthcare delivery. Clearly this is only the beginning and we now need further investigation and research, which we plan to embark upon. We close by encouraging other researchers to also delve deeper into this imperative healthcare research area.

References

Afuah, A., & Tucci, C. L. (2000). *Internet business models and strategies—text and cases*. McGraw Hill Irwin.

Alavi, M. A., & Leidner, D. E. (2001). Review: Knowledge management and knowledge management systems: Conceptual foundations and research issues. *MIS Quarterly, 25*(1), 107-136.

Feeny, D. (2001). Making business sense of the e-opportunity. *MIT Sloan Management Review, 42*(2), 42.

Gargeya, V., & Sorrell, D. (2005). Moving toward an e-hospital. In N. Wickramasinghe, J. Gupta, & S. Sharma (Eds.), *Creating knowledge-based healthcare organizations*, (pp. 50-64). Hershey, PA: Idea Group Publishing.

Glaser, J. (2002). *The strategic application of information technology in health care organizations* (2nd ed.). San Francisco: Jossey Bass.

Hendersen, J., & Venktraman, N. (1992). Strategic alignment: A model for organizational transformation through information technology. In T. Kochan, & M. Unseem (Eds.), *Transforming organisations*. NY: Oxford University Press.

Hofer, C. (1975). Toward a contingency theory of business strategy. *Academy of Management, 18*(4), 784-810.

La Monica, M. (2000, October). Building trust into e-business models. *InfoWorld*, *22*(28), 3.

Lyytinen, K., & Rose, G. M. (2003). The disruptive nature of information technology innovations: The case of internet computing in systems development organizations. *MIS Quarterly*, *27*(4), 557-595.

Porter, M. (1980). *Competitive strategy*. New York: Free Press.

Porter, M. (1985). Competitive advantage. New York: Free Press.

Porter, M., & Teisberg, E. (2004). Redefining competition in healthcare. *Harvard Business Review*, 65-76, June.

Sharma, S., & Wickramasinghe, N. (2005). e-health with knowledge management: areas for tomorrow. In N. Wickramasinghe, J. Gupta, & S. Sharma (Eds.), *Creating knowledge-based healthcare organizations* (pp. 110-124). Hershey, PA: Idea Group Publishing.

Sharma, S., Wickramasingeh, N., Xu, B., & Ahmed, N. (2006). Electronic healthcare: Issues and challenges. *International Journal of Electronic Healthcare*, *2*(1), 50-65.

Van De Ven, A., Angle, H., & Poole, S. (2000). Research on the management of innovation. Oxford: Oxford University Press.

Von Lubitz, D., & Wickramasinghe, N. (2006). Healthcare and technology: The Doctrine of Networkcentric Healthcare. *International Journal of Electronic Healthcare* (IJEH, in press).

Wickramasinghe, N., & Lamb, R. (2002). Enterprise-wide systems enabling physicians to manage care. *International Journal Healthcare Technology and Management*, *4*(3/4), 288-302.

Wickramasinghe, N., & Silvers, J. (2003). IS/IT: The prescription to enable medical group practices to manage managed care. *Health Care Management Science*, *6*(2), 75-86.

Wickramasinghe, N., Fadlalla, A., Geisler, E., & Schaffer, J. (2005). A framework for assessing e-health preparedness. *International Journal of Electronic Healthcare* (IJEH), *1*(3), 316-334.

This work was previously published in International Journal of Healthcare Information Systems and Informatics, Vol. 1, Issue 4, edited by J. Tan, pp. 68-81, copyright 2006 by IGI Publishing, formerly known as Idea Group Publishing (an imprint of IGI Global).

Chapter XX

From Theory to Practice:
Healthcare Technology Management (HCTM) Conceptualization, Measures, and Practices

George Eisler, BC Academic Health Council, Canada

Joseph Tan, Wayne State University, USA

Samuel Sheps, University of British Columbia, Canada

Introduction

The challenge of conceptualizing healthcare technology management (HCTM) construct begins with an extensive literature content analysis to generate a set of definitions and attributes of the technology management (TM) concept, which was eventually extended to HCTM. To move from a theoretical framework to understanding best practices in HCTM, a critical step is the development of an instrument through a formal design process involving expert panel review, pilot testing, and instrument refinement and field-testing in order to extract and measure HCTM performance indicators. This metric that was generated for its formalization was then used to assess HCTM best practices. This chapter, which discusses the flow of HCTM theoretical framework into best practices, provides insights into the status of HCTM practices in Canadian teaching hospitals.

Business strategists, analysts and researchers as well as economists have pointed to technology innovation as a catalytic change agent in the structure of industries and competition. Indeed, technological innovation can shift the competitive balance within an industry and create opportunities for growth. A technology management (TM) problem arises when business strategy development does not fully incorporate technology-based threats and opportunities. Countries around the world are recognizing that the global competitiveness of their industries depends on their focus on TM. Technology has become a competitive tool in national and corporate survival, especially in an environment of global and more intense competition (Perrino & Tipping, 1989; Sharif, 1994).

Until today, the history of digital computing and automated information processing technology has only been with us for a brief period of about six decades. In the last decade, we witness a gradual convergence of computing, telecommunications, and web-based services. This trend has now been augmented by high-speed global access to an explosion of information on the Internet and increased global competition (Ramanathan, 1990; Ulhoi, 1996; Geisler, 2000). A key challenge here is to unravel how the management of technology innovation can impact on business and operational performance of healthcare organizations in today's competitive environment. Andersen et al. (1994), for instance, noted that the issues are similar in the public service arena in that, "Public expectations for the level and quality of government services... have grown while satisfaction with their fulfillment has steadily declined. In the past few years, it has become evident that cutting fat, eliminating waste, and preventing abuse is not nearly enough. Government needs to rethink its methods and restructure its approach to public services."

As identified by Canadian healthcare CEOs, for the health services sector, the task of managing healthcare organizations and systems is particularly complex. It demands that the healthcare executive masters many different skills, including, government relations, community liaison, human resources, finances, patient care, research, and teaching. Communication skills, culture management, creativity, shared leadership, and alliance building rank among the top (Armstrong, Brunelle, Angus & Levac, 2001). HCTM, therefore, adds another dimension to these challenges.

Background

More recently, increasing attention has been focused on the need to diffuse HCTM practices and expertise in developed countries (e.g., Japan and countries in Europe and North America) as well as developing nations (e.g., Singapore and China). The World Health Organization (WHO), for example, had alluded to serious shortcomings in the performance of health systems around the globe (WHO, 2000). Unfortunately,

WHO's attempts to introduce components of a HCTM-like system in the late 1980s into countries and regions around the world had not been very successful.

HCTM Framework

The lack of a working HCTM framework and the shortage of TM training, knowledge and expertise among workers in developed as well as developing countries were identified as serious limitations. Without an accepted HCTM model, TM component functions and activities, such as technology planning, life-cycle management, assessment, and performance assurance had no lasting infrastructural support and impact. Even outside of the healthcare sector, deficiencies in TM skills point to the crucial need to align technology strategy and business strategy in organizations across many business industry sectors (Kauonides, 1999; Neumann et al., 1999). The strengthening, linking, and aligning of technology planning and business planning in healthcare is the essential purpose of HCTM.

Accordingly, this discussion concentrated on understanding the status of HCTM practices among Canadian teaching hospitals. For this purpose, we have to address the following key questions:

- How can TM and HCTM be conceptualized?
- What are key and specific dimensions and performance indicators of the HCTM construct and how can these be determined empirically?
- How can HCTM performance indicators be measured? How can these measures be aggregated, grouped appropriately, and developed into a reliable and valid instrument for easy and convenient administration on the Web?
- Where are potential "weaknesses" and "specific performance gaps" among HCTM measures as applied to Canadian teaching hospitals?

Essentially, the complexity of the healthcare environment, the multitude of forces that shape technology decisions, and the uniqueness of the healthcare environment is part of the justification for the promotion of the academic discipline of MMT (management of medical technology) as separate and unique from MOT (management of technology) in general. Compared to other industry sectors, such as banking, housing and transportation, the healthcare environment is seen not only as more complex, but also more emotionally charged (Geisler & Heller, 1996; Tan, 2002). This environment is characterized not only by the complexities inherent in the development and maintenance of a seamless system spanning the continuum of healthcare delivery, but also by the complexity of relationships between provider organizations, service and product vendors, third-party payers and insurers, patients (consumers), the general public, regulators, researchers, and educators.

In a 2005 *Communications of the ACM* publication, Tan et al. (date) pointed to characterizing the present day healthcare and services delivery systems as "Complex Adaptive Systems." The need for understanding of the strategic TM concept in such a modern, complex system environment is clearly warranted. The healthcare industry is an industry in transition, driven by such factors as changing population demographics, technology trends, and global economic shifts. These pressures have resulted in changes to structure, process, financing, and human resource management. These challenges may be summarized as attempts to ensure timely access to quality and cost-effective healthcare services facilitated by technological innovation. Healthcare systems in Canada, the U.S., and other OECD countries are expected to continue on this road of cost reduction and quality improvement. Technology can play a vital strategic role in healthcare, as it does in other knowledge-based service industries like banking, entertainment, and other professional and technical fields. This is particularly true for information technology (IT) and communications technology, which can impact significantly to improved management, cost effectiveness, customer service and support. These applications have strategic implications, creating opportunities for new services or for delivering existing services in new ways.

MOT, MMT and HCTM

A survey of the field of MOT finds that it is based on an evolving concept about the role of technology in organizations. Technology and its management have long been seen as critical factors to an organization's success and survival, particularly in competitive environments (van Wyk, 1988; Morton, 1991; Badawy, 1996). As we noted, in public sector environments, MOT concepts are equally relevant because these help organizations to provide better services within available resources, to optimize seamless access and quality, to address special needs, societal problems, and/or for fulfilling political purposes.

In the past, many industries see IT as playing only supportive roles, thereby contributing simply to overhead costs. In short, these technologies are not central to corporate goals and objectives. Today, new perspectives are being championed: emerging technologies are seen as significant core-enabling assets with major strategic implications for business survival and success. The power of integrative and converging technologies is blurring the boundaries between administrative and core business assets. Many CEOs now believe that such enabling technologies, if managed appropriately, can contribute significantly to the achievement of organizational objectives. As well, they may change fundamentally the way an organization functions and the way it relates to its industry sector, its sponsors, suppliers, and, perhaps most importantly, its customers and clients.

A common case example is that of the Internet and related Web services. Many companies, realizing the power of the Internet have set up shops online. From a marketing perspective, such unpredictable and rapid technological development creates a volatile technology push on the input side of organizations. For example, companies such as CVS Pharmacy and Rite Aid have gone online to withstand its chain stores from losing customers to its growing list of competitors that have virtual storefronts. On the output side, customers expect reliable, consistent, safe, effective, and efficient services. The convenience of online shopping means that they can change their royalty to companies more easily and faster than queuing up at the retail store counter waiting to pay for their purchases. To these e-consumers, the technology and its applications should be seamless. The challenge then is for executives, in the face of increasingly difficult internal and external constraints, to employ management strategies to enable the organization to continuously transform the turbulent technology input into a customer-focused and appropriate output (Tapscott & Caston, 1993; Tapscott, 1996).

According to McGee & Thomas (1989), what has been missing "is a comprehensive view of how technological change can affect the rules of competition, and the ways in which technology can be the foundation of creating defensible strategies for firms." Driven by the need to compete more aggressively and efficiently in global markets, a new way of doing business has emerged, including shared responsibilities and programs restructuring, buyouts and takeover campaigns, and various forms of online collaborative and joint venture arrangements. Studies have indicated that levels of companies' investments in technology may explain international differences in productivity and in shares of world markets.

In contrast to the disciplinary tradition of MOT, very little attention has been given to the more recent work on MMT. In an attempt to develop a new intellectual space, Geisler and Heller (1998a; 1998b) were among the firsts to suggest the application of the TM construct to the healthcare field. The scope of MMT advocated by Professor Eli Geisler encompasses both clinical and administrative technologies (and functions) of the healthcare system. The premise is that owing to economic pressures, the health services delivery system is in crisis unless it can further, and more substantially, benefit from the increasing role that technology has played. It is, therefore, argued that proper and better management of medical technology is critical in overcoming the challenges faced in future healthcare. Even so, the terminology and constructs in the MMT field are still poorly understood due to varied interpretations of the individual components of these constructs and the lack of commonly accepted definitions of the constructs. Before measures for these constructs can be established, Geisler (2000) argued that clear definitions and indicators have to be determined.

THE HCTM Construct

"Health," as defined by the WHO, refers to a state of total physical, mental, and social well being, not just the absence of disease or infirmity. It is now recognized that population and individual health has many determinants not traditionally associated directly with the healthcare system. Correspondingly, the concept of "healthcare technology" includes applications of know-how's, methods, tools and techniques that influence the environment, health information dissemination, healthy lifestyle, care protection and disease prevention. It goes beyond technologies applied in modern acute care systems or for direct medical care. In this context, it applies broadly to facilities, information, devices, processes, and drugs, from the simplest to the most complex, along the entire continuum of healthcare. Technologies that may contribute to quality or sustainability of healthcare systems could be associated with direct patient care, infrastructure, or business processes. Therefore, it seems appropriate to refer to the management of these various and diverse forms of technologies as healthcare technology management (HCTM).

Notwithstanding, our content analysis of current MOT literature leads to the conclusion that there still is no commonly accepted definition of the TM construct, much less the HCTM construct. On the one hand, Anderson (1993) infers that the lack of agreement on a definition might be a barrier to the growth of the TM concept even though it is expected that a set of favored definitions will emerge over time. On the other hand, there has been some agreement that MOT is a multi-faceted discipline, linking engineering, science and management concepts and theories in a holistic, systematic, and integrative fashion, and that TM should shape and support organizational strategic goals and objectives.

Following a review of the literature across several industry sectors, we found that the multi-faceted TM concept yields a number of general but important observations (IJHISI paper reference): (1) TM forms the basis for a technology strategy; (2) TM is characteristics of a technology-ready organization; and (3) TM encompasses the responsibilities and capabilities of the chief technology officer (CTO).

1. *TM forms the basis for a technology strategy; the technology strategy is based on:*

    - The competitive environment, the organization, and technology; consideration of firm-specific factors, environmental factors, and customer preferences; creation of strategic advantage, technological expertise, the decision-making process, and organizational capabilities; comprehensive rethinking and readjustment of job descriptions, information systems, organizational structure, incentives, and decision-making processes

    - Organizational structure is one of the most important issues; policies hold together a decentralized, virtual workplace with direct access to global information; in addition to flexible organizational structures, management emphasizes information flow, incentives, and different performance assessment schemes; centralization versus decentralization is one of the single biggest organizational issues

2. *TM is characteristic of a technology-ready organization; technology-readiness strategy is characterized by:*

- Top management vision, foresight, and entrepreneurial spirit; leadership is the most critical aspect; commitment to knowledge acquisition rather than product development; alignment with strategic planning and integration of related functions; management must know what it wants, given the difficult-to-quantify costs and benefits of new technologies and attributes like flexibility; set the goals, understand the product/market interactions, being clearly aware of resources, constraints, and risks

- Decisions and attitudes are based on analysis of competitive position, market intelligence, technical preferences of customers and internal capabilities; focus on the customer replaced organization-centered approaches; emphasis is on market pull rather than technology push

- Management systems focus on an integrated enterprise; coordination across functional boundaries has priority over efficiency-driven divisions within functions; cross-functional approaches facilitate convergence of divergent views between technical- and marketing-oriented individuals; full and meaningful worker and customer participation in the production process is assured

- Process management has replaced product management; focus is on flexibility, adaptability, responsiveness, and effectiveness rather than efficiency and costs; competitive advantage comes from technology and strategy, not from savings in labor costs; able to change, to adapt, and to avail itself of new opportunities; effectiveness is considered with efficiency

3. *TM encompasses the responsibilities and capabilities of the CTO; characteristics of the CTO include:*

- Being responsible for visionary leadership, organization, funding, alignment with objectives, bridging between and among operational units, planning, resource allocation, development of standards, rapid reorganization when necessary, leading adoption and implementation of fundamental organizational change; must also be steward of inter-networked leadership, be close to the business front line, and build an invisible enabling infrastructure

- Assures that promises made on behalf of technology are kept; builds a viable, productive, and flexible technology asset base; gets back to basics and delivers the goods; takes responsibility for managing technology-driven organizational change, for learning what can be done and how to apply it, and for acting as a change champion

- Capabilities include managing in an environment of decentralized decision making with a high level of inter-functional coordination; must have commitment, technical competence; capable of skills to effect and manage change; conversant in business and organizational matters, as well as with technical information; understands the importance of systems that provide a competitive edge and the need for systems that support the goals of the organization

Methods

The study reported here was conducted in three phases. Phase I, content analysis, concentrates on identifying the constructs and related critical MOT capabilities and attributes. Phase II, the instrument development, emphasizes the selection of items, expert panel review and metric refinement and validation. Phase III, the national survey, involves the administration of the field-tested instrument via a Web survey of hospital executives.

Content Analysis

A rigorous content analysis was used to develop and contribute to a definition of TM construct and to identify related critical MOT capabilities and attributes. Lewis (1993) refers to the methodology of "content analysis" as a "common technique employed in the social sciences to draw inference from text; it is executed by objectively and systematically extracting attributes from written communication and by analyzing those extracted parts." Essentially, a broad and comprehensive review of both published and unpublished sources forms the basis of this methodology.[1]

The database of 255 articles and dissertations was searched for the sampling unit "defin*" (for definition) in its abstract or full text, to locate discussions of the definition of "technology management." 30 such articles were found, which were in turn scanned to eliminate those that did not in fact discuss or contain a definition, leaving seven articles. Although only one dissertation contained the root word 'defin*' in its abstract, eight more dissertations with discussions about the definition were located by detailed reading of 47 dissertation abstracts.

A summative definition of the conceptual TM construct emerged from this exercise:

Figure 1. Technology management framework

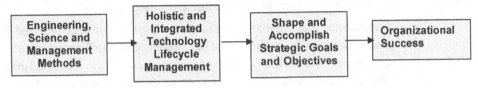

Technology management can be defined as a holistic and integrated application of engineering, science, and management capabilities to strategic lifecycle management of new and relevant product and process technologies in order to shape as well as accomplish the goals and objectives necessary for organizational success.

From this definition, a schematic diagram for the TM Framework emerges, as shown in Figure 1. Organizational success in healthcare could, for example, be expressed as improved patient care within given resources or as protection of the principles of the *Canada Health Act.*

Instrumentation

TM is a complex, multifaceted process with interlinked activities, clearly containing more than one indicator. Following an abstraction ladder approach to metric development, the goal was to create a hierarchy of major dimensions, of variables that described the dimensions, and of indicators that gave shape to the variables. The measurement instrument itself was constructed from an exhaustive list of individual attributes, which were the result of the literature content analysis.

A long list of indicators was initially formed. These were grouped and regrouped iteratively until an intuitively sensible and comprehensible list of 26 indicators emerged. The list of indicators was far more detailed than similar reported attempts in the literature, although, it became apparent, that the indicators could be grouped into variables comparable in name to ones referred to in the literature.

The Pilot Test

Using the Delphi approach, senior healthcare administrators and management consultants were asked to rank and validate the attributes of the HCTM construct from the perspective of Canadian teaching hospitals, with a focus on the responsibilities at the corporate or executive level. This pilot process constituted an expert panel review and a more specific content validity assessment.

In order to qualify as expert, an individual had to have been involved in healthcare management at senior levels for more than 10 years. Their collective professional backgrounds were to cover technical, administrative, and patient care arenas. They were provided with a draft survey and were asked to critique it from the perspectives of clarity and understandability. These experts were also asked to recommend unambiguous descriptors for the state of implementation of each statement category in the survey. The positions held by these experts at some point in their career were: deputy and assistant deputy minister, CEOs, VPs, and CIOs of hospitals, directors and executive directors of Canadian health industry organizations.

The experts were informed about the national character and the expected target audience of the study. They were presented with the prototype questionnaire including 42 indicators, and were asked to:

- Complete the survey keeping any familiar large healthcare organization in mind
- Identify if and how specific statements should be altered
- Add statements that they thought were important but not included
- Express concerns they may have about the appropriateness of the three main domains and the categories within each domain of the survey
- Identify examples of additional real and practical evidence or indicators that could be used to support statements about the extent of implementation in the various categories (strategic plans, job descriptions, budgets, etc.)

At this stage, the objective was to test the comprehensiveness and comprehensibility of the metric.

The Field Test

For further refinement of the HCTM metric, a field test was undertaken, incorporating feedback from the pilot study. It was targeted at institutions that would not be included in the survey of teaching hospitals. Senior managers of four regional referral organizations, who represented a variety of administrative responsibilities, participated.

The CEOs of four medium-size BC health service organizations provided the e-mail addresses of their executive teams and the individuals reporting to the executive team members (VPs, CEOs). A total of 64 senior managers, representing eight different areas of responsibility, received a cover letter serving as the consent form designed and based on recommendation of the respective Human Investigative committees (HICs) as well as the survey instrument. With 33 responses from 64 individuals on the e-mail list, the overall response rate was 52% and varied between 43% and 64% for the four participating institutions. As in the pilot test, respondents were asked to comment on content, wording, and structure of the instrument. No changes to the instrument were suggested. The importance of the HCTM topic itself was confirmed by a consistently high average rating from each organization. On the 6-point Likert scale, average ratings for each organization ranged from 5.6 to 5.9, where 5 means 'great importance' and 6 means 'very great' importance.

In addition to the Likert ratings for each indicator, a single measure was established to capture each respondent's perception of the "gap" between the ideal extent of implementation (reflected in a rating of 6 on the Likert scale) and perceived extent of implementation (1-6 rating) for each of the 26 indicators. Gap scores were weighted using the respondent's assessment of the importance of the respective indicator.

The result is a new variable (gap score) calculated by the formula

$$GS = (6-E) \times B, \text{ where}$$

GS = gap between ideal and perceived implementation

6 = ideal implementation rating

E = rating for perceived extent of implementation

B = rating for the perceived benefit/importance of implementation

A gap score (GS) was therefore calculated for each respondent. The term $(6 - E)$ can be interpreted as an indication for 'room for improvement,' as an E score of '6' would indicate full implementation. The factor B becomes a weighting factor relative to the perceived importance of the item. For example, perceived full implementation of an indicator would yield a gap score of zero:

$$GS = (6 - 6) \times B = 0 \qquad GS = (6 - 1) \times 6 = 30$$

A rating of '1' (meaning: not at all) for implementation would yield the highest gap score if the indicator was also rated as '6' for importance (meaning: very great).

The possible range for gap scores is, therefore: 0 to 30. An average gap score (average of responses from a particular organization) of less than 8 for an indicator can be interpreted to mean that this indicator has been implemented to a high level and would not require additional attention for improvement. This could be either because the indicator has been well implemented (rating of 5 or 6) or because the importance was rated lower than other indicators (4 or less). Field test results

Table 1. Distribution of Indicators by Gap Score Range

Average Gap Score Range (high, low)	Indicators			
	Organization 1	Organization 2	Organization 3	Organization 4
6-10 (low)	none	none	1,3,10,11,12,13,14, 20,21,22,24	2,3,4,6,10,14,16,25
15-19 (high)	4,8,15,19,20,21,26	3,4,11,13,17,18,2 1,23,25,26	none	9,13,18,19,23,26

indicated that the resulting metric and the gap score measure seemed to capture differences in perception between senior managers from different organizations with some consistency.

As summarized in Table 1, responses from organizations 1 and 2 did not result in an average gap score of less than 10 for any of the 26 indicators in the metric. Results of the pilot test on the individual indicators (numbered 1 to 26) for computing average gap scores are shown below. For example, organizations 1, 2, and 4 had average gap scores of 15-19 on 8, 10, and 6 indicators respectively, while none were recorded at the higher gap score for organization 3.

One could also interpret Table 1 as indicating that compared to organization 3, organizations 1 and 2 are not performing well in the eyes of their senior managers. Also, senior managers in organization 4 have a less consistent view of their organization's performance. Organization 3 seems to have reached a high level of HCTM performance. Coincidentally, organization 3 is nationally recognized for its quality management system.

National Survey Administration

The resulting survey design was influenced by the choice of a Web-based delivery system. The survey was presented in a logical sequence according to the overall model laid out for participants in the cover letter. Given that the target audiences for the survey were highly experienced and knowledgeable individuals, it was deemed unnecessary and probably not helpful in this study to scramble the sequence of the statements.

The Executive committee of the Association of Canadian Academic Health Organizations (ACAHO) had enthusiastically endorsed this research and acknowledged its importance. Executive members, the CEOs of some of Canada's largest teaching hopitals, shared the view that HCTM approaches in the Canadian healthcare system could and needed to be strengthened. Their support and active promotion of this project presented an invaluable opportunity to attract participation from senior managers in Canada's teaching hopitals. Following the decision of the ACAHO's Executive committee, which included the CEOs of six of Canada's largest health-care organizations and ACAHO's executive director, to sponsor this survey, letters were sent to the CEOs of member organizations asking for their organization's participation.

The list of ACAHO member organizations was compared with the list of organizations ranked by number of 'technology intensive beds' from the Canadian Health Assotiation guide. This list indicated that ACAHO member organizations provided a national target audience of the majority of highly technology-intensive organizations. It was felt that the senior managers of these organizations were best positioned to assess HCTM practices in Canada.

Web-Survey Administration

E-survey was chosen in this study because:

- Senior hospital administrators are expected to have access to Web-based technology
- The spirit of the HCTM topic warrants an application that would better serve the customers; speed of data collection, convenience for the recipients, ease of data handling and online data analysis are among the key influencing factors on making this choice

Interestingly, the most time consuming aspect of the process was determining and iteratively correcting hundreds of e-mail addresses. The process of developing and posting the survey on to the Web involved a number of additional steps. The e-survey content was developed as a Microsoft Word document, including all associated notes and rating scales. The Web pages with forms to accept data input were designed with Dreamweaver 4.0 Web design software.

The decision to design the Web-survey tool rather than to use purchased software was based on the ability to design a more professional look and the need to create data files of submitted responses that could easily be exported directly into the Microsoft Excel program for convenient storage and rapid analysis. The e-survey was tested internally and externally before it was posted live on the British Columbia Institute of Technology (BCIT) server via the BCIT School of Health Sciences Web site. It was sent electronically with the cover letter allowing convenient links to the e-survey URL to hundreds of senior managers for whom e-mail addresses had been secured and verified.

Finally, a "thank-you" page was generated and sent automatically upon receipt of a survey response to the Web server. The participating organization and individuals were assured of the privacy of their identities and that any published reports would not identify and link organizations, individuals, or responses.

Findings

Owing to space limitation, issues of instrument validity, consistency, and reliability are only highlighted here prior to discussing the study results.[2] First, content validity was optimized through the iterative process in which the instrument was developed. Content analysis informed the metric development and expert opinions in pilot and field test stages refined the instrument.

Furthermore, validity and reliability of the metric was strengthened through:

- Supporting the instrument development process with a comprehensive literature review and content analysis (face/content validity)
- Refining the metric based on initial faculty suggestions and on comments and suggestions received from experts in the two-stage pilot and field testing (content validity)
- Clustering items on the instrument following expert panel review on its content as well as on comprehensibility, understandability, clarity, and structure of the instrument (construct validity)
- Factor analyzing responses during repeated testing of the instrument for key dimensions (construct validity)
- Triangulating the results via a comparison of findings with a performance review of the same institutions using a completely different metric, which was conducted completely independently (concurrent validity)

Lastly, the Cronbach's alpha coefficient was also computed to determine internal consistency of the metric. It was applied to each of the dimensions resulting from the factor analysis. The reliability of the instrument was assessed for each of the indicators according to the factors established by the factor analysis. Reliability was high for all indicators with alpha ranging from .79 to .94.

Survey Responses

Thirty-three ACAHO member organizations were invited to participate in this project. The offices of the CEOs invested considerable energy in putting these lists together. In the end, approximately 850 individuals in 28 organizations received the survey; of these, 324 individuals responded, representing an average response rate of approximately 38% per participating institution with a range of 24% to 58%.

As indicated in Figure 2, 317 out of 324 (98%) rated the topic's importance as great or very great. No respondent rated the importance as less than 4 (some) on the 1-6 rating scale.

As noted, owing to privacy and confidentiality concerns, participating organizations were coded from 1 to 33. This is how the individual organization will be identified for the remainder of the discussion. For example, organization 1 submitted 36 responses, reflecting a 33% response rate relative to the number of senior managers who received the survey. Of these respondents, 6 executive members had patient care responsibilities (VP Nursing, VP Medicine, etc.) and 7 did not (VP Finance, VP Support Services, etc.). Of the responding managers reporting to VPs, 8 had patient care responsibilities and 15 did not. The respondents were first asked to rate the importance of the topic of the survey (1- 'not at all,' 2- 'very little,' 3- 'little,' 4- 'some,' 5-'great,' and 6- 'very great').

One of the key questions to be answered by this research was the ability of the metric to differentiate between organizations relative to their HCTM approach. As no significant differences in gap scores between the categories of respondents were

Figure 2. Topic importance rating

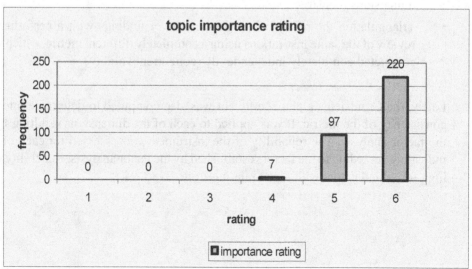

found, it indicated that all responses from the same organization could be grouped for the purpose of testing for significant differences between organizations. The 20 organizations that supplied five or more responses were included in this part of the analysis. Based on ANOVA and the resulting p-values, significant differences ($p < 0.01$) were found in the way in which senior managers across the 20 organizations perceived the state of HCTM in their organization. This suggests the need to further investigate the possibility that senior managers with direct patient care responsibilities responded differently from those that did not have direct patient care responsibilities. The same applies to the question of whether executive team members (VPs, CEOs) would respond differently from those senior managers reporting to VPs.

Factor analysis was applied to identify variables that reflect some common underlying factor or dimension. Table 2 shows three underlying factors (or 'latent variables') on which the 26 indicators 'loaded': (a) strategic management; (b) management of change and innovation; and (c) organizational management

Table 2. Model of indicators

A) Strategic Management	B) Management of change and Innovation	C) Organizational Management
Technology Strategy 1. Tech and business strategies aligned 8. Technology linked to customer needs **Chief Technology Officer** 3. Executive member formulates technology strategy 4. Executive member administers/manages technology strategy **Knowledge Management** 5. Vision re technology through routine scanning 6. Environmental factors re technology strategy identified	**Customer Focus** 9. Line managers responsible for customer service 13. Performance management based on customer satisfaction **Change Management** 10. Senior management participates in change management 11. Corporate learning culture prevails 12. Senior management promotes organizational vision/direction 19. Organization has strategy to respond to change **Integration of Innovation Chain** 14. Communication system promotes technology 15. Innovation system integrates R&D/operations 20. Organizational design uses multi-functional teams **Human Resource Management** 17. HR development/planning key to technology capability 18. Accomplishments formally recognized 21. Skilled employees seek innovative opportunities	**Effectiveness and Flexibility** 2. Key technology supported by infrastructure 16. Technology diffusion/transfer encouraged **Operations Management** 22. Organization uses sound project/process management 23. Technology lifecycle systematically managed **Assessment and Evaluation** 24. Technology related risks evaluated 25. Technology assessment informs technology decisions 26. Performance due to technology management evaluated

Cluster analysis was used to group 'like' hospital organizations based on their responses ('like' based on indicator gap scores) to optimize the comparison and identification of differing HCTM practices and capabilities. A practical three-cluster solution resulted out of the 20 organizations with more than five responses:

- **Cluster 1:** Organizations 1, 2, 3, 5, 6, 7, 9, 11, 13, 14, 17, 18, 19
- **Cluster 2:** Organizations 4, 8, 10, 12, 16
- **Cluster 3:** Organizations 15, 20

Testing for significant differences in-between clusters indicated that there was a statistically significant difference ($p < 0.01$) between the cluster mean gap scores for each of the three dimension variables. Since cluster 3 consisted of only two institutions with comparatively fewer responses, further comparative analysis was focused on the differences between clusters 1 and 2. The significant differences between the two clusters of organizations, based on senior managers' perception, are influenced by some variables more than others.

Table 3 lists the 26 variables in the survey in the order of the percent difference between cluster 1 and 2 mean gap scores. As illustrated, it shows that the average gap scores for each and every indicator were lower for cluster 2 organizations. Percent differences range from 6.54% to 56.62%. The two indicators 3 and 4 with the highest percent difference were also the ones with the highest variability on a national basis.

The data revealed what constituted the major difference among managerial responses between the two clusters of organizations. On the one hand, cluster 2 managers rated their organization very highly (low gap score) in the following three areas:

- **Indicator 3:** Executive member formulates technology strategy
- **Indicator 4:** Executive member administers/manages technology strategy
- **Indicator 12:** Senior management promotes organizational vision/direction

On the other hand, cluster 1 managers rated their organization particularly low (high gap scores) in the areas:

- **Indicator 8:** Technology linked to customer needs
- **Indicator 19:** Organization has strategies to respond to change
- **Indicator 26:** Performance due to technology management evaluated

Table 4 portrays the distribution of indicators in the 4 quartiles of the gap score range. Apparently, cluster 1 managers rated none of the indicators in the lowest quartile of gap scores compared to 4 indicators for cluster 2 managers. In contrast, 7 indicators were rated in the highest quartile for cluster 1 as opposed to none by cluster 2 managers. It is interesting to note that indicators 8, 19, and 26 were also the ones that were deemed to need the most attention based on the overall national average. They also top the list of indicators needing attention in cluster 1 organizations. The largest differences in reported perception based on implementation ratings and gap scores between cluster 1 and cluster 2 managers related to indicators 3 and 4 of our HCTM model.

It can be concluded that the resulting metric is able to distinguish between differences in perception by senior managers about their organization's HCTM standard. Significant differences between clusters of organizations can be identified consistently

Table 3. Gap score differences between clusters 1 and 2

Indicator	Difference	% Difference	Cluster 1	Cluster 2
7	0.61	6.54	9.33	8.73
22	0.80	7.50	10.73	9.93
10	1.24	13.15	9.43	8.19
9	1.53	13.53	11.31	9.77
25	1.89	14.26	13.25	11.36
17	2.00	15.85	12.62	10.62
8	2.34	16.03	14.60	12.26
2	2.15	16.17	13.30	11.15
14	2.83	17.58	11.55	8.72
21	2.33	17.72	13.15	10.81
20	2.36	18.50	12.76	10.39
23	2.58	18.57	13.89	11.31
15	2.59	18.82	13.76	11.16
24	2.20	19.00	11.58	9.38
6	2.49	20.66	12.05	9.56
19	3.27	21.48	15.22	11.95
11	2.54	21.77	11.67	9.13
18	3.34	24.38	13.70	10.36
16	2.94	25.28	11.63	8.69
1	3.93	28.98	13.56	9.63
13	4.02	28.98	13.87	9.85
12	2.69	29.89	9.00	6.31
5	3.98	31.37	12.59	8.61
26	4.86	31.52	15.42	10.55
4	5.71	48.15	11.87	6.15
3	7.29	56.42	12.92	5.62

Table 4. Indicator distribution

Gap score quartiles	Cluster 1 indicators	Cluster 2 indicators
6.0 - 8.4		**3,4,12**,10,
8.5 - 11.0	12,10,22	16,14,11,24,6,1,9,13,22,18,20,26, 17,21
11.1 - 13.5	9,14,24,16,11,4,6,5,20,3,21,25,2,1	2,15,23,25,19,8
13.6 - 16.0	18,15,13,23,**8**,**19**,**26**	

across all three dimensions of the HCTM construct. In particular, the perceived presence of 'chief technology officer' roles in the organization seems to contribute strongly to the differences in mean gap scores between clusters. Other 'strategic management' and 'change management' variables seem to be perceived as being implemented to a greater extent in cluster 2 institutions. Improvements seem to be possible along all three dimensions.

The Hay Group Study

As indicated, the purpose of studying HCTM status is to assess its impact on health organizational performance in terms of alignment of IT goals with the strategic business goals and objectives of the organization. For a private sector organization, this may be expressed as competitive advantage, market share, profit, return on investment or other such measures. What would be the metric that would indicate organizational 'success or survival' of our study hospitals? What difference would it make that one cluster of hospitals seems to manage technology better than another cluster?

Fortunately, ACAHO provided independently generated information about operational efficiency and clinical efficiency of the same study hospitals (and others not included in the study) on a confidential basis. The Hay Group in Toronto compiled the data in an annual report entitled *Benchmarking Comparison of Canadian Hospitals*. The Hay study was commissioned by the hospitals in an effort 'to improve the efficiency, effectiveness and quality of their care processes.' The comparisons were based on CIHI hospital separation data, on accounts and statistics reported to ministries of health, and other data provided by the hospitals.

In order to determine if there was any association between the HCTM performance of the two clusters of hospitals identified in this study and other measures of performance, the Hay study outcomes for the same two clusters were analyzed. The following two summary measures, as defined in the report, were used:

Figure 3. Hay study comparison

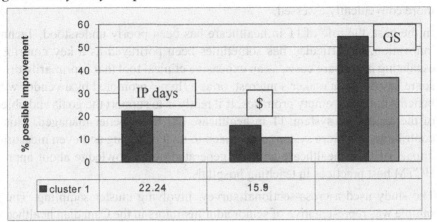

- The measure for the overall clinical efficiency of a hospital is the percentage of inpatient days that can be reduced if a hospital were to achieve benchmark levels of performance; the smaller the percentage, the more efficient the hospital.

- The measure for the overall operational efficiency of a hospital is the potential reduction in operating cost to the 25th percentile performance, including direct care, administrative, and support functions. Subject to some caveats, the hospital with the smaller potential reduction can be considered more efficient with respect to the areas examined in these comparisons.

If an average gap score of 6 (over all responses and all indicators for each organization) was considered as the benchmark target, the potential HCTM improvement could be calculated and expressed in terms of potential percent reduction. This measure is used in the comparison. As demonstrated in Figure 3, the Hay Study Comparison results provide independent validation of our findings with respect to organizational performance of the two clusters of hospitals studied and at the same time provide support of the concurrent validity of our HCTM metric.

Conclusion

Altogether, there has been recurring and increasing interests between both the academic and practitioner communities about the potential impact of HCTM on healthcare organizational performance. Like the management of other key strategic resources, such as health human resource and financial resource management,

HCTM should and could become a more easily understood concept and its impact more conveniently assessed.

In the past, the role of IT in healthcare has been poorly understood. Technology innovation, in particular, has sometimes been portrayed as a key contributor to escalating healthcare costs, as an expensive clinical tool that is primarily driven by some key decision maker's interest, or as a 'hype' promoted by a vendor with few benefits but many empty promises. If it really is to support the goals and objectives of the healthcare system, IT in healthcare has to be better managed. This study contributes to a more systemic approach to understanding and even measuring the impact of IT in healthcare and has generated new knowledge about appropriate HCTM best practices in teaching hospitals.

The study used a cross-sectional survey, involving cluster sampling. The target sample was representative of senior administrators in the Canadian healthcare system. We studied executive team members of the 40 largest Canadian teaching hospitals. Selected individuals from this group responded to a newly developed HCTM metric. Factor analysis and cluster analyses were the two key statistical inference methods applied to the resulting data set. Major clusters of respondents were those associated with individual organizations. These responses were analyzed to identify systemic differences in HCTM practices among different clustering organizations. For in-depth analysis of the data, the Analysis of Variance (ANOVA) technique was applied. It assumed that respondents from within each organization could be treated as one cluster. Unfortunately, field test analysis was inconclusive on this question due to limited sample size. Yet, the outcome of this study provided new thinking on HCTM, recognizes and bridges a multi-disciplinary science base with the broad modern concepts of healthcare, technology, and management.

A new definition for the construct 'technology' was not developed. Rather, the perspective of technology as *extension of human and organizational ability* was adopted from the literature. Based on an extensive literature content analysis, the study does propose a new definition and a theoretical model for the HCTM construct. The major critical dimensions of the HCTM metric include: (a) strategic management factors, (b) management of change and innovation factors, and (c) organizational management factors. Interestingly, two indicators (indicators 3 and 4 of our metric) that focused on the function of a chief technology officer (CTO) were found to be the largest differences in reported perception based on implementation ratings and gap scores between high performing and low performing teaching hospitals. Indicator 3 states: "A designated member of the executive team is responsible for the formulation of the organization's technology strategy" while indicator 4 states: "A designated member of the executive team is responsible for the administration and management of the organization's technology strategy." This result strongly confirmed the message from the literature about the necessity of executive attention and leadership for HCTM. Along with providing leadership, coordination, and facilitation, the responsibilities of the CTO include such activities as gate-keeping, advocacy, funding, sponsorship, policy and procedure development, promotion, capacity building, and overseeing the technology management system. Not all hospitals have a CTO, in which case the responsibilities discussed here are either taken up by the CEO or, more likely, delegated to someone else such as the chief financial officer or chief operations officer. This person job is to understand the strategic business issues, the customers, and the technology. S/he should be an effective leader and command the respect of his or her employees, managers, and peers. Our finding implies that a good CTO is key to differentiating among clustering organizations as to their HCTM status.

Another set of indicators that were shown to be critical for poor-performing hospitals and presented the highest need for improvement on a national, system-wide basis is the set of Indicators 8, 19, and 26. Indicator 8 states: "Technology is linked to clearly-identified customer needs and priorities." Indicator 19 states: "The organization has strategies to respond flexibly and rapidly to technological change." Finally, indicator 26 states: "The organization's performance as a function of TM activities is routinely evaluated and benchmarked." A high gap score on indicator 8 implies a lack of ongoing access to information about current and future needs and priorities of customers and staff. Indicator 19, similarly, addresses how quickly the organization responds to shifts in technological trends. A high gap score here implies that the organization ignores "market pull" strategies as part of its customer relations policy, essentially going along with "technology push." Product development times, innovation cycles, and overall cycle times for putting ideas and innovations into practice are longer than expected relative to industry norms. Lastly, a high gap score for indicator 26 implies a lack of systematic performance reviews for different aspects of HCTM. These might include their impact on overall organizational goals, objectives, and customer service, including, for example, annual performance evaluations of the executive fulfilling the CTO role. Apparently, our results tell us that poor performing hospitals must pay particular attention to these factors.

In summary, our findings indicate that there are key differences in HCTM sophistication among Canadian teaching hospitals. Major differences occur in areas of strategic technology management, followed by change management, and to a lesser extent, organizational management. The perceptions of senior managers are not significantly influenced by their area of responsibility relative to patient and non-patient care, or by their position in the reporting structure. Improvements are needed generally in all areas addressed by the HCTM metric. A further question relates to the impact of HCTM sophistication on organizational performance and success. This study was able to explore to some extent the relationship between clinical and operational efficiency and HCTM performance. It did not address the more strategic impact of HCTM performance on customer satisfaction and customer service levels relative to customer needs.

Future Research

This work was built on earlier research in the areas of MOT and MMT. An outcome of this study is the enhancement and the expansion of the current research agenda for the MOT and MMT disciplines. Research in this area should be focused on development of more specific measurement items, refinement of the measures and applications of these measuring tools. For example, an expanded application of our HCTM metric is go beyond teaching hospital settings.

Another stream of research could further explore the metric relative to particular health systems issues at national, provincial, and institutional levels of management. While knowledge could undoubtedly be expanded in each of these facets, some examples of priority research questions for HCTM metric refinement include:

•   Who are the customers in healthcare, what are their needs, and what order of priority is attached to those needs?

•   While senior managers in teaching hospitals provided their perspectives on HCTM, how can IT contribute to clinical and operational efficiencies, quality and levels of care, and customer satisfaction?

•   The study results are based on perceptions of senior managers. How can follow-up case studies be designed to compare perceptions with reality?

•   Case studies would also be useful with respect to the real, rather than perceived differences between some cluster 1 and cluster 2 hospitals. To what extent are CTO functions explicitly established, given the large difference in perception between the clusters on this point?

Last but not least, the metric could be used to probe into the strengths and weaknesses of an individual institution. A case study with full management and staff participation would allow further statistical validation of the instrument. The motivation for undertaking this study was that in Canada's healthcare organizations, technology was not managed well enough, neither tactically or strategically. The CEOs of some of Canada's largest teaching hospitals expressed support for this notion when they agreed to promote and support this study among their peers. Of the 324 surveyed senior managers, a vast majority of 317 confirmed the importance of HCTM for Canadian healthcare managers by rating it as 'great' to very great (between 5 and 6 on a 6- point scale), the remaining managers rated it as being of 'some' importance (rating 4).

Finally, other key research questions emerging from this study are issues related to the definition and identification of customers, customer groups, and customer needs in healthcare. Organizations like teaching hospitals are faced with competing customer interests (provincial services, community services, research and education services). Resource planning of any kind, human, technology, or financial, is difficult under circumstances where the primary customers and their needs are not well defined. Lately, with the emergence of e-health, a whole new scenario of customer-consumer relationships is unfolding with significant implications for providers and agencies of healthcare services.

References

Anderson, P. (1993). Toward exemplary research in the management of technology—an introductory essay. *Journal of Engineering and Technology Management, 10*(1-2).

Andersen, D., Belardo, S., & Dawes, S. (1994). Strategic information management: Conceptual frameworks for the public sector. *Public Productivity & Management Review, XVII*(4), 335-353.

Armstrong, R., Brunelle, F., Angus, D., & Levac, G. (2001). The changing role of Canadian healthcare CEOs: Results of a national study. *Healthcare Management Forum Supplement.*

Badawy, M. (1996). A new paradigm for understanding management technology: A research agenda for 'technocologists'. *International Journal of Technology Management, 12*(5-6), 717-732.

Geisler. (2000).

Geisler, E. (2000). *The metrics of science and technology.* Westport, CT: Quorum Books.

Geisler, E., & Heller, O. (1996). *Managing technology in healthcare.* Boston, MA: Kluwer Academic Publishers.

Geisler, E., & Heller, O. (1998a). Management of medical technology (MMT): Research, education, and practice. *International Journal of Technology Management, 15*(3-5), 196-210.

Geisler, E., & Heller, O. (1998b). *Management of medical technology: theory, practice, and cases.* Boston, MA: Kluwer Academic Publishers.

Kaounides, L. (1999). Science, technology, and global competitive advantage. *International Studies of Management & Organization.*

Lewis, B. (1993). *The information resource management concept: Domain, measurement, and implementation status (technology planning).* Unpublished doctoral dissertation, Auburn University, UMI Dissertaton Services.

McGee, J., & Thomas, H. (1989). Technology and strategic management progress and future dire. *R & D Management, 19*(3).

Morton, M. (1991). *The corporation of the 1990s: Information technology and organizational transformation.* New York, NY: Oxford University Press.

Neumann, L., & et al. (1999). Achieving success: Assessing the role of and building a business case for technology in healthcare. *Frontiers of Health Services Management.*

Our IJHISI paper

Perrino, A., & Tipping, J. (1989). Global management of technology. *Research Technology Management, 32*(3), 12.

Ramanathan, K. (1990). Management of technology: Issues of management skill and effectiveness. *International Journal of Technology Management, 5*(4).

Sharif, N. (1994a). Integrating business and technology strategies in developing countries. *Technological Forecasting and Social Change, 45*(2), 151-167.

Tan, J. (2002). HCTM: Presentation.

Tan, J., Wen, J., & Awad, N. "Healthcare and Services Delivery Systems as Complex

Tapscott, D. (1996). *The digital economy: Promise and peril in the age of networked intelligence.* New York, NY: McGraw-Hill.

Tapscott, D., & Caston, A. (1993). *Paradigm shift: The new promise of information technology.* New York, NY: McGraw-Hill.

Ulhoi, J. (1996). Towards a theoretical and methodological corporate technology management framework. The strategic perspective. *International Journal of Technology Management, 12*(2), 199-209.

van Wyk, R. (1988). Management of technology: New frameworks. *Technovation, 7*, 341-351.

World Health Organization. (2000). *The world health report 2000: Health Systems: Improving performance.* Geneva, Switzerland: World Health Organization.

Endnotes

[1]   Readers interested in the details of this methodology should also consult Lewis [27].

[2]   Interested readers may refer to the original IJHISI article: Eisler et al. [date from paper].

About the Contributors

Joseph Tan, Dip, BA, MS, PhD, holds a professional diploma in civil engineering from Singapore Polytechnic, an undergraduate degree in mathematics and computer science from Wartburg College, IA, a master's degree in industrial & management engineering from the University of Iowa, and a PhD in management information systems from the University of British Columbia (UBC). He has been a tenured associate professor, teaching in the Department of HealthCare & Epidemiology at UBC for many years prior to serving as Professor and Head of Information System and Manufacturing (ISM) department, School of Business, Wayne State University. Joseph publishes widely in numerous computing, ergonomics, information systems, health informatics, health education, e-health and e-business journals and has served as guest editor and member of various journal editorial boards. He sits on key organizing committees for local, national, and international meetings and conferences. Professor Tan's research, which has enjoyed significant support in the last several years from local, national and international funding agencies and other sources, has also been widely cited and applied across a number of major disciplines, including healthcare informatics and clinical decision support, health technology management research, human processing of graphical representations, ergonomics, health administration education, telehealth, mobile health, and e-health promotion programming.

* * *

James Anderson, earned a BES in chemical engineering, MSE in operations research and industrial engineering, MAT in chemistry and mathematics, and a PhD in education and sociology from Johns Hopkins University. He is the former director of the Division of Engineering of the evening college at Johns Hopkins University. At Purdue, he has served as assistant dean for analytical studies of the School of Humanities, Social Sciences and Education (1975-1978), director of the Social Research Institute (1995-1998), and co-director of the Rural Center for AIDS/STD Prevention (1994-2006). He is the author/co-author of five books including *Evaluating the Organizational Impact of Health Care Information Systems* (Springer, 2005); *Ethics and Information Technology: A Case-Based Approach to a Health Care System in Transition (*Springer, 2002); and *Evaluating Health Care Information Systems: Methods and Applications* (Sage, 1994).

Ioannis Apostolakis was born in Chania of Crete and studied mathematicsat the University of Athens. He holds a MSc in informatics, operational research and in administration in educational units, and a PhD in health informatics.For several years he has been scientific researcher in the Department of the Clinical Therapeutics at the University of Athens. He had been teaching at the University of Athens and at the Polytechnic University of Crete. Today he teaches in the post-graduate program of the National School of Public Health and at Panteion University.

Andrew Balas serves as the dean of the College of Health Sciences and professor of community health at Old Dominion University in Norfolk, Virginia. His areas of expertise include development of policy priorities for the production of new scientific knowledge responsive to public health needs, and application of advanced information technologies to improve health outcomes. He is a member of the Healthcare Information Technology Advisory Panel of JCAHO and the board of directors of the American Medical Informatics Association. He is an elected member of the European Academy of Sciences and Arts and the American College of Medical Informatics. As a congressional fellow, Andrew Balas worked on healthcare legislation for the Public Health and Safety subcommittee and his contribution has been acknowledged in the records of the United States Senate. The credentials of Andrew Balas include over 100 publications, including reviews and editorials in the *Journal of the American Medical Association (JAMA)*, *British Medical Journal*, *Archives of Internal Medicine* and other periodicals. During the last ten years, he has been responsible for over 10 million dollars of externally-funded research as principal investigator/project director. Prior to his current position, he served as dean of the School of Public Health at St. Louis University, director of the Missouri European Union Center and well distinguished professor of health policy at the University of Missouri-Columbia. He obtained degrees in medicine (MD), medical informatics (PhD), and applied mathematics.

John C. Beachboard joined the computer information systems faculty at Idaho State University in 2001. He completed his PhD in information transfer and his MS in information resources management at the school of information studies, Syracuse University. He holds an MS in business administration from Boston University and a BS in public administration from the University of Arizona. Dr. Beachboard has taught graduate courses in research methods, project management, and IT use in business, and undergraduate courses in IT management and systems architectures. He has held staff and management positions developing, implementing and operating information and telecommunications systems for the Department of Defense. He is keenly interested in the development, application and effectiveness of information technology management policies in the private and public sectors.

Anol Bhattacherjee is a professor of information systems in the College of Business at the University of South Florida. His research interests are diffusion and use of information technology innovations, applications of information technology in healthcare, and knowledge transfer in social networks. His research has been published in *MIS Quarterly, Information Systems Research, Journal of MIS, Decision Sciences*, and various other journals. Dr. Bhattacherjee holds PhD and MBA degrees from University of Houston, and MS and BS degrees from Indian Institute of Technology (India). He also serves on the current editorial board of *MIS Quarterly*.

Melanie L. Braswell is a clinical assistant professor in the Purdue University School of Nursing. Her areas of interest include information technology, surgical site infection reduction, and undergraduate education. She has a doctorate of Nursing Practice degree from Purdue University. Her doctoral project involved the implementation of the guidelines related to surgical site infection reduction from the Institute for Healthcare Improvement. She also maintains a collaborative agreement with a Midwestern hospital system where she is a clinical nurse specialist with a peri-operative focus to improve patient outcomes in the surgical setting. She currently teaches peri-operative nursing, senior leadership and capstone courses.

Karen Chang is an assistant professor and the director of information technology (IT) at Purdue University School of Nursing. She is also a medical informatics fellow at the center of excellence for implementing evidence-based practice, Roudebush Veterans Administration Medical Center, Indianapolis, Indiana. Her main interest is to use IT to improve the quality of patient care and nursing education. Her research studies and publications are related to the development and evaluation of using mobile computing devices (Pocket PC, Tablet PC, and wireless Pocket PC) for patient care and nursing education and the evaluation of using tele-health technologies to manage patients with diabetes at home and using insulin decision support system to manage patients in the hospital with hyperglycemia.

Neset Hikmet is the director of the Center for Research in Healthcare Systems and Policies and an associate professor of information systems in the College of Business at the University of South Florida. His research interests include the use of information technology and the economics of information technology investments in healthcare organizations. His research has been published in *Information Systems Management, Journal of Computer Information Systems, Communications of the ACM, International Journal of Medical Informatics*, and various other journals. Neset holds PhD and MBA degrees from the University of Rhode Island and a BS degree from Middle East Technical University, Ankara, Turkey.

Kyle Lutes is an associate professor of computer and information technology at Purdue University. He has authored/co-authored numerous papers, many of which were presented at national conferences or published in trade magazines/journals as well as two college textbooks. His teaching and scholarly interests cover all areas of software development, including programming languages, mobile computing, software engineering, client/server information systems, Web application development, user interface design, and rapid application development. Kyle has been writing software professionally since 1982. Prior to his current appointment at Purdue, he held various software development positions in industry and has worked on projects for such industries as banking, telecommunications, publishing, hospitals, medical schools, retail, and pharmaceuticals.

Arlyn Melcher is a professor of management at Southern Illinois University. He has an MBA from UCLA and a PhD from the Graduate School of Business at University of Chicago. He has written widely on organization and strategic management issues. Currently, his central research focus is on how to design and manage high performance organizations, supply chain management and methodology of complexity theory.

Jacqueline Nielsen is a clinical assistant professor at the Purdue University School of Nursing. She also maintains a collaborative agreement with a Mid-western hospital system where she is an oncology clinical nurse specialist, focusing on outcomes in the clinical oncology setting. Her teaching and scholarly activities include oncology nursing, interdisciplinary oncology care, medical-surgical nursing and patho-physiology. She participates in a number of consortiums and interdisciplinary projects. She has a strong emphasis for the integration of information technology into clinical practice and education. She has integrated the use of the Pocket PC and the Tablet PC into her students' practice at the clinical site and has incorporated Web-based technology to enhance students' learning.

Phillip Olla is an associate professor at the school of business at Madonna University in Michigan, USA. His research interests include knowledge management, mobile telecommunication, and health informatics. He received his PhD from the department of information systems and computing at Brunel University, UK. Phillip is a member of the editorial board for the *Industrial Management & Data Systems Journal* and is currently the book review and software review editor for the International Journal of Healthcare Information Systems and is also a member of the Editorial Advisory & Review Board for the *Journal of Knowledge Management Practice*.

David Parry is a senior lecturer in the Auckland University of Technology School of Computing and Mathematical Sciences New Zealand. His PhD thesis was concerned with the use of fuzzy ontologies for medical information retrieval. He holds degrees from Imperial College and St. Bartholomew's Medical College, London and the University of Otago, New Zealand. His research interests include Internet-based knowledge management and the semantic Web, health informatics, the use of radio frequency ID in healthcare and information retrieval.

Edmund Prater is an associate professor of operations management in the College of Business Administration at the University of Texas-Arlington. He is director of the Texas Health Resources/University of Texas Arlington Medical Mini-MBA program. He received his PhD in operations management from the Georgia Institute of Technology. He also holds a BS in electrical engineering from Tennessee Technology University and MS degrees in both electrical engineering and systems analysis from Georgia Tech.

Lela D. Pumphrey is currently a professor of accounting at Idaho State University in Pocatello, Idaho, USA. She is licensed as a certified public accountant (CPA) in Idaho. In addition to being a CPA, she is a certified government financial manager (CGFM), certified management accountant (CMA), and certified internal auditor (CIA). She served a five-year term on the Idaho State Board of Accountancy (1999-2004), where she served as chair 2003-2003. Currently, she serves as a member of the NASBA's Examination Review Board. She was selected by the Idaho Centennial Chapter of AGA as the government financial manager of the year in 1992 and 2000. She has received the Chapter Service Award twice—in 1986 by the Little Rock Chapter and in 1990 by the Idaho Centennial Chapter. In addition, in 2000 she was selected by the Idaho Chapter as the 50th Anniversary Member.

Christopher G. Reddick is an associate professor of public administration at the University of Texas at San Antonio. Dr. Reddick's research interests include e-government, public budgeting, and employee benefits. Some of his publications can be found in *Public Budgeting & Finance*, *Government Information Quarterly*, and the *E-Service Journal*.

C. Ranganathan is assistant professor of information systems at the Liautaud Graduate School of Business, University of Illinois at Chicago. His current research interests include e-business transformation, strategic management of information systems, management of IT outsourcing and business value of IT investments. Ranganathan holds a doctorate from the Indian Institute of Management of Management, Ahmedabad and a master's degree from BITS, Pilani, India. Ranganathan's papers have appeared in several journals including *Communications of the ACM, Decision Sciences Journal, Information & Management, Information Systems Management, International Journal of Electronic Commerce, Journal of IT, Journal of Strategic Information Systems*, among others. Ranganathan has consulted and researched for several national and multi-national corporations across the globe. He is the winner of the Best Doctoral Dissertation Award and the Best Teaching Case Award at the International Conference on Information Systems and he is also a two-time winner of the SIM's Paper Awards Competition.

Dana Schwieger is an assistant professor of management information systems in the Donald L. Harrison College of Business at Southeast Missouri State University in Cape Girardeau. She holds a PhD in management information systems from Southern Illinois University–Carbondale. Her current research interests include adaptive structuration theory, health management information systems and e-business strategy.

Marion Sobol is professor of information technology and operations management at the Cox School of Business at SMU. She received her PhD from Michigan in economics (statistics). She also holds a BA from Syracuse and an MA from Michigan. At various times, she has been on the editorial board of *Management Science, Interfaces, IEEE Software*, and *Decision Sciences*. She has published extensively on healthcare issues and headed *Decision Sciences'* Healthcare division for several years.

Ken Trimmer is an associate professor of computer information systems at Idaho State University. He holds a PhD in management information systems from the University of South Florida. His research focuses on information systems issues in healthcare organizations, pedagogical approaches to systems analysis and design, group processes in systems development teams, and information system issues in small to medium enterprises.

Periklis Valsamos graduated from the department of computer science and telecommunications, University of Athens. He also holds a MSc degree in advanced information systems from the same department. He graduated with honors from the National School of Public Administration (greek government's authorized institute for the training of public administration's managers-executives), with a specialization in healthcare management. He has a permanent staff position in the Greek Ministry of Health and Social Solidarity. Currently, he is working for the Managing Authority of Operational Program (Information Society). His research interests include medical informatics, distributed and wireless systems and Web technologies.

Iraklis Varlamis is a post-doctoral researcher in the computer science department of Athens University of Economics and Business. His research interests vary from data-mining and knowledge management to virtual communities and their applications. He has written and presented several articles in international conferences, concerning the design and implementation aspects of virtual communities. For more information visit: http://wim.aueb.gr/iraklis.

H. Joseph Wen is chairperson and associate professor of management information systems,department of accounting and management information systems, Harrison College of Business, Southeast Missouri State University. He holds a PhD from Virginia Commonwealth University. He has published over 100 papers in academic refereed journals, book chapters, encyclopedias and national conference proceedings. He has received over six million dollars in research grants from various State and Federal funding sources. His areas of expertise are Internet research, electronic commerce (EC), transportation information systems, and software development. He has also worked as a senior developer and project manager for various software development contracts since 1988.

Dr. Carla Wiggins' doctorate is in health services research, policy, and administration from the University of Minnesota. She is an academic fellow of the American College of Healthcare Executives (ACHE), and an active member of the Association of University Programs in Health Administration (AUPHA) where she serves on the board of directors and Undergraduate Review committee. Dr. Wiggins' teaching, research, and speaking emphases are in healthcare management, management career success factors, and in rural health organizations' use of technology and information systems.

Vance Wilson is an information systems faculty member at the University of Toledo. His research focuses generally on human-computer interaction in organizational contexts with significant publication streams in the areas of e-health, computer-mediated communication, and decisional guidance.

Index

A

abbreviated injury score (AIS) 95
adaptive structuration theory (AST)
    164, 166
American Health Information Management
    Association (AHIMA) 299
artificial neural network (ANN) 93
artificial neural network (ANN) systems
    109
artificial neural networks (ANNs) 108

B

baby boomers, use of Internet 69
blood donor recruitment (BDR) 17
blood donor recruitment (BDR) project 17

C

Center for Education and Research in
    Information Assurance and Security
    (CERIAS) 146
Clinical Information access program
    (CIAP) 331
code-division multiple-access (CDMA) 8
code division multiple access (CDMA) 8
communication-level security protection
    principle 45

competitive forces, modeling of in e-health
    381
computerized order entry systems (CPOE)
    203
computerized physician order entry
    (CPOE) 185, 361
computerized physician order entry
    (CPOE) systems 273
computer systems used, LAN vs. non-con-
    nected 259
consent requirement principle 45
continuing medical education (CME) 143

D

data-level security protection principle 44
deep vein thrombosis (DVT) 109
demonstration: assistance in rural training
    (DART) project 209
differences between boomers and seniors
    72
digital literacy 25, 92, 108, 164, 224,
    392

E

e-commerce paradigm 346
e-health, competitive forces 375
e-health, definition of 345

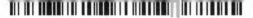
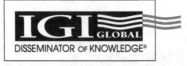
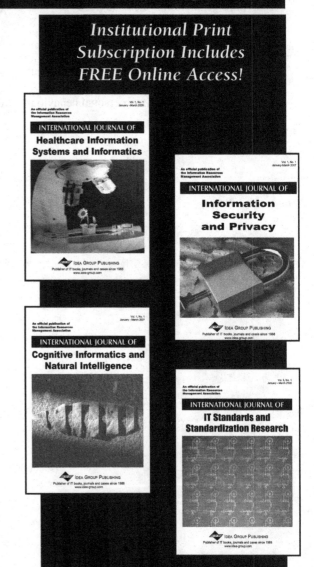